Man Against Cancer

BY THE SAME AUTHOR:

novels:

THE TWINS
HIGH MOON
STRANGERS IN FLORIDA
THE DOVE ON HIS SHOULDER
THE BLOW AT THE HEART
GALLERY OF WOMEN
THE LIEUTENANT
HERO'S WALK
GIRL ON A WING
THE BRIDES
NICHOLAS
A VERY SPECIAL AGENT

for younger readers:

RADAR COMMANDOS
ALL ABOUT THE HUMAN BODY
ALL ABOUT BIOLOGY

MAN AGAINST CANCER

BERNARD GLEMSER

Funk & Wagnalls
NEW YORK

Copyright © 1969 by Bernard Glemser
ALL RIGHTS RESERVED
Published by Funk & Wagnalls, A *Division of* Reader's Digest Books, Inc.
Printed in the United States of America

Illustrations by Shirley Baty

*This book is dedicated
with respect and admiration
to all cancer researchers,
everywhere*

Foreword

I first met Dr. Martin Sonenberg at a New Year's party in Manhattan several years ago. He was a tall, good-looking young man with a very shy manner. During dinner our host, who had recently undergone an operation, became unwell; a drug that had been prescribed for him could not be obtained because all nearby drugstores were closed; and Dr. Sonenberg offered to go to his hospital, where supplies of the drug were available. It seemed unfair to let him drive alone across snowy Manhattan, and I offered to accompany him. I had no knowledge, then, what he meant by "his hospital."

A little while later I found myself walking through the children's leukemia ward in Memorial Hospital for Cancer and Allied Diseases. I had never before, as far as I can recall, met a child who was suffering from leukemia. Here there were about thirty. The ward was gay with Christmas and New Year decorations, but it was strangely quiet. I remember very vividly that soundlessness, the lack of movement. Dr. Sonenberg paused to say hello to some of the children and introduced me to them. They were all near death.

As we left the ward he asked me if I would care to look at some of the work he was doing, and I replied politely that I would be greatly interested. I have often wondered whether I sounded as nervous as I felt. He explained that he was working on some gland or other, and in the laboratories attached to his office in the Sloan-Kettering Institute for Cancer Research he showed me a number of animals he had used for his experiments. There were rabbits, rats, mice; and some of them had grown to an absolutely prodigious size. It was like a scene in a science-fiction novel.

The gland Dr. Sonenberg was investigating was, of course,

the pituitary, the so-called master gland, which among its many functions has a responsibility for growth. Broadly speaking, a tumor is a growth of a special kind; and Dr. Sonenberg was seeking to control tumors by acting upon the pituitary in some way. He was in fact collaborating with scientists in Europe to develop techniques for operating on the gland—a cherry-sized organ (in human beings) situated at the base of the brain, approximately in the center of the head. It could hardly be more inaccessible.

We returned with pills for our host; they helped him considerably. But something else had now been started; and Dr. Sonenberg continued to talk to me and to answer my questions not only about his own work but about some of the other work in progress at the Institute. I began to realize that he was living in a world where the most extraordinary events were taking place. It was not just a secluded world of test tubes and beakers and microscopes. This was a world of enormous intellectual ferment, where the innermost mysteries of life were being probed in order to find means to overcome a grim, almost incomprehensible disease.

The conversation continued, on and off, for several days. Then, with Dr. Sonenberg's encouragement, I applied for permission to attend Sloan-Kettering as an observer, with the ultimate intention of writing a book about what was happening there. I was received with the greatest kindness, and I went to the Institute nearly every day for about ten months.

But I soon found myself at an alarming disadvantage. My profession was writing. I knew very little about physiology, about biology, about organic chemistry, about medicine in general; and consequently I was often hopelessly at sea, literally unable to comprehend what all these brilliant scientists were saying to me and to each other. This had to be remedied; and I did so in the old-fashioned way, by burning the midnight oil. A practical result was that I wrote a book for children on the workings of the human body which is now used in many schools all over the country and has been translated into a dozen languages; soon afterwards it was followed by a similar introduction to biology.

FOREWORD   ix

This book arrived at its present form after consultations with many friends and many editors. At the outset it became apparent that a book about current cancer research should not be confined to the activities of a single institution, or even to a single country. But no book intended for the general reader could possibly describe everything that is happening everywhere. The National Cancer Institute supports more than 2,000 research and training projects in the United States alone.

So this book describes ideas, projects, controversies, that have been collected from countries all over the world. It is not a book about cancer (which could only be written by an expert); it is not a history of cancer research and it is not a treatise on cancer research. Rather, it is an account of a novelist's excursions, poking his nose into all sorts of strange places where few novelists have gone in the past, trying to understand and explain what is happening out there, engaging in all sorts of improbable conversations and taking them down on a tape recorder so that they could be studied at leisure afterwards. *Improbable* is not a word I use lightly. The most inventive writer could never have devised the dialogue that occurred, for example, during my interview with George Mathé—the turning of rats into mice, monkeys into men; or the incredible problems described by K. D. Bagshawe arising from a more or less fortuitous encounter with a woman suffering from an "hysterical state of overbreathing"; or the account of Denis Burkitt's tumor safari through tropical Africa.

I doubt if any reader will find this an alarming book, although there is a reference to cancer on virtually every page. I think it is a hopeful book—not necessarily hopeful about the disease, but certainly hopeful about human beings; and it was a very exciting book to write. I have tried to keep it as simple and free of technicalities as possible; and wherever technical terms were unavoidable I have tried to clarify their meaning.

Many people helped to make this book possible, and I owe all of them an immense debt of gratitude. They are named here in some sort of chronological order, that is, as I met and conferred with them from Day 1.

C. Raphael, my host at the New Year's party, whose temporary indisposition started everything.

Dr. Martin Sonenberg.

Dr. Cornelius P. Rhoads, who allowed me to attend the Sloan-Kettering Institute for Cancer Research, and many members of his staff, particularly Ruth Abramson (now Mrs. Gilbert Cant), Director of Public Information; Helena Curtis; Betty Pezzoni (now Mrs. Polykarp Kusch); Shirley Baty; and Mrs. Miriam Adams.

Many officers of the American Cancer Society, who opened innumerable doors to me not only in the United States but all over the world: Dr. Richard P. Mason, Senior Vice President for Research, advised me where to go and whom to see; Mrs. Mildred Allen, who has since retired, gave me the benefit of her years of experience as head of the Foreign Desk. Clifton Read, Theodore Adams, Harry Milt, and Gerry Schramm were encouraging and helpful at all times.

Dr. Kenneth M. Endicott, Director of the National Cancer Institute, Bethesda, Maryland; James F. Kieley, Chief of the Research Information Branch; Mrs. Norma Golumbic; Dr. Ian A. Mitchell.

Joseph W. Hotchkiss, Kenneth Wilson, and June Wilson, who have a special place in the book's history.

Hobart Lewis and Walter W. Hitesman, Jr., who most generously made available to me the world-wide research and organizational facilities of the Reader's Digest Association, Inc.

James Monahan, who gave me valuable assistance throughout the time this book has been in preparation.

James Whitmore, who died in a tragic accident soon after the first chapters were written.

I am particularly grateful to all the scientists who received me so courteously, and who took such pains to increase my understanding: Dr. Ernest L. Wynder, Dr. Charlotte Friend, Dr.

FOREWORD

Chester M. Southam, of Sloan-Kettering Institute, who were the first to be interviewed.

In London, Professor Sir Alexander Haddow; Professor Sir Peter Medawar; Dr. J. T. Boyd. On a later visit, Professor Peter Alexander, Mr. Ronald W. Raven, Dr. I. Hieger, Dr. R. J. C. Harris, Dr. K. D. Bagshawe, Dr. M. A. Epstein, Dr. Francis J. C. Roe. I deeply regret that, on two occasions, snowstorms caused the cancellation of interviews with Dr. Richard Doll.

In Paris, Professor George Mathé; Dr. Eva Klein and Dr. Jan Stjernswärd in Stockholm; Professor Dr. Herwig Hamperl in Bonn and, on a later visit, Professor Dr. H. Druckrey in Freiburg im Breisgau; at the World Health Organization in Geneva, Dr. Joseph Handler, Professor Albert Tuyns, Dr. William I. B. Beveridge, Dr. Gregory T. O'Connor; in Milan, Professor Pietro Bucalossi (who is not only a renowned cancer scientist, but the Mayor of Milan, and whom I interviewed in the magnificent Palazzo Marino), Professor Giuseppe Della Porta, Professor Umberto Veronesi, Dr. Gianni Buonadonna; in Rome, Professor Ambesi Impiombato, Dr. Carlo Nervi, Professor Romano Zito, whom I interviewed at the Istituto Regina Elena; in Bombay, Dr. V. R. Khanolkar, Dr. Ernest J. Borges, Dr. (Mrs.) Satyavati M. Sirsat, Dr. Beatriz M. Braganca and Dr. L. D. Sanghvi. In Tokyo, during the Ninth International Congress of the *International Union Against Cancer,* many scientists kindly agreed to interviews, despite the pressure of conference business: Dr. John Higginson; Mr. Denis P. Burkitt; Dr. Dennis Wright; two charming scientists from the Soviet Union, Dr. N. I. Perevodchikova and Dr. Galina I. Deichman; and Dr. Shooichi Miyata. Dr. Grant N. Stemmermann in Hawaii; Mr. Earl Glover, Dr. F. R. Senti, and Dr. Calvin Golumbic at the U. S. Department of Agriculture. In Grand Rapids, Michigan, I had a second and very lengthy interview with Mr. Denis Burkitt; and in New York, at the Sloan-Kettering Institute once again, I spoke to Dr. Joseph H. Burchenal. The final interview in this series was with Dr. Sidney Farber in Boston.

I must also express my thanks to my friend Mrs. Phyllis Jackson; to Roger Donald and Peggy Wriedt; to Peter Glemser, Sheila Pike and Susie Colclough in London, who were efficient beyond belief at arranging and enforcing schedules; Nena Sundstrom in Stockholm; Erika Ferrari in Milan; Titti Campanelli in Rome; Lily and T. Parameshwar in Bombay, and T. R. Ramachandran; Teo Mui Seng in Bangkok; T. Stanley Holt, Lin Tai-yi and Sybil Wong in Hong Kong; and a host of friends and helpers in Tokyo, including Seiichi Fukuoka, Roy Otake, Kozo Kaito, Sen Matsuda, Howard Candlish, Robert Austin, and my personal guide and assistant, Motoko Iwabuchi.

It would be almost impossible to list all the books and papers I have consulted. Direct references will be found throughout the text. I would like to pay a special tribute, however, to the writings of Dr. Michael B. Shimkin; to that classic of cancer literature, *The Riddle of Cancer*, by Professor Dr. Charles Oberling; and to two books published more recently, *The Biology of Cancer*, edited by Professor E. J. Ambrose and Dr. F. J. C. Roe, and *The Prevention of Cancer*, edited by Ronald W. Raven, F.R.C.S., and Dr. F. J. C. Roe. Special thanks are due to Dr. Roe, who read my manuscript with care and great understanding. In all interviews except one, the engineer in charge of the recording equipment was my wife, Violetta Constance Glemser.

Contents

FOREWORD vii

1
Search and Accomplishment
ONE *The African Children* 3

2
The Nature of the Problem
TWO *The Scene* 27
THREE *A Galaxy of Problems* 59

3
World Around Us
FOUR *Of People and Places* 91
FIVE *More of People and Places* 109
SIX *Visit to a Sub-Continent* 127

4
Burkitt and Others
SEVEN *The Implications of Mr. Burkitt* 159
EIGHT *Stalking Horse* 179

5
Today and Tomorrow

NINE   *Villejuif—London—Boston*   205

6
Defense

TEN   *But Immunologists Speak Only to Immunologists*   243

7
The Hidden Toxins

ELEVEN   *". . . A New Kingdom of Medicine"*   275
TWELVE   *The Case of the Depraved Turkeys*   293
THIRTEEN   *The Case of the Tumorous Trout*   305

8
Finale

FOURTEEN   *The Best of Hopes*   325

INDEX   351

1

Search
and Accomplishment

ONE

The African Children

Some three years ago there was a conference about the Burkitt tumor in Kampala, and Dr. Burchenal invited us to attend it. We had never seen a patient with this disease; we had never seen the actual clinical situation. Have you ever seen a Burkitt patient? Oh, it is terrible, terrible.

Burkitt showed us pictures, one after another; then he went out and came back with about fifteen children, and sat them on the table. They were the children whose pictures he had shown us, suffering from the tumor. Now they were completely healthy. Everybody—all the scientists—were deeply moved.

It's very nice to work here in this Institute in Stockholm. One doesn't see patients, and so the problems are on the whole theoretical. But then you go out to Africa, and see these children, and you want to do anything possible to help them. When we were in Nairobi I didn't go out anywhere, I didn't even see a giraffe, because I was trying to think what I could do about this tumor. . . . Now I cannot sleep. I lie awake at night thinking about my work. I neglect my children and my home. I keep thinking about those unfortunate children in Kampala.

DR. EVA KLEIN
interviewed in her laboratory in the
Karolinska Institutet, Stockholm

In my day I have attended many hundreds of scientific meetings. Yet never have I been more inspired than by the symposium held in Kampala on the Burkitt lymphoma of African children, arranged by the Chemotherapy Panel under the effective chairmanship of Dr. Burchenal. There we considered the pathology and epidemiology of this tragic disease, but also learned that some 16 per cent of cases are miraculously amenable to cure by chemical means alone. We saw such African children; and the father of one of them said to the physician, "I will be your servant all my days."

PROFESSOR SIR ALEXANDER HADDOW Director
Chester Beatty Research Institute
London

From the early sixteenth century, when medicine began to assume the aspect of a science rather than a black art, it has been customary to name a newly-found anatomical feature after the physician or scientist who discovered it. Names derived in this way are called eponyms. One thinks, at random, of the Fallopian tubes, named for Fallopius (or Fallopio), a pupil of Vesalius; of the canal of Schlemm, the islets of Langerhans, the fissures of Rolando and Sylvius, the organ of Corti, Purkinje cells, Malpighian bodies. Similarly, diseases were commonly named after the physician who first described them: Bright's disease, Addison's disease, Parkinson's syndrome, Charcot's joints, Bell's palsy; and, in the field of cancer, Hodgkin's disease, Wilms' tumor, Ewing's sarcoma, and so on. Operations or medical procedures were also named in the same way. The practice, of course, was not in any way confined to medicine: it ranges over all human experience and activities—the Bunsen burner, Newton's rings, Audubon's warbler, the Seckel pear. The Hellenic race was named for Hellen, son of Deucalion, the Americas for Amerigo Vespucci.

But—at least in medicine—there has been a change in recent years. Attaching the name of a physician to a disease is not particularly informative and may lead to errors in communication; and the Committee on Tumor Nomenclature, formed by the International Union Against Cancer[1] to select names for

[1] The International Union Against Cancer (also known as L'Union In-

tumors which would be acceptable throughout the scientific world, stated in its illustrated manual (published in 1965), "In accordance with agreed international conventions it has been decided that all designations based on personal names should be rejected and replaced by appropriative descriptive terms, but, to avoid misunderstanding, the name by which some such tumor has been known in the past is now printed in brackets." Thus, the preferred name for Hodgkin's disease is lymphogranuloma, conveying the information that the disease is characterized by a certain kind of tumor occurring in lymph nodes; Wilms' tumor (discovered by Max Wilms, a German surgeon who lived from 1867–1918) is more comprehensible as embryonic nephroma, a kidney tumor arising from embryonic tissue. A minor problem is that nearly everybody concerned with these afflictions continues to call them Hodgkin's disease or Wilms' tumor. The new names have not yet caught on.

In the past decade, however, there has been one outstanding discovery—a disease that affects young children in certain parts of Africa (and less frequently elsewhere)—which has been named for the man who first described it in detail. The disease is known popularly as Burkitt's tumor; and the man whose name was given to it is Denis P. Burkitt. A brilliant young pathologist, Dr. Dennis Wright, who worked closely with Burkitt, explained to me, "One reason it was called Burkitt's tumor was to give credit to Mr. Burkitt; and we are all very glad about that. But another was that the pathologists couldn't agree what else to call it. At a conference in Paris, the French wouldn't even agree that it was a lymphoma (that is, a cancer of lymphatic tissue); and some of the Americans weren't even certain that it was a malignant tumor; so they ended up by calling it Burkitt's tumor, because any lump can be called a tumor."

---

ternationale Contre le Cancer, or UICC) is a non-governmental voluntary organization with member organizations in sixty-seven countries. It strives to achieve its aim—in the words of its manifesto—"by facilitating the exchange of information between national cancer organizations, holding international cancer congresses and conferences, standardizing nomenclatures and classifications, and by stimulating national efforts against cancer." Its headquarters are in Geneva.

"Subsequent work," Mr. Burkitt wrote recently,[2] "has clarified the picture, and the more meaningful term, lymphoma, is often used, instead of tumor." It affects most frequently the jaws, salivary glands, kidneys, adrenals, liver, ovaries, and long bones of children from two to fourteen years of age; the rate of growth is greater than any other human tumor, parts of the tumor doubling in size in a single day; and the face of a child suffering from a tumor of the jaws or salivary glands becomes horribly distorted. Patients who receive no treatment, or fail to respond to treatment, die in six to twelve weeks after the tumor first appears. Few people in Europe or America are likely to encounter Burkitt's tumor as such (the exceptions are very significant); but it may prove to be of paramount importance in the understanding and eventual control of forms of cancer which people outside equatorial Africa or New Guinea see, unfortunately, too often. Unquestionably, the story of Burkitt's tumor is the most dramatic and the most intriguing in cancer research today.

Denis Burkitt does not fit one's concept—however vague—of a cancer researcher. It is difficult to picture him confined to a laboratory. There is a good reason for this: he is not by profession a cancer researcher or in any other way a laboratory scientist. He was trained as a surgeon (and therefore, in accordance with British medical etiquette, he is addressed as Mr. Burkitt rather than Dr. Burkitt). Additionally, he is not a man who would be happy working day in, day out, in a laboratory. By nature he is very active, very brisk, bursting with energy: a tall, sparely-built man with a bright face and eager eyes. ("He's a tremendous traveler," I was told by Dr. M. A. Epstein, a scientist who has done some extremely important work on the tumor: "He likes to go everywhere." And, again in the words of Dr. Epstein, he is apt to describe himself as a bush surgeon, or an up-country surgeon.) He is profoundly religious: he speaks of God providing him with direction, and

[2] *Abbottempo*, London, December, 1967.

he means it. God is close to him in all his work, and this is particularly striking in an age of agnosticism and in relation to a disease which, to many people, appears to be an expression of pure evil. Others, looking at the mystery of cancer, are distressed by the apparent absence of God, the absence of any sign of Divine responsibility. Burkitt is supported by the abundant presence of God, at all times and presumably in all circumstances.

Denis Parsons Burkitt was born in Enniskillen, Northern Ireland, in 1911. His father, an engineer in charge of all the county roads, had (Burkitt told me in the course of one of our conversations) "a little hobby which none of us took very seriously. He was very interested in birds. I believe he was the first man ever to plot geographically the territories of birds, and he did this in our garden at home—I still have his little pencil drawings. After he died, the great ornithologist David Lack was asked to select the seven people who had done most in research on bird habits at any time in the world, and he named my father as one of the seven. It's rather like the work I'm doing, a generation later."

At Dublin University he first studied engineering, then switched to medicine; and it was here that his future course was determined. "I was brought up in a Christian home," he said in response to a question about the part played by religion in his upbringing, "but I don't think my Christian faith really crystallized until I was at the University of Dublin and got in with a crowd of men whose lives were motivated and enriched by a faith in Christ. I owe more to these men—other than to my family and home, I suppose—than to any other influence in my life."

For three years after he qualified in 1935 he did what he calls "ordinary house surgeon's jobs in Dublin and in England." Then, in 1938, he completed his surgical training in Edinburgh, taking the degree of F.R.C.S. (Fellow of the Royal College of Surgeons). During this period he shared rooms with Dr. Guy Timmis, each paying two guineas a week (a little more than ten dollars at the time), a sum that Burkitt considered exorbitant. Subsequently, Dr. Timmis ("my oldest friend," Burkitt calls him) went out to Africa, spent fifteen years in government service, and then opened a leper settlement for a mission in Tanzania. Many of Burkitt's friends followed a smiliar pattern; and later this was to prove of vital significance in the study and investigation of Burkitt's tumor.

For a while Burkitt was unsure about his personal destiny. He signed on as ship's surgeon on a cargo boat, the *Glen Shiel* of the Blue Funnel Line, and sailed off on a five month voyage to Manchuria. "The crew was Chinese," Burkitt said. "There was really no work to do—I pulled a few teeth out, nothing more. We went to Penang and Singapore, Shanghai, Hong Kong, and so on, and I have never regretted it, it was invaluable. I had time to read, and be myself, and see places, and I had an opportunity to think."

"What did you think about?"

"What I should do next. And I felt increasingly that I should go overseas and not join the rat race at home. I first applied to the Colonial Service in 1940, and I felt in all honesty that I ought to say what my motive was; and I gave my surgical qualifications and added that I wanted to go out with something of a missionary motive. I think that frightened them a bit. I also mentioned that when I was a little boy of eleven, I lost an eye in an accident; and they turned me down on the pretext that I hadn't enough sight, although I have very good sight in the other eye."

"How did you lose it?"

"A chap threw a stone at me, broke my glasses."

If the Colonial Office was unable to use a surgeon with one eye and a burning missionary fervor, the British Army most certainly could. World War II was in progress and there was an urgent need for men who were expert at patching up broken bodies. Almost as if it were complying with the instructions of an even higher authority, the Army sent Denis Burkitt precisely where he had hoped to go: East Africa. He served in Kenya, in Somaliland, then in Ceylon; and, on furlough, he made a trip to Uganda. "I saw the need there," he said later: "I liked the people, and I felt perhaps this was the place I ought to come back to, and lend a hand."

As soon as he was released from the Army he made a new application to the Colonial Office for overseas service. This time he was accepted. Acceptance meant that he was totally in the hands of the Colonial Office administrators: they could send him anywhere they pleased, to carry out any duties they chose for him. When they asked, "Will you do anything we want you to do," he could only answer, "Yes," since this was the vocation he had chosen.

They sent him to Lira, in Northern Uganda.

Lira is about a hundred and fifty miles north of the equator and about three and a half thousand feet above sea level. It is north of a vast complex of lakes that, among other things, feed the Victoria Nile; and, not unexpectedly, this is one of the most highly malarial districts in Africa. Burkitt could scarcely have asked for a more challenging assignment: the hospital had less than a hundred beds, his only assistant was an African doctor, Dr. B. Kununka, and he found himself acting as surgeon, physician, gynecologist, and public health administrator for more than a quarter of a million people in territory that was largely tropical jungle. Ten sub-dispensaries were run from the main hospital, staffed by aides who had received a minimum of medical training, and Burkitt or Dr. Kununka would visit them once a week, taking out fresh stocks of drugs, escorting patients home from the hospital or bringing patients to the hospital from the sub-dispensaries.

Life in Lira, as Burkitt now describes it, had an old-fashioned colonial flavor. "It was part of an era that has now gone. There were about a dozen European families. The British community lived in little bungalows around the golf course, which was kept up by labor from the local prison. The District Commissioner was a sort of father to the whole area. We played tennis almost every day."

Tennis and tea parties were only a small part of the story. There was a desperate need for medical services in this area.

Half of the children died before they reached the age of five. In the first year of Burkitt's administration the number of major operations went up from 17 to more than 600. Emergencies resulting from accidents, fights, strangulated hernias, were the common rule. The hospital and its sub-dispensaries were overrun with cases of malaria, hookworm, malnutrition, and an exceedingly painful testicular disease called hydrocele, which in some parts of the territory afflicted one-third of the men. There were always six patients for every available bed.

Burkitt remained in Lira for fifteen months. Then the Colonial Office decided to move him. Presumably he could have been sent anywhere in the British Commonwealth; but the curious pattern remained unbroken, and he was posted to Mulago Hospital in Kampala, the capital of Uganda. Mulago is the teaching hospital of East Africa, attached to Makerere College Medical School; and here Burkitt was very happy. "I had the blessing, the joy, and the privilege of growing up with the Department of Surgery, with the best colleagues in the world. I had a far more exciting surgical career than if I had stayed in England, and to me it is an illustration that if you follow what you feel is right you do not lose on it. I didn't, anyway." It was spiritually rewarding; and suddenly, after ten years, it became spectacular.

Early in 1957 the senior consultant physician at the hospital, Dr. Hugh Trowell, asked Burkitt to look at a boy, about seven years old, who had something wrong with both sides of his lower jaw and both sides of his upper jaw. Burkitt, like Dr. Trowell, was puzzled. The condition made no sense as a tumor —he had never heard of four symmetrical tumors appearing simultaneously; and it made no sense as an infection.

A few weeks later when he was visiting the district hospital at Jinja, about 50 miles east of Kampala, he happened to glance through the ward window and caught sight of a child with a swollen face, like the boy in Mulago Hospital. He hurried outside to examine the child and saw that the condition was the same—symmetrical tumor-like swellings in the upper and lower jaws. He took several photographs (he always carried two cameras, one for color, one for black and white), and began to think seriously about this strange malady.

In the past he had often seen children at Mulago Hospital with large ugly tumors of the jaw. He had *seen* them, he said later, but he had not *observed* them. "We called the tumors 'sarcomas,' and we cut them out. It was butchery, it was useless, and it was wrong."[3] No child with this tumor lived very long after surgery, or for that matter without surgery. The malignancy grew at a tremendous rate, doubling itself in 48 hours, and the average life expectancy after the tumor was first noticed was about three months.

Burkitt now set himself to investigate these tumors more carefully, and he soon discovered that whenever he saw a jaw tumor he could generally find another tumor somewhere else in the child's body. It then became clear that the jaw tumor was only one tumor in what seemed to be a sort of multiple tumor arising in various parts of the body and coming to the surface in different places. Thus, it might appear as a tumor of the jaw, or the internal organs, or the eye, or the long bones. All were manifestations of the same disease, in Burkitt's words "like an actor coming on to a stage with a different mask for each play in which he appears."

At this time Burkitt met A. G. Oettlé, head of the Cancer Research Unit of the South African Institute for Medical Research. Oettlé looked at Burkitt's photographs, studied Bur-

---

[3] One of the earliest medical missionaries, Sir Albert Cook, kept meticulous records of all his cases at the hospital he established in East Africa, and these show clearly that the cancer pattern there has not changed since the beginning of the century. In 1902, he reported in the *Journal of Tropical Medicine,* "Sarcoma is common in East Africa, particularly sarcoma of the jaws," an eloquent and memorable phrase which Dennis Wright used to open his M.D. thesis more than fifty years later. It might be noted that many of the old textbooks (according to Dr. Wright) claim that cancer does not occur in Africans; and even Albert Schweitzer wrote that when he went first to Lambaréné, in what was then French Equatorial Africa, cancer was very rare, but over the years he had gradually seen it appearing, a state of affairs which he attributed to the white man coming to Africa. Schweitzer, for all his professed reverence for life, was curiously embittered; and this observation is not only spiteful but inaccurate.

kitt's notes, and commented, "This tumor doesn't occur in South Africa," a statement which was to have extraordinary repercussions, for it led Burkitt to ask himself, *"If it doesn't occur in South Africa, and it's common here in Uganda, where does it stop? It must stop somewhere."*

Burkitt now obtained his first research grant. It came from government funds and amounted to £15. Most of this money was used to pay the cost of printing a thousand leaflets carrying photographs of the tumor; and these were sent to hospitals all over Africa with a questionnaire asking whether the medical officers had seen this tumor in their locality.

The answers indicated that it was found in a belt across tropical Africa, with a tail that seemed to run down the east coast. Strangely, there were areas *within* the belt where the tumor was unknown.

The next step was to attempt to find a dividing line (Burkitt called it "an edge") separating areas where the tumor occurred and where it did not occur. If such an edge were found, it would obviously be the place to seek the answer to another question: *Why does the tumor occur on this side and not on the other side?*

For a year Burkitt worked on plans to go in search of this theoretical edge. He obtained a second research grant, this time from the British Medical Research Council, for about £150. Adding £50 of his own to this sum he bought an old Ford station wagon which had already done eight years of service in the Congo, and prudently filled it with spare parts.

Two colleagues were chosen to accompany him. One was an English missionary doctor, Ted Williams, who "with his own hands" had built a mission hospital near Arua, Northern Uganda, even making his own bricks. More to the point (according to Burkitt), he was an expert at repairing old cars and could change the engine bearings while you were having a cup of coffee. The third member of the team was a Canadian, Dr. Clifton Nelson, who was just leaving government service to become a mission doctor.

A detailed schedule was made of dates and times for visiting each hospital; and early in October, 1961, the three men set off on the great tumor safari which was to cover more than 10,000 miles in ten weeks, passing through Uganda, Tanganyika, Northern and Southern Rhodesia, Nyasaland, South Africa, Mozambique, Swaziland, and Kenya.

Inevitably they ran into troubles galore. There were times when they found themselves driving the wrong way. Rivers had fallen so low that the ferries had stopped running, or were so swollen by unprecedented rains that no ferry could get across. Often rivers had to be crossed by what Burkitt calls Irish bridges—"where the road went *under* rather than *over* the water." Roads marked on the map faded out into rough tracks that even the tough old Ford could not follow; and on some occasions they had to leave the roads altogether and travel by freight train or lake steamer.

Nevertheless, they were able to visit fifty-six hospitals. They held staff conferences, gave lectures, spoke individually to doctors, nurses, medical assistants, and made contact with hospitals which were off their route. The purpose of all this was to discover the *localities* from which the patients came, rather than the hospitals where the condition was recognized. The localities in which the cancer occurred were of primary importance.

Burkitt returned to Kampala in December with some remarkable information. About the reality and the prevalence of the disease there was no doubt at all: where it was prevalent it comprised more than half of all childhood cancers. At Lourenço Marques in Mozambique one doctor had seen forty children suffering from the disease in the past four years (and had been so impressed by it that he had arranged with the curator of the city museum to make plaster models of children with the tumor). A hospital in Tanganyika had reported six cases in the past three months; another, in Nyasaland, had admitted five patients in six months. What was impressive, too, was that in South Africa and various other countries the disease was to all intents and purposes unknown.

Most important, one of the principal objectives of the safari had been accomplished. Burkitt had learned where the tumor stopped—an unexpected and startling finding.

In central Africa, near the equator, the tumor occurred *no higher* than 5000 feet.

In Nyasaland it occurred *no higher* than 3000 feet.

In Swaziland it occurred *no higher* than 1000 feet.

Burkitt had found, apparently, not an edge but an *altitude barrier*. Up to a certain altitude, which varied with the locality and the closeness to the equator, the tumor might be common. *But above that altitude the tumor never appeared.*[4]

This seemed at first to be utterly without reason. Why should a malignant tumor of young children be dependent upon the altitude at which those children lived?

Alexander Haddow,[5] director of the Virus Research Institute at Entebbe, near Kampala, provided part of the answer. He recognized that the altitude barrier was actually a *temperature* barrier. The tumor stopped at a temperature of about 60°. In areas where the temperature commonly fell below 60°F, children did not develop this cancer; in areas where the temperature was generally above 60°, the tumor was likely to occur.

For the first time in medical history a malignant tumor had been found to be dependent upon climatic temperature—an extraordinary discovery.

Burkitt now went across the continent to West Africa.

In the southern areas of Nigeria the tumor was seen nearly everywhere. Yet in the heavily populated area around Kano in northern Nigeria it was almost unknown. The same peculiar pattern was evident in Ghana: the tumor was common almost everywhere, except around Accra, on the coast.

[4] One of Burkitt's comments about this discovery is of interest: "In retrospect I realize that relating the tumor to altitude was the result of the unhurried discussions possible on road travel but denied to the air traveller. I would almost certainly have missed the point had I travelled alone." *Abbottempo*, London, December, 1967.

[5] It is a coincidence that two scientists named Alexander Haddow appear in this chapter. They are not related.

Clues to this new puzzle were provided by maps and statistical tables from the government Lands and Surveys Department. The rainfall in southern Nigeria and neighboring Ghana is from 200 to 400 inches a year. Kano, on the fringe of the Sahara Desert, is in a sort of rain shadow: its rainfall is only 10 to 20 inches a year. Accra has the same meager rainfall and is the driest part of the entire West African coast.

Thus the tumor appeared to be dependent on rainfall as well as temperature. It was another surprise. Burkitt's tumor was proving to be something utterly unique in medical history.

One might assume that Burkitt would have concentrated all his energy now on further research; but, of necessity, research had to be carried on in addition to his other duties. He was in charge of a full surgical unit where the normal condition was an emergency every hour on the hour. There were also the small but inescapable human emergencies, like the eleven year old African boy who had to have an eye removed. Burkitt, only too aware of what this meant, sent frantic pleas to every hospital in East Africa until he found a matching glass eye; so that the boy, instead of being handicapped and possibly an outcast, became something of a legend in his community.

And, of course, there was an oppressive shortage of money for research. Dr. Epstein told me of visiting Burkitt in Kampala and seeing the map of East Africa on which Burkitt plotted the incidence of the tumor, in the usual way, by means of colored pins. But the hospital could not provide colored pins. They were a luxury, not included in the budget. Consequently Burkitt had obtained plain pins and had painted colors on them himself. Money was lacking, too, for experimental drugs. Again, Burkitt overcame the difficulty by coaxing the representatives of various drug companies to give him free supplies. "I suppose I nagged at people a bit," Burkitt told me cheerily. "When you're enthusiastic about something, you can't help driving away at it."

This map, or one similar to it, enters the next phase of the story, in a scene that has the primitive charm of certain pages of J. D. Watson's *The Double Helix.*

"I had a map of Africa in my office with the tumor plotted on it," Burkitt explained to me, "and one day Alec Haddow of our Virus Research Institute looked at it and asked himself, *Now, what must I do to Africa to get that map?* He knows all the factors about climate and insects and so on; and he found that if he rubbed chalk all over a map of Africa and then took a handkerchief and wiped off those areas where the rainfall was below thirty inches and the temperature fell below 60°F, he was left with an almost exact duplicate of my tumor map, simply on these factors of temperature and rainfall.

"Naturally, we then began to look around to see whether we could find any insect map of Africa which might fit our tumor map. It's difficult to get a map of mosquitoes; but we found the old tsetse map in Buxton's book on tsetse flies; and the tsetse—before it was eliminated—fits extraordinarily closely.

"Now, we didn't think of the tsetse in terms of the tumor, but at least we'd found *one* insect which was limited by the same factors. We had, therefore, at least a *suspicion* that we might be dealing with something which in some way or another was insect-dependent."

Next, a colleague of Burkitt, Dr. J. N. P. Davies, suggested that the same pattern applied to yellow fever; and this was one of the most striking hypotheses to come out of cancer research in many a long day. The tsetse fly carries the trypanosome (a single-celled organism) which is responsible for sleeping sickness. Yellow fever, however, is carried by mosquitoes, which are only active in warm, moist areas; and the organism responsible for this disease is a virus.

Another demonstration of this pattern was provided by the outbreak in 1959 of a disease called o'nyong-nyong fever. ("The name means broken bones," Burkitt explained to me: "You don't die of it, but you feel as if all your bones are broken.") The epidemic raged across northern Uganda, affecting 98 per cent of the population; it went around Lake Victoria and into Tanganyika; and it was apparently limited everywhere to the same geographical boundaries as Burkitt's tumor. O'nyong-nyong fever, too, is caused by a virus carried by mosquitoes. "It proves nothing," Burkitt said, "but it's interesting."[6]

Here, in other circumstances, the story of Denis Burkitt and Burkitt's lymphoma might be expected to come to a conclusion. We have an upright and God-fearing man, trained as a surgeon, who goes out to work in East Africa because he is convinced it is God's will that he go there; who finds young African children suffering from tumors which one of his colleagues has described as "appallingly malignant"; who is revolted by the mutilating surgery which was customarily performed on these children with little hope of curing them or even of extending their lives by a few months; and who then, with incredible energy, pursued the disease up and down and through the mountains and jungles of tropical Africa with the result that for the first time in medical history a cancer was related to geographical conditions of temperature and rainfall and—almost certainly—to an infective organism (which may or may not be a virus) carried by an arthropod (which may or may not be a mosquito). The long-term value of this discovery is obviously enormous; and Burkitt's lymphoma stands out as one of the major landmarks in cancer research.

What is extraordinary—and would not be tolerated in any contemporary novel or motion picture, because it is so far removed from the bounds of possibility—is that having discovered Burkitt's lymphoma, Mr. Burkitt then proceeded to find means for curing a significant number of children suffering from Burkitt's lymphoma.

Up to this time cancer (with one rare exception) could be cured only in two ways: the excision of all cancerous tissue

[6] More evidence was provided some time later (1967) by studies carried out by M. C. Pike, E. H. Williams and B. Wright, showing that cases of the tumor do not occur in a random manner but spread year by year from one part of a district to another. This phenomenon—the clustering of patients and the shifting of clusters annually—strongly suggests that an infectious process is at work.

by surgery, or the destruction of all cancerous tissue by radiation. But total cure was always dubious because the surgeon or the radiologist could never be absolutely sure that all cancerous tissue had indeed been eliminated, that not a single cancerous cell remained to re-establish the malignancy.

Burkitt had found that surgery could do nothing for this lymphoma because it was a condition characterized by multiple tumors. Radiotherapy was not then available in tropical Africa, and its efficacy in treating these tumors was, in any case, uncertain. And, hitherto, the hope that cancer could be cured by chemotherapy—that is, by the use of drugs—had not been fulfilled. Drugs might, as in leukemia, produce dramatic remissions of the disease, but the remissions were not maintained permanently.

In January, 1960, a group of scientists from Sloan-Kettering Institute for Cancer Research went out to East Africa to treat patients suffering from a variety of cancers. One purpose of the expedition was to try out some promising new drugs and techniques. In this group were Dr. Joseph H. Burchenal and Dr. Herbert F. Oettgen; and one of the drugs they had brought with them was methotrexate, manufactured by Lederle Laboratories and widely used in the treatment of leukemia.

Dr. Burchenal said later, "I thought I had seen all children's tumors in Memorial Hospital (New York), but I had never seen anything like these." He gave Burkitt a supply of methotrexate, and Dr. Oettgen advised Burkitt on the use of the drug. Lederle Laboratories also provided Burkitt with methotrexate, after he persuaded their representative in Nairobi that here was a "golden opportunity" to test out their drugs on patients who had not been treated with deep X-rays. (Radiotherapy may affect the patient's immune response, and therefore it hinders accurate evaluation of a drug's anti-cancer capabilities.) Burkitt's own account of what happened deserves to be quoted in full.

"Very, very fortunately," he told me, "about the time I became involved with the tumor, therapy also became available. The Uganda government didn't provide it—we're a poor government; but I received gifts of drugs from different sources.

I first treated patients with methotrexate. Later I went on to cyclophosphamide (also known as Endoxan and Cytosan); later I treated a series of patients with vincristine.

"It was very encouraging. The tumor proved to be incredibly amenable to treatment. Some of the first patients we ever treated, more than six years ago, are still alive and well, and—I believe—cured. Our experience over these years has shown that the tumor is exceedingly sensitive to cytotoxic drugs (that is, cell-poisoning drugs); and if you give a patient not too big a course of treatment he does better, I believe, than if he is treated to toxicity (the state of being poisoned) which is the normal approach. The normal approach, in other words, is to give the patient all the drugs you can without killing him, to try to destroy all the malignant cells. Now, I had no training in chemotherapy; I was very busy—I had a whole surgical unit to look after; and so I wasn't treating patients as intensively as an expert would. Just the same, my patients did extraordinarily well. I continued to treat them badly—according to the experts—and I got very good results. In fact, some of those patients who ran away from the hospital before their treatment was completed sometimes did best of all."

This remark required an explanation. He said, "At the best of times African children hate being in a hospital—it's a very alarming experience for them. I can think of one little girl who I thought would be a very favorable patient to treat—she was to have three courses[7] of methotrexate. After she had one course out of her three I did the rounds one morning and I found, as so often happens in Darkest Africa, that the mother had come in during the night and taken the child home. I was so disappointed: I had felt that this child might respond to treatment; and it seemed as if we'd missed the opportunity.

"But about a year later one of our African workers came across this little girl in her home in the bush; and since then I've seen her often. She's perfectly well, six years later, and I believe she's entirely cured."

Mr. Burkitt, in a statement that is remarkable by any stand-

[7] A full course consists of a hundred milligrams divided into forty pills, given at the rate of eight pills a day for five days.

ards, went on to enlarge upon this theme. He said, "Subsequently, I repeatedly gave patients a single injection and saw not only total clinical regression but total radiological recovery of diseased bone (that is, as shown by X-ray photographs); and my policy was that when I saw total regression on one dose I did not give a second. We have seen patients go along to what we believe to be total cure after one dose; but this depends on seeing them early. *In my experience, if you saw an early jaw tumor you could expect to get total clinical remission, which would not recur at that site, in the large majority of cases, from a single dose of a cytotoxic agent.*"

"Is there any explanation for this?"

"The very fact that we see long term remissions—which we believe to be cures—following what would normally be considered totally inadequate therapy means, I believe, that the drug helps to stimulate the patient's own defenses. I believe the real clearance of malignant cells comes from a host response against the tumor, in the same way that the body's responses tend to eliminate a bacterial infection. If you over-treat the patient you may knock out more cells initially; but because at the same time you knock out his defense mechanisms you lose more than you gain. From ordinary observation I would suggest that the minimal dose consistent with clinical elimination of the tumor is the best dose, and to go on giving more drugs does more harm than good. And, of course, this approach to cancer of trying to enhance and enrich the body's response against tumor cells looks to me as far more promising and happy than cutting out more and more of the patient. . . . I know that you are hardly allowed to claim a cure for chemotherapy—you're not allowed to say a patient is cured until he's dead. I am claiming cures on this ground: that if the patient is symptom free after a year, some—but very, very few—ever get into trouble again. And therefore the patient who is symptom free after a year is, I think, nineteen times out of twenty going to go on living, and he will not die from this tumor."

"What is the future of Burkitt's lymphoma in Africa? Are you going to be able to eliminate it completely?"

"No," Burkitt said. "I think that if you see it early you can now almost guarantee a cure. But it's only the jaw tumor that you will ever see early. The abdominal tumor isn't detectable until it's relatively late.

"If it could be determined that the tumor is caused by a virus, and if the virus could be isolated, there might then be the possibility of immunization against it. But I don't think that would be a practical proposition in Africa, because cancer there is so unimportant compared to the million and one other problems, and vaccination wouldn't be worth the effort.

"Of course, if one could find a virus and develop an immunization technique against these lymphomas, there would be the hope that this might lead the way toward finding a virus and establishing immunization against leukemia. And that would be quite something in the Western world."

It is a remarkable experience to attend a lecture given by Denis Burkitt to an audience of cancer specialists. He has a decided military bearing—the result, perhaps, of his five years of service in the British Army, or of having grown up in Enniskillen which is renowned (he will tell you proudly) as the home of two great regiments. His voice has an Irish lilt, and he cannot resist making a joke or two as he tells about his work in Kampala.

Then the color slides come on the screen. About half are photographs of his African children, with grotesquely distorted faces or swollen bodies, resulting from the tumor which has been given his name. *But each color slide showing a child with a tumor is followed by another color slide showing the same child without a tumor*—cured by a handful of pills or a single injection. The last color slide shows a long line of these children, attired in their bright East African robes, standing in a sunny little street and gazing solemnly at the camera. They are clear-eyed and, as far as any human being can tell, in perfect health. It is moving and impressive, and it invariably brings Burkitt an ovation.

Almost exactly ten years after Dr. Hugh Trowell consulted

him about the puzzling case of the little boy with swellings in all four jaw quadrants, Burkitt wrote,[8] "Scarcely a week passes without the publication of a new paper on some aspect of this tumor. . . . The volume of interest focused on the tumor reflects the widespread belief that its unusual characteristics and behavior may not only throw light on some problems of cancer etiology (the causes of cancer) but also give guidance in therapy. Why this sudden interest in a condition that has long been prevalent in tropical Africa? The answer lies in the happy combination of several factors. . . . Doctors and other scientists trained in different specialties have each played their complementary and distinctive roles, and each has contributed from his particular experience. . . . The story of this tumor is evolving daily. Fragments of new information are being added constantly and are reminiscent of a jigsaw puzzle tackled by many people simultaneously. The final picture may give information that will help to place the missing pieces in some other cancer jigsaw puzzle. Whatever happens, credit will be equally shared among many workers, and not only those whose work has appeared in print."

Denis Burkitt is unique. There is nobody quite like him in the history of cancer research. The implications of his work are discussed more fully in a later chapter; but this chapter might well conclude with some comments made about him by two distinguished cancer scientists.

The first is Dr. R. J. C. Harris, Director of the Imperial Cancer Research Fund, who said in the course of an interview in London, "By and large, cancer research is a closed field. You don't expect people who have spent their lives doing surgery to erupt into it suddenly. But that's what Denis did. He burst into cancer research more or less like an atom bomb." Dr. Harris suggested several reasons for Burkitt's success. One was his remarkable talent as an observer. Another was that he never allowed himself to be discouraged by experts who disputed

[8] *Burkitt's Lymphoma: A Study in Medical Detection*, by Denis P. Burkitt, M.D., F.R.C.S., *Abbottempo*, London, December 1967.

his findings. Still another arose from his deep religious beliefs and the special relationships he established with medical missionaries throughout Africa, who cooperated fully in his work. And, finally, there was Burkitt's love for those unfortunate children afflicted with the disease he was investigating. "I worked with Denis in Kampala and I've been on safari with him several times," Dr. Harris said. "The second time I went out there was one boy in the hospital who was in a dreadful state. The poor little chap obviously had no future at all—he was far beyond help. But whenever Denis could get away from his surgical work, he'd put this boy in his car and drive him around the town, just to give him an outing."

An equally generous tribute was paid to Mr. Burkitt a couple of days later during an interview with Professor Peter Alexander. "I think he is a fabulous character," Professor Alexander said. "He has shown that there is no substitute in cancer research for brains, good observation, and exploiting good fortune. Cancer is not an incurable disease. A lot of cancer is cured. The remarkable thing about Burkitt's tumor is that one can cure it at such an advanced state, when the experts would have said any possibility of a cure was hopeless and crazy. The beautiful thing is he has shown us all to be wrong, and I think this is absolutely marvelous."

2

The Nature of the Problem

TWO

The Scene

We live in an age which has seen man triumph over most of his ancient maladies. Not only in the so-called highly developed areas of the world but in many underdeveloped areas, life expectancy has gone up during the past twenty-five years, in some countries to a striking degree, and the incidence of disease—with a few exceptions—has greatly diminished. Many of the old terrifying epidemic diseases have virtually disappeared. Bubonic plague, the grisly Black Death which once menaced the whole of civilization, has gone almost completely in Europe and North America—an occasional case puzzles young doctors who have never encountered it before (although there are signs that it may return as a result of the war in Vietnam); smallpox, which killed (very horribly) one person in ten not so long ago in Europe, is now scarcely known there; tuberculosis, once our second most deadly disease, has dropped to thirteenth place; cholera, malaria, yellow fever, sleeping sickness, are now generally associated with exotic, far-off places. We have not quite run out of diseases yet; Nature still has a few unpleasant surprises for us up her sleeve; and the relatively sudden extension of life expectancy all over the world is providing man with a staggering new problem on which to exercise his ingenuity—how to support all those who may now live twice as long as their forefathers and are thus enabled to produce larger families who, in turn, may produce even larger families.

Sooner or later, of course, we must each of us die of something; and of the old-fashioned epidemic diseases the most severe will probably continue to be influenza, in its ever-changing forms, until medical science comes to our aid with some new kind of vaccine. It is worth bearing in mind that influenza, which we call by a sort of pet name and tend to consider nothing much more than an over-sized cold, is possibly the most ferocious of man's contemporary enemies. In the pandemic of 1918–19, literally half of all the people in the world contracted the disease and it killed twenty-one million of them. The outbreak of Asian 'flu in 1957–58 was nearly as widespread, but it was less deadly because antibiotics reduced the number of fatalities from bacterial pneumonia, which is a common complication of influenza and adds materially to its lethality.

In terms of man's mortality, nearly all other infectious diseases are more or less under control, a cheery assertion that rarely comforts those who contract measles or hepatitis or rheumatic fever; and in the Western Hemisphere people tend to die more and more of what physicians call the chronic degenerative diseases, those ailments which come with the later years and the breakdown of our physical resources. The leading cause of death now is heart disease; the second is cancer; the third is cerebral hemorrhage; the fourth is not a disease but the sum total of the accidents that befall us—motor vehicle accidents and, in nearly equal numbers, other kinds of accidents, particularly accidents in the home. These, the four mid-twentieth century riders of the Apocalypse, account for about 72 per cent of all deaths. The remaining 28 per cent is made up of influenza and pneumonia, certain diseases peculiar to early infancy, suicide, ulcers, hernias, and items listed as "other and ill-defined."[1]

[1] These figures are for the United States in 1965. A few statistics, in this particular instance, help to tell the story more clearly.

Heart disease puts an end to the lives of twice as many human beings as its nearest competitor, yet it does not inspire mass terror, it is not a national obsession, it seems to be accepted as an appropriate way for our affairs to terminate. What occurs is comprehensible in purely mechanical terms, similar to the troubles that afflict the best of machines after six or seven decades of constant use: the main structure becomes slack, the valves no longer open and close with their original precision, the fuel pipes are encrusted with deposits so that the flow of fuel is diminished, the electrical circuits are erratic, and sooner or later the mechanism falters and comes to a halt, or it comes to a sudden stop and gives up the ghost. A mechanical flaw—the rupture of a blood vessel in the brain—is the cause of a cerebral hemorrhage, and this too is something we understand: the occurrence is unfortunate but it is not beyond reason. Accidents are simply the combination of ill-chance and human fallibility—the skidding car, the broken ladder, the cake of soap in the bathtub, the bolt of lightning in the orchard, hazards that raise only a few remote philosophical speculations. And this is true, with one exception, of the rest of the fifteen leading causes of death: they are comprehensible, they do not outrage the mind, effect follows cause, vital organs suffer severe injury and consequently cannot continue to function, with the final result that the whole organism is no longer able to sustain itself and cannot stave off its destruction. The sole exception is, of course, cancer, which to most people appears totally mysterious, totally inexplicable, and totally evil, a concept which is not altogether correct.

In 1965, the total population of the United States was 192,700,000:

Live births	3,908,000
Deaths	1,825,000
Deaths from diseases of the	
Heart	706,010 [38.8%
Cancer	296,320 [16.2%
Cerebral hemorrhage	203,330 [11.1%
Accidents	106,900 [5.9%

It is noteworthy that for every American who died, two new Americans came into existence.

Cancer afflicts, as far as we know, all living things.[2] Plants are subject to it; the tiny fruit fly may have cancerous tumors, so may whales, so may cattle, and so may birds. It is an ancient disease, much older than man: paleontologists have found evidence of it in the bones of dinosaurs who inhabited the earth millions of years ago. Two thousand years before the birth of Christ, Indian physicians treated it with a paste containing arsenic, and there is a reference to it in the Ebers Papyrus, found at Thebes and dating back to 1550 B.C. Hippocrates, who was born in 460 B.C. and according to legend lived for 109 years, knew the disease well: he is said to have cured a cancer of the neck by cauterization, and taught that treatment for the disease should begin early. On the other hand, John of Arderne, who was born in 1307 and is reputed to have been the first English surgeon, urged physicians to have nothing to do with patients suffering from the disease for their reputations would be jeopardized since it was incurable. He charged enormous fees, cheated the nobles whom he served, and may have been the original of Chaucer's Doctor of Physic: "In all this world there was none like him to speak of physik and surgerye, for he was grounded in astronomye," a description which is not really applicable to most present-day surgeons.

There are only a few outstanding figures in the history of cancer before the twentieth century. Percival Pott, who lived from 1714 to 1788 and was a surgeon at St. Bartholomew's Hospital in London, has won immortality for observing and describing the first occupational malignancy—cancer of the scrotum which he found in young chimney sweeps. Thomas Hodgkin (1798-1866), a pathologist at Guy's Hospital in London, recognized a malady marked by "certain morbid alterations of structure" which was later named after him, Hodgkin's disease. For its treatment he proposed "the utmost protection from the inclemencies and vicissitudes of the weather, to employ iodine externally, and to push the internal use of caustic potash as far as circumstances might render allowable." The German pathologist Rudolf Virchow (1821-1902) began his

[2] With the possible exception of one-celled organisms, the Protozoa.

career at the age of twenty-five with the discovery of "white blood," and in the words of Charles Singer, "set in motion the now familiar idea that the body may be regarded as a state in which every cell is a citizen; and disease is a civil war, a conflict of citizens brought about by the action of external forces."

The modern era in cancer research opened with two discoveries, widely separated in time and space. In 1915, a Japanese scientist, Professor K. Yamagiwa, aided by a colleague, Professor K. Ichikawa, induced cancer in rabbits for the first time by dabbing the skin of the ear with coal tar every day for more than six months. Scientists familiar with the finding of Percival Pott had attempted to induce cancer in animals by applying coal tar, but they had failed for two reasons: they had not been fortunate enough to select the rabbit, which is particularly sensitive to tars, or they had not been as patient as the two professors at Tokyo University. Fifteen years later, Sir Ernest Kennaway and his colleagues at the Royal Cancer Hospital in London synthesized the first chemical carcinogens—substances capable of inducing cancer—and succeeded in isolating from coal tar a chemical in it which induces skin cancer: 3,4-benzpyrene. This is further described in scientific terminology as a polycyclic aromatic hydrocarbon, and it occupies a special niche in the history of cancer research. The significance of the discoveries made by Yamagiwa, Ichikawa and Kennaway is that they enabled controlled tests to be made on laboratory animals, so that cancer scientists now had possession of their first important research tool. They could experiment, they could observe, they could measure. In passing, it might be mentioned that 3,4-benzpyrene is a ubiquitous carcinogen found in many foods, particularly in smoked meats and fish, and it is present in tobacco smoke and polluted air.

Progress after Kennaway's discoveries was slow, for many reasons. But toward the end of World War II medical science flexed its muscles and began preparations for a massive effort which, if it went as expected, might solve the problem of cancer with the same finality that the problems of many infectious diseases had been solved (with the notable exception, then, of polio). The demands and the pressures of warfare have always stimulated man's inventiveness, and this particular war had seen some quite extraordinary exploits resulting from the collaboration of scientists and technicians. Huge air fleets and huge armadas of cargo-carrying ships had been built at incredible speed; enormous armies had been provided with equipment far more efficient than anything used in previous wars; and, most striking of all, an unprecedented concentration of scientific and technological brainpower had provided the United States with a superweapon, the atom bomb, which swiftly ended the war with Japan and, at the time, was virtually guaranteed to end any future wars just as swiftly. In medicine there had been at least one outstanding accomplishment, the production (near the end of the war) of adequate supplies of penicillin; and as a result of all these successes a number of scientists were confident that with enough money, enough equipment, enough manpower and enough pressure, a speedy solution to the riddle of cancer might be found. One heard an echo of that brave old Churchillian phrase, "Give us the tools and we will finish the job." This overflowing optimism found expression during a press conference held on Thursday, August 7, 1945, in the New York offices of the General Motors Corporation, when reporters were given details of a new building planned for construction on East 68th Street, adjacent to Memorial Hospital, to be called the Sloan-Kettering Institute for Cancer Research.

Purely by chance the press conference was held the day after the first atom bomb was dropped on Hiroshima, and several of the overwrought journalists at the meeting wanted to know whether there was any connection between the development of the bomb and the creation of the new Institute. The answer, given by Dr. Cornelius P. Rhoads who had been appointed Director of the Institute, was that no direct connection existed beyond the fact that the principles of atomic physics are basic principles that apply to any sort of productive research, and the principle on which the atom bomb worked might be used both to cause cancer and to cure it. An unexpected connection developed months (and even years) later, for several scientists who helped to design the bomb asked to be permitted to work at the Institute (as they explained) for reasons of conscience, as if taking part in cancer research was an act of penance.

Speeches at press conferences announcing plans for new research centers, no matter how eloquent, rarely linger in the memory, but on this occasion something quite new and intriguing was revealed: the entry of a large industrial organization —perhaps the largest in the world—into the field of medical research. Any direct involvement was specifically denied; nevertheless, the projected institute was named for two of the top executives of General Motors, Alfred P. Sloan, Jr., Chairman of the Board, and Dr. Charles F. Kettering, head of the research division. "This," Dr. Rhoads explained, "represents a unique advance in medical science inasmuch as the plan essentially provides the extraordinarily competent technical skills and knowledge of industrial science as a co-worker with the more limited skills of medical and biological science. We know the problem is much more difficult, more time-consuming, more complex than it was ever dreamed to be. However, we feel certain that this type of development is going to be ideally suited to obtain the desired end."

Precise details of the plan were not revealed, but it was described in broad terms by Dr. Kettering: "I think that in this set-up here, all we are going to do is to become assistants to the doctors. Our work has got to be done through the medical profession. We are going to bring them, through types of instrumentation, the technique which we know. We are going to lay it on the table; and they will have to decide whether or not the thing is useful in their particular problem. We have no desire to dictate a procedure. That belongs to the medical profession and it has got to be done through them. But we can bring them and lay on the table things which we have used in other types of research, which may or may not be useful to them."

Also present was Frank Howard, of Standard Oil of New Jersey, another of this breed of exceedingly wealthy industrialists who were devoting themselves to the cause of human welfare. In due course he was to serve for ten years as President of the Institute and for an additional five years as Chairman of the Board of Trustees. He, too, was stirred by the projected union of science and industry. "The thing that struck me about this program from the beginning was that through you (Mr. Sloan and Dr. Kettering) there is being brought into medical research a new viewpoint of industrial research. It is that viewpoint which, in the hands of the Government, produced this miracle (the atom bomb) that we are talking about today. Things are moving very fast, and thinking in the field of research is moving faster. It has moved faster in the field of industrial research than in the field of pure science. Directness and willingness to amass large funds, large resources, and large personnel on a single objective, on a very limited objective, to go right at it and get it done—that method of approach is really quite different from the characteristic scientific approach. Mr. Sloan and Dr. Kettering are going to try to use that approach in medicine, and that I think is the important news of this development."

The atom bomb was referred to frequently. "Do you think," a reporter asked, "there is any *analogy* between the development of the atomic bomb and this research program?" The reply given by Dr. Rhoads expressed very clearly what was in the minds of those who had planned the Institute: "In the development of the atomic bomb as in other military projects it was possible not only to spend money but to acquire any essential personnel and facilities. As Mr. Sloan pointed out, personnel is just as important as money; we need it to make the job a success. . . . *I think no one would doubt that if there were put at the disposal of the cancer problem the same personnel, the same funds, the same facilities made available for the study of the atomic bomb, the progress would be very rapid.*"

Cornelius Packard Rhoads was apparently born to take command of the Sloan-Kettering Institute for Cancer Research; the Institute apparently came into existence to be ruled by Dr.

Rhoads. His energy was incredible. His ambition was boundless. He was big, handsome, brusque, irritable, and he did not suffer fools gladly. When, at our first meeting, I told him that I wanted to write a book about the Institute, he looked at me with deep suspicion and snapped, "I've already asked John Steinbeck to write it." One of his aides, showing me around the new laboratories, said, "You don't want to write a book about all this. Do a book about the Director. *He's* what counts here." You had the sense when you were with him that he was absolutely determined that the cure for cancer was going to be found in his institute and nowhere else. His energy and dedication were tremendously impressive, but also somewhat alarming because only a few human beings could possibly keep pace with him.

Rhoads could not help making enemies, partly because of his nature, partly because of his position, and from the beginning it was said of him by some people that he had cunningly inveigled Alfred P. Sloan and Charles F. Kettering into providing him with a magnificent research organization by convincing them that he would apply techniques devised by General Motors to the search for the cure for cancer, implying that if such a cure were found, to General Motors would go much of the glory. It was a Machiavellian scheme, his critics claimed, which the two General Motors executives could not resist. "Rhoads was fully aware," a scientist told me, "that General Motors couldn't contribute anything to help research, except money."

There is probably little truth in this allegation. From the record it is apparent that Sloan and Kettering were genuinely eager to play whatever part they could, as individuals and not as company men, to alleviate human suffering. "When you come to consider the amount of money that is being spent on tackling this thing (cancer) from a research point of view," Mr. Sloan said at the press conference, clearly speaking with very deep feeling, "it is just a drop in the bucket in comparison with what it ought to be. In an organization like General Motors we do not hesitate at all in approving a research project involving the expenditure of a million dollars a year. We might have to conduct that experiment for quite a number of years. That would not mean anything to us if we thought it would contribute to a result we were trying to get. And yet here is the most terrible affliction that any human being can have, and the aggregate amount of money spent on it is really inconsequential compared with what is spent on a single industrial product. It was appalling to me when I realized that." Kettering, a hard-headed engineer, had his own idea of what was involved. "It may be a two- or three-generation job, but some generation has to start it. . . . If anybody is under the impression that when this building is completed you are going to get the answer quickly, he is wrong. You may get it in a week, you may get it in a year after the building is up, but that would be a pure accident. If it follows the normal course, this thing will not come as a brilliant discovery like the atomic bomb (Dr. Kettering was obviously not aware of the agony that had gone into producing the atom bomb) but it will come as a slow, steady addition to the improvement of the facilities that you have; and finally, after X number of years, the thing will gradually disappear and nobody will know exactly what happened. These biological things happen that way." Despite this simple approach, Kettering was familiar with certain biological "things." For some time he had been supporting a research group which, as he phrased it, was trying to find out why grass is green—or, in other words, was attempting to learn more about chlorophyll, a biological project of great importance.

How it came about may never be known precisely, but as a result of the generosity of these two men, Dr. Rhoads found himself in charge of a lavishly endowed institute with funds guaranteed for ten years and an implicit guarantee that, if necessary, funds would be made available for an additional period of ten years. There was also a provision, emphasized by Mr. Sloan, that "if the problem should be solved—we take that optimistic point of view—the institute will be carried on . . . and it will devote itself to other medical research. There will always be a necessity for research in the medical area, just as there will always be a necessity for research in all areas of scientific development."

The new institute was to be housed in a thirteen-story building constructed on a plot of land valued at two million dollars which had been donated by the Rockefeller family. Adjoining it on one side, and connected to it, would be Memorial Hospital for Cancer and Allied Diseases, which—under the plan—was itself to be enlarged considerably. Adjoining the institute and connected to it on the opposite side would be a second large cancer hospital constructed by the city and named for a famous cancer scientist, Dr. James R. Ewing. The Sloan-Kettering Institute for Cancer Research would thus be the center of a large medical complex concerned solely with one disease, drawing material for study from the two adjoining hospitals while its staff assisted to a certain extent in the treatment of patients. There was little chance that the institute would become an ivory tower: every scientist employed in it would at all times be close, stimulatingly close, to the realities of the disease he, or she, was investigating.

So a powerful assault was mounted against the most formidable of mankind's enemies. Nothing remotely like it had occurred in medical history. Dr. Rhoads, with his overwhelming energy and ambition, was burning to lead an army of dedicated scientists into battle; and his troops seemed to thrive under his ceaseless exhortations to fight on, to work harder and still harder. The Sloan-Kettering Institute for Cancer Research, the largest and wealthiest and best-equipped cancer research center in the world, hummed with excitement, with unquenchable enthusiasm. It is told that some General Motors technical experts *did* appear on the scene, *did* attempt to impart their famous know-how; but one is forced to conclude that the medical scientists did not make them too welcome, or perhaps General Motors' know-how was not the kind of know-how that was required. Soon the men with micrometers ceased to come and the men and women with microscopes and microsomes had the laboratories to themselves.

At the outset Dr. Rhoads estimated that the annual budget

for the support of the institute would *eventually rise* to about $500,000, an immense sum at that time, similar to that received from the Federal government by the National Cancer Institute; it is interesting to note that in 1966 the institute's operating expenses were more than $9 million. No estimate was originally given of the staff to be employed by the institute but, again in 1966, the professional staff—that is, with the degree of M.D. or its equivalent—numbered more than 250, with an additional 100 Fellows in Training, many of whom had come from overseas. This was a vital part of the original concept: the institute and its two great hospitals were to serve not simply as a national center but in a much wider sense as an international center. Reginald G. Coombe, one of the nine trustees, stated this principle clearly: "I think you will see coming here a great many European doctors who for four years[3] have been kept back and repressed, concentrating entirely on war activities and unable to pursue this kind of work (in cancer research) who will come here for training. We already have a good many doctors who have come up from South America." A trip around the world talking to cancer specialists twenty years later confirmed the value of this program and the goodwill it engendered: one met men and women everywhere who spoke warmly, and with pride, of their training at Sloan-Kettering.

The American people—those who were aware of the institute's existence—clearly felt, from the beginning, great confidence that it would succeed in its task. This was the way Americans had become accustomed to seeing things done: the concentration of enormous resources, an all-out effort, relentless pressure, leading to total victory in the shortest possible period of time. But the institute's first years were inevitably exploratory; the territory was unknown, the work done in the past quarter of a century did not provide adequate guide lines for the future. New programs had to be laid out for the investigation of many different aspects of cancer and its treatment. In a sense, a magnificent theatre had been built, the stage had been set, the actors had been engaged, but

[3] The reference was to the period of World War II, actually (by European standards) nearly six years.

the play—or, at least, the greater part of the play—remained to be written. The settling-in period was bound to be long and difficult.

Yet in the early 50s, rumors spread of new miracle drugs that had been developed at the institute, of miracle life-saving operations. A national magazine, in a blaze of publicity, paid all expenses for a baby girl, suffering from retinal tumors in both eyes, to be flown from Nebraska for "miracle" treatment. Nothing could have been more cruel. There was not the remotest possibility of saving her or of ameliorating her condition. The same week a young soldier was flown in from Memphis on an Army transport plane, with his wife and mother, because he had been assured by his doctor that "those fellows at Sloan-Kettering" had perfected a miracle life-saving operation for his disease. No notification was sent to the institute; no records, no X-rays accompanied him; he simply arrived. Embarrassed officials in New York could not turn him away, for again there had been extensive publicity and a refusal to admit the young man and make the life-saving operation available to him might have led to a national outcry. A room was found for him in Memorial Hospital, but his wife and mother —who were totally without money—refused to leave his bedside and camped in his room, although the director of social services offered to provide funds for them to stay at a hotel. After two days the man said to his wife, "I don't want to have any operation," and his wife dutifully answered, "If you don't want to have it, honey, you don't have to have it." He was far beyond help, with widespread cancer of the lung; the miracle operation, excision of the pituitary gland, would not have done him the slightest good; and he died soon after he was flown back to Memphis.

C. P. Rhoads died suddenly and unexpectedly of a heart attack in August, 1959. He was only sixty-one years old, and there can be little doubt that his work at Sloan-Kettering, furious and unremitting, shortened his life. He helped to extend the lives of a great many people; he initiated work of vital importance; but he did not live to see a cure for cancer.

Charles F. Kettering had died the previous year, also of a heart attack. He, too, did not see a cure for cancer, nor the solution of the mysteries of chlorophyll and photosynthesis. Frank Howard died, of a heart attack, in 1964. Alfred P. Sloan, Jr., was hospitalized for the first time in his life in 1965 at the age of eighty-nine, for a minor ailment. One year later he was hospitalized again, and died within a day or so of a heart attack. He left $10 million to the Sloan-Kettering Institute for Cancer Research and $10 million to Memorial Hospital for Cancer and Allied Diseases. Before their deaths, both Sloan and Howard might have been aware that the first cures by means of chemotherapy had occurred (that is, by the use of drugs), as distinct from cures by surgery or radiation therapy. A number of women had been cured of a rare form of cancer called choriocarcinoma which sometimes follows pregnancy; a number of children in equatorial Africa had been cured of cancers which sometimes affected the jaws, sometimes affected the viscera. A number of children had experienced long-term remissions—five years or more—of leukemia. Altogether, the total of chemotherapy cures from 1945 up to the time of Alfred P. Sloan's death in 1966 was rather less than five hundred.

One has no way of knowing what went on in the minds of the trustees and the staff of the Sloan-Kettering Institute for Cancer Research at the time of Dr. Rhoads' death, apart from the sense of shock and loss; nor the reaction some six years later when Alfred P. Sloan died. Undoubtedly there was much searching of hearts; thoughts must have gone back to 1945, and the high hopes these remarkable men had expressed so eloquently, and the astonishing energy with which they set to work. Only a fool would say that the institute they founded had failed in its task; it had done well, establishing a great store of new knowledge, developing new techniques, finding new drugs, training new young men and women to continue the investigation of cancer. But the cure, the ultimate cure which would relieve mankind of the pain and the mutilation and the uncertainties and the dangers of surgery and deep X-rays had not been found after twenty years of intensive search: a fact that was inescapable, distressing, and possibly alarming because it suggested that a cure might be forever out of man's reach.

The scene can be surveyed from another vantage point.

In 1913 an organization called the American Society for the Control of Cancer came into existence with the aim of encouraging cancer education and carrying out some limited forms of cancer research, chiefly in the field of statistics. The Society was supported, not too lavishly, by public contributions—cancer was still in many minds considered to be a twin of leprosy, depressingly unpleasant and unmentionable in polite company. In due course the organization changed its name to the American Cancer Society, and today it is the greatest voluntary agency of its kind in the world (as distinct from the National Cancer Institute, a governmental agency). The financial support provided by the public has become almost phenomenal, amounting to nearly $60 million in 1968; the programs in cancer education and cancer research have become equally phenomenal. Some 68,000 volunteers interviewed more than a million people, obtaining cancer data which has been coded and processed by computers so that it is immediately available for special studies; 158,000 volunteers prepared 16,000,000 surgical dressings for use by cancer patients; trained volunteers went to the aid of cancer patients who had suffered particularly disabling operations—psychologically disabling, for example, in the case of breast surgery, physically disabling as in removal of the larynx. Public education is carried out on a huge scale, with armies of volunteers moving from house to house and city to city, backed by hundreds of thousands of posters, brochures, films, filmstrips, radio and television programs, adapted whenever necessary to the needs of the local population, who may speak English, Spanish, Polish, Yiddish or Chinese, but who are equally vulnerable to the disease. Education on the highest professional level is also provided through special programs for nurses, medical students, dentists, physicians, and through conferences which are designed to give research workers the opportunity of benefiting from discussions with outstanding scientists. Without a doubt, the Society's work is of immense importance to the American people and, by extension, to the world at large. In an age of ugliness and mischief, the evidence of such widespread human charity is heartwarming.

At about the same time that the Sloan-Kettering Institute was founded, in 1945, and perhaps as the outcome of similar thinking and similar pressures, the Society started an expanded cancer research program. A "Committee on Growth" was set up (*Growth* here refers not so much to the expansion of physical or spiritual attributes but rather to growth, benign or malignant, of tissues), and this committee appointed nineteen advisory panels of experts in specialized areas of research. In turn, these panels were to guide the Society in the development of its activities in three directions, which were defined elegantly but ambiguously as:

> The support of investigations, both basic and clinical, directed toward the uncovering of essential new information not only in the specific field of cancer but also in the field of phenomena of growth fundamental to it;
> the encouraging of young students through the award of fellowships;
> the formation of strategies for the ultimate assault on the problem of human cancer.

A curious situation had now developed—curious, that is to say, to the unaligned observer. Several years earlier, in 1937, the Federal Government had established through an Act of Congress an agency for research on the cause, diagnosis and treatment of cancer, known as the National Cancer Institute. By the same Act of Congress a National Advisory Cancer Council was created, consisting of twelve "non-Federal scientists and persons prominent in public affairs," as well as ex-officio representatives of the Department of Defense and the

THE SCENE 43

Veterans Administration. The function of this council was—
and still is—to advise the Surgeon General on all aspects of
cancer research—the needs, the programs, the policies. The
Institute is now one of nine Institutes and four Divisions that
comprise the National Institutes of Health, which are under
the direction of the Department of Health, Education, and
Welfare. The scale of these various undertakings can be
assessed to some extent by their budgets. The Department of
Health, Education and Welfare for fiscal year 1969 received
$15,861,342,800; for the National Institutes of Health as a
whole the appropriation was $1,170,399,000; while for the
National Cancer Institute the appropriation was $185,149,500
—more than three times the income of the American Cancer
Society.

Thus, from 1945, the Society found itself faced by formidable competition. Superficially the programs of both agencies, particularly in research, appeared to run along parallel
lines; and there was a clear and present danger that the public
might be disinclined to contribute twice to this worthy but
seemingly duplicated cause—through taxes for the support of
the Institute and voluntarily for the support of the Society.
At every opportunity, therefore, and with great force, the
Society pressed the case for the voluntary agency which could
"draw on the broad support of millions of individual citizens
and thousands of private corporations . . . which could complement the government's activities and join with it to provide
a broad and balanced program of cancer research support."
The theme was capable of endless variations: "It is precisely
in this area (of personal involvement and personal commit-
ment) that the most important distinction between the Society
and governmental agencies—no matter how benevolent and
well-financed—is revealed. For it is we of the Society who
can effectively organize the resources, tap the potential, of
countless dedicated citizens in all parts of our land. The value
of this resource, the power of this potential, is incalculable."
The theme was expressed in more earthy terms by Mary
Lasker (Mrs. Albert D. Lasker), Honorary Chairman of the
Board of Directors of the American Cancer Society, a lady

of legendary charm and iron resolve who has done as much for the cause of public health in the United States as anyone alive. "Don't for a moment believe the government can cure the nation's diseases alone. It has done a great deal to influence the whole health picture. But the private agency is absolutely vital—to keep interest high, actively alive. And to give the problems fresh air. No government agency should be empowered to be alone in a field of such life-and-death importance. The American Cancer Society gave publicity to the national needs and laid the foundation for getting money from Congress. Without the ACS *nobody* could have gotten much money. No one else could have done the Society's pioneering work on cigarettes and lung cancer. The ACS supports ideas and provides lines of research that the Cancer Institute might never think of . . ." It would be an error to construe these remarks as showing a bias in favor of the American Cancer Society, for, as well as serving on the Board of Directors of the Society, Mrs. Lasker was one of the twelve appointive members of the National Advisory Cancer Council, which helps to guide the affairs of the National Cancer Institute.

Public support for the Society has not, of course, been diverted; it has increased encouragingly year by year. But at the end of her statement, which appeared in the Annual Report of the American Cancer Society for 1965, Mrs. Lasker struck an unexpected note. Usually the concluding sentences in a statement of this kind, marking the twenty years of activity since the Society's great leap forward in 1945, tend to express certain noble abstractions, such as hope, faith, confidence, the future, the horizon. The difference here was significant. "Tremendous advances have been made in the laboratories," Mrs. Lasker said, "but there hasn't been enough clinical progress, in my opinion. . . . We have started around the edges—against choriocarcinoma, Wilms' tumor, retinoblastoma and remissions in other types of cancer with various drugs. There has been great progress in treatment, in education. I must admit, twenty years ago I thought we would have ended it by now. What we need is that extra push.

There's an awful lot of information that might bring cures if it were energetically followed. I'm not discouraged. I *know* cancer will be wiped out . . . but we've got to get cracking."

The following year the Board of Directors of the Society announced that a special committee had, from February, 1964, to November, 1965, carried out a nationwide survey to analyze the Society's performance and policies. Committee members had interviewed research scientists in medical schools, universities, institutes and industrial laboratories throughout the country. A study had also been made of recent scientific literature: an endless outpouring of scientific papers, usually written in a brain-chilling style that can only be termed researchese, tells in detail the story of the progress of cancer research.

The findings, evidently, were not altogether encouraging. To some people, indeed, they may have appeared grim and dismaying.

Large sums of money (one restrains oneself from saying gigantic sums of money) are spent by the National Cancer Institute and the American Cancer Society on research project grants, grants to institutions such as hospitals and universities, grants for the training and support of men and women who are specializing in cancer research, and long-term grants to outstanding scientists who are thereby enabled to plan far-reaching projects without the ever-present fear of running out of funds. Without these grants, of course, cancer research in the United States would virtually come to a halt. A few examples will serve to show the extent of the support provided in recent years by the larger of the two principal agencies.

In 1965, the National Cancer Institute negotiated an agreement with the Sloan-Kettering Institute for Cancer Research which provided *an annual grant* of approximately $4,300,000 for five years, nearly half (47 per cent) of Sloan-Kettering's annual operating budget. The University of California received $2,626,382 (these and the following figures are as of

June 30, 1964); the University of Texas, $2,483,651; Roswell Park Memorial Institute, $2,383,722; the University of Wisconsin, $1,986,958, and five other institutions received more than a million dollars. About two thousand grants were made in 1965 for research, research fellowships, and training, totaling about $72,750,000, while some $46 million was spent on research carried out under contracts to the National Cancer Institute.

The American Cancer Society total income in 1968 was some $60 million; out of this, one-third—$20 million—was allocated for research grants. Altogether, since its inception, the Society has provided research funds that exceed $180 million.

These statistics are important, but they are nothing but *statistics*, conveying no information beyond amounts and numbers. Theoretically, every project supported by a grant is of potential value; whether that value will be realized is often unpredictable and can be decided only when the project is completed. In general it can be assumed that 90 per cent of all scientific research is only of indirect value, adding nothing more than a fragment of knowledge to what is already known. "Untold millions of dollars have been spent on research into the nucleic acids," a scientist with a high reputation in another branch of research said to me recently, "without extending the life of a single cancer patient by one day." Yet there is the possibility that nucleic acid research *might* come up with information, some time in the future, which could have profound effects upon cancer therapy. Dr. Charles B. Huggins, who was awarded a Nobel Prize in 1966 for his work on hormone therapy in the treatment of cancer of the breast and of the prostate, received from the American Cancer Society alone grants amounting to some $2,000,000 over a period of fifteen years. Denis Burkitt began research which has had extraordinary results with an initial grant of $45, followed two years later by another grant of $400 which went toward the purchase of an essential research tool—an ancient station wagon. No comparison between Dr. Huggins and Mr.

THE SCENE

Burkitt is intended—this is merely an illustration of how, in medical science, things happen.

The preliminary report of the special committee surveying current cancer research and the special role of the American Cancer Society was presented in October, 1965. Certain historical facts had considerable bearing on the report: they can be stated briefly.

At the beginning of the twentieth century, cancer was almost invariably fatal. The possibility of a cure—by any definition—was remote.

By 1937, one out of four cancer patients survived five years or longer after treatment by surgery or radiation.

By 1955 the cure rate (five years or longer) had risen to one out of three.

There was every hope that in the next ten years the cure rate would continue to rise, with one out of two cancer patients surviving five years or longer after treatment. This had not occurred by 1965. The cure rate remained where it had been in 1955.

Beginning in the 1940s and continuing into the first half of the 1950s there had been exciting advances in chemotherapy and hormone therapy. Important breakthroughs seemed imminent. These breakthroughs did not take place.

Hope had been high that leukemia and possibly the lymphomas would be conquered before 1960. These hopes (as late as 1968) had not been realized.

To even the most ardent well-wisher it seemed that the attack on cancer, so promising ten years earlier, had lost its momentum. There had been a great accumulation of knowledge about the disease, but this knowledge was far from complete. There had been great improvements in methods of treating the disease, but new cures had not been discovered. Furthermore, there were no high priority projects in progress that offered substantial promise for the *immediate* future. Some scientists had difted away, disheartened, to other fields of research.

Aroused by this somewhat bleak picture and, presumably, by the results of its nationwide investigations, the committee made a number of unusually sharp recommendations, preceded by a few nebulous remarks that are inescapable in reports of this kind. The committee agreed, for example, on the need for accelerating the research effort against cancer; it also agreed that the cancer problem despite the best efforts of everybody was far from being solved; and so on. The report then urged:

> that the Society should assume a more positive role in achieving its research objectives, taking initiative for choosing research undertakings and for planning and supporting their development;
> that the Society should direct attention to the major unsolved problems of human cancer, both at the clinical and basic research levels;
> that the Society should launch a new program of strategic research focused on specific objectives;
> that there should be greater emphasis on the unsolved clinical problems of cancer.

These were strong words, the words of hawks. They were in fact an admonition to the Society to come down to earth, to do something, and to do it now.

Recommendations of a similar sort, but expressed in even more pointed language, had been made in a twenty-one-page document addressed to the Society by Dr. Richard E. Shope, Professor and Member of the Rockefeller University and one of the renowned figures in cancer research. Shope was the first scientist to isolate a virus in mammalian tumors, as long ago as 1931, and the virus was, appropriately, named after him: the Shope rabbit-papilloma virus. He had also done outstanding work on influenza viruses, and, all in all, he has an assured place in the history of medicine.

The document, according to the Society, was written under "terrific emotional pressure" and it is classified as highly confidential. Dr. Shope was suffering from cancer at the time he

THE SCENE

wrote it, and he died a few months after it was submitted, at the early age of 65. The title of the paper is "An Attempted Classification of Research Currently Supported by the American Cancer Society with Comments on Deficit Areas and an Appraisal of What Needs to be Done," and in his summing-up Dr. Shope stated: "The program is deficient because it fails to support research in a number of important areas; also because even in areas where support appears reasonably adequate, the nature of the research supported is either not sufficiently oriented to the human cancer patient or it leans toward obtaining more or less obvious answers." The plea here is not greatly different from that made in the report by the special committee—*the need to direct attention to the major unsolved problems of human cancer.*

Without singling out the Society, Dr. Shope asserted that at the heart of the problem was the "passive" manner in which the large granting agencies in the field of medical research traditionally made their awards. "There is no discipline," he wrote, "no strategy, no tactics," and apparently a lack of direction toward specific objectives. "The time has come," Dr. Shope concluded, "when intelligent direction and leadership will have to be introduced into cancer research to assure that we hew to the line of fixing our objectives of solving human cancer problems more closely than in the past."

Dr. Shope was considerably more outspoken than the Research Survey Committee. "No discipline, no strategy, no tactics. . . . The time has come when intelligent direction and leadership will have to be introduced into cancer research. . . ."[4] Was he really implying that up to now there had been an absence of intelligent direction and leadership in cancer research? One cannot say: the document is secret. But his criticism, and the criticism expressed by the research committee, took effect. On October 20, 1966, the Board of Di-

[4] A distinguished British scientist commented about this statement that it applies just as readily to British cancer research. It applies, indeed, to all cancer research everywhere, for the simple reason that cancer scientists are still in the process of penetrating the mysteries of this extraordinary disease.

rectors of the American Cancer Society "voted to reorganize the Society's research program, and to establish within that program a new function and a new unit to execute it. The new function is development of research strategy for a focused attack on key research objectives." The new unit, called the Department of Research Analysis and Projection, "will search out significant leads which have been inadequately pursued and proceed to implement their exploitation. It will also strive to enhance the development of new insights and new lines of inquiry in critical areas where progress has been slow or has come to a standstill entirely."

The American Cancer Society then made a gesture that deserves commendation for courage and public responsibility. It distributed a sixty-page booklet entitled "New Directions in Cancer Research" in which it gave an account of the events that led to the decision to reorganize its research program. The quotations above have been taken from this booklet. Only the main body of the Shope document was withheld, for the reason given—that it was confidential. But the willingness of the Society to submit to harsh criticism, to acknowledge the criticism publicly, and above all to act on that criticism when it is justified, is admirable and reassuring.

The National Cancer Institute is located with its sister Institutes and Divisions on a 306-acre tract of land in Bethesda, Maryland, a suburb of Washington, D.C. A booklet published by the Public Health Service of the U. S. Department of Health, Education, and Welfare, gives a broad description of the Institute's multifarious activities: "Studies on the causes of cancer and methods of preventing or treating it are conducted in its laboratories and clinics at Bethesda and under contract with other research organizations.

"In the Institute's laboratories and clinics over six hundred scientists, physicians, nurses, technicians, and assistants are joined each year by visiting scientists and by scientists in training, known as research fellows and clinical associates.

"A strong clinical program involves the cooperation of almost 1,000 cancer patients admitted annually to the Clinical Center, the 516-bed hospital shared by seven of the nine Institutes of the National Institutes of Health.

"A Board of Scientific Counselors composed of outstanding scientists serves as an advisory body to the Institute on all aspects of its 'intramural' research program carried out by the in-house staff.

"Certain types of research, such as the identification of environmental causes of cancer, the development of new diagnostic techniques, and the synthesis and testing of new drugs, which require laboratory and animal resources unavailable at Bethesda, are carried out under contract as designed and supervised by National Cancer Institute scientists.

"Cancer research conducted in many non-Federal institutions in the United States and in other parts of the world are [*sic*] supported by Public Health Service grants administered by the National Cancer Institute. Applications for grants are first evaluated by committees of scientists serving as consultants. They are then reviewed by the National Advisory Cancer Council which makes final recommendations to the Surgeon General, who has the authority to award grants with the approval of the Council.

"Approximately half of the Institute's annual appropriation is allocated to support of research through grants to individuals and organizations. At present about 2,000 grants for cancer research are in effect."

Since the Institute is the chief source of support for cancer research in the United States and also provides support for research in other countries, its power is formidable and far-reaching. At its disposal are funds sufficient to permit the development of certain selected research schemes on a scale that is impressively grandiose.

For example, the testing of chemical substances which may be helpful in the treatment of cancer is exceedingly laborious and consequently exceedingly costly. From 1955 to 1966 the Institute spent $257,685,000 of Federal funds on this work, screening some 257,000 materials. The average cost of testing each substance, therefore, was very conveniently about $1,000.

But—again very conveniently—only one out of about every thousand substances tested was judged suitable for carrying on to the all-important stage of clinical evaluation (that is, for testing in the actual treatment of patients), raising the cost of each *prospectively useful* chemical substance to about $1,000,000.[5]

An optimistic appraisal would suggest that perhaps 25 of all the substances tested might be found to have some anti-cancer value when applied to human beings, bringing the cost of each *useful* substance to about $10,000,000. Perhaps five of these would eventually be found to be of considerable value in cancer treatment, bringing the cost of each *valuable* anti-cancer substance to about $50,000,000. If, of course, after all this agony only *one* drug was found with wide-ranging curative properties, at the cost of a mere $257,685,000 it would be a marvelous bargain, and there would be dancing in the gray streets of Bethesda.

In December, 1966, I visited the National Cancer Institute and interviewed the Director, Dr. Kenneth M. Endicott. Pressed for time because he had to attend a hearing (where, he explained cheerily, "I shall be asking for more money,") Dr. Endicott answered all questions with complete frankness and equanimity. Some of his remarks appear later in this book; here, however, is a verbatim report of the first two or three minutes of the conversation.

> Q: Your appropriation this year [1966] is $163 million, and you have requested a slightly higher amount for 1967. . . . Do you have any idea how much money the National Cancer Institute has received since it was founded in 1937?
> ENDICOTT: Including this fiscal year, about $1.3 billion.
> Q: The bulk of that money has gone toward cancer research?
> ENDICOTT: Yes. The principal other expenses have been for

[5] The precise number of suitable substances was 275. Participating in the clinical tests were nearly 1,200 physicians, 64,000 patients and 300 hospital services throughout the country. The figures are taken from a report by the National Advisory Cancer Council, *Progress Against Cancer*, 1966.

training of personnel, for construction of research facilities and, to some extent, for cancer control programs in the United States.

Q: The question I would like to ask is—it's a very obvious, brutal, journalistic question—do you feel there has been an adequate return for this huge amount of money?

ENDICOTT: I'll tell you very frankly what I think. We who are in the field of medicine and biology are unaccustomed to dealing with the kind of figures—the kind of money—that is really going to be required to answer some of the problems of cancer. Our colleagues who concern themselves with space exploration, or with atomic energy, or with military hardware, don't boggle at spending ten billion dollars a year. We've hoped for some miracle to happen which would solve the problem inexpensively. But it isn't, in my opinion, that kind of problem. We'll probably spend ten times as much as we have already spent before we get it completely solved—if we ever get it completely solved.

Q: You are the topmost figure in this entire pyramid of cancer research. What I am trying to learn is whether you think it should be better organized, whether it is more organized than it appears to be, or whether it would in fact be a bad thing to attempt to organize it too much.

ENDICOTT: I think the academic approach, which is one of finding able men, providing them with the necessary resources and encouraging them to do what they think is best, is an excellent device for uncovering fundamental knowledge which may, and hopefully will, be applicable to the solution of practical problems. Without this fundamental knowledge we could never really expect to solve the problem.

But the difficulty has been that most of us in this field—and, indeed, in almost every field of health research—have been prone to conclude it was all that had to be done, and that somehow a solution to all these problems would arrive if we had enough men working on enough problems, each following his own nose.

It is my firm conviction that to solve practical problems of large magnitude requires organization, planning, and (in the applied developmental field, certainly) a considerable amount of control.

So our strategy is to have two programs: one, an external program, the other an internal program, in which we select good men and encourage them to follow their noses. The external program we support through grants. The internal program we support simply by employing first-rate scientists and letting them work in our laboratories as they see fit.

But, in addition, we have organized a number of applied and developmental programs which are aimed directly at practical targets, in which very large numbers of scientists work together under planned central control. They are organized in two general areas. One is aimed at the management of the patient who has cancer. The other is aimed at discovering causes of cancer which can be eliminated, thus preventing the disease in the first place. We're investing heavily (and I hope in the years to come even more heavily) in identifying cancer-causing substances and eliminating them from the environment.

A second approach is more of a gamble. This is a very hard-hitting program to attempt to determine whether or not viruses cause cancer in man. We're gambling a lot of energy, money, and resources on this.

As regards therapy—that is, treatment of the disease—we have concluded that although some small gains can be expected in the fields of surgery and radiation therapy, the one area which seems to offer an opportunity for major gain is chemotherapy, the use of drugs. You must be aware that over the past ten years we have spent a quarter of a billion dollars on the search for more effective drugs.

As for the future, obviously we shall go on training scientists, supporting individual scientists, and developing and managing large, organized enterprises. I think there's a change which is already becoming apparent—at least, as far as therapy is concerned—and that is, we're beginning to organize programs tackling a specific kind of cancer. Instead of talking in general terms of the chemotherapy of cancer, we're now beginning to study drugs; to develop drugs; to seek drugs effective against a specific kind of cancer.

The first effort of this kind was the creation of the Acute Leukemia Task Force. Within the past year we've developed another task force, in breast cancer. And at least for the next decade or so this may be the most significant change in our attitude to the problem—to attack it disease by disease.

First, we have to get some leads. There are a number of kinds of cancer against which we can't design an attack because one has nothing to hold on to. . . .

The Manhattan Project was started in 1940: the atom bomb was ready for use within five years. The American space program began in earnest about 1948: the first American astronaut circled the earth in 1962.

It is clear that the great assault on cancer which opened in 1945 has not achieved comparable success. One recalls Cornelius P. Rhoads's statement: *I think no one would doubt that if there were put at the disposal of the cancer problem the same personnel, the same funds, the same facilities made available for the study of the atomic bomb, the progress would be very rapid.* Those means were made available; but nearly a quarter of a century later the largest cancer institute in the world is still hard at work on the problems of cancer; the largest voluntary cancer organization in the world has gone through a long and painful reappraisal of its research philosophy; the Director of the largest governmental cancer agency in the world talks of spending billions of dollars on future research and of the difficulty of designing an attack on a number of kinds of cancer that *one has nothing to hold on to*. And it is not a conspicuously *American* failure. The great cancer research establishments of Great Britain, of Europe generally, of the USSR, of Japan, have not progressed any further than the United States. "There are no secrets in cancer research," a famous German scientist remarked during an interview: "We are all one family."

In the Istituto Regina Elena in Rome, Dr. Carlo Nervi, a young cancer surgeon, suddenly said to me with deep feeling, "We will never find the cure for cancer, *never*. It will be more and more possible to *treat* the disease. But a *cure*—that is impossible." In an office of the World Health Organization in Geneva, Dr. William I. B. Beveridge, a Consultant in Comparative Medicine, said when I spoke of the recent progress in cancer research, "I think, personally, that I am rather more impressed by our lack of progress. It's interesting to reflect that during this century medical research has made tremendous strides in mastering the infectious diseases (that is, diseases caused by microorganisms); but in the chronic degenerative diseases, in which I include cancer, progress has really been very meager." To my question, "Do you see any hope of this progress accelerating in the future." Professor Beveridge replied pleasantly, "One always hopes. One wouldn't be in research if one didn't hope."

The scene, then, is restless and shifting—a typical contemporary scene, without absolutes. There are countless successes to match countless failures. There is hope, there is gloom. Man's accomplishments in the search for an answer to the problem have been brilliant, astounding; and every new discovery seems to accentuate our ignorance. One of the pioneers of nucleic acid research, Dr. James D. Watson, who was awarded a Nobel Prize at the age of thirty-four,[6] has written, "Many intelligent biochemists hold the view that now is not the time to work seriously on the biochemistry of cancerous cells. They argue that, even though cancer cells are the cause of enormous human suffering, nonetheless it does not make sense to put a disproportionate share of our scientific effort into trying to meet an unripe intellectual challenge. They compare the current situation with the desire to understand the nature of solar energy at the time of Newton." Dr. Watson adds, "I suspect, however, that this pessimism may not be justified;" and it is interesting to note that in February, 1968, he became the director of a famous laboratory (the Cold Spring Harbor Laboratory of Quantitative Biology on Long Island, N.Y.) which, in the words of *The New York Times,* he hoped to convert into a major center of basic cancer research and training.

---

[6] The Nobel Prize in Medicine and Physiology was awarded in 1962 jointly to J. D. Watson, Francis Crick, and Maurice Wilkins. The quotation is from *Molecular Biology of the Gene,* W. A. Benjamin, Inc., New York, 1965.

Pessimism and optimism are not really relevant here. The problem *must* be pursued; there is no alternative; and the large scale investigation of cancer proceeds all over the world with enormous vigor.

THREE

A Galaxy of Problems

The previous chapter may have left an impression that cancer research is at an impasse, that progress has slowed down, that the future is clouded. An impression of this kind is not altogether true, nor is it justified by the facts. An impasse *may* have been reached, but it can be circumvented by a change of direction—like the paramecium the cancer scientist can back away and approach his target from another direction. Progress *may* have slowed down, but it has by no means stopped—papers reporting new findings by researchers pour off the presses and mimeograph machines at the rate of a thousand a month. The future *may* be clouded, but bright new hopes constantly present themselves. "Cancer is not an incurable disease," Professor Peter Alexander said to me recently in London: "It is steadily being eroded away. A lot of cancer is being cured—40 per cent, if you include skin cancer. But the subject is incredibly difficult. To make any worthwhile contribution one has to dig hard. And if one finds something giving, one concentrates on that."

The cancer researcher is not only involved in a subject of incredible difficulty: he is reminded every moment that the subject is a grim reality to a vast number of people, including himself and his family; and as he goes about his work he is under constant physical and emotional pressure. The day after Christmas, 1967, *Le Figaro* in Paris published the results of a survey carried out by a hundred *experts internationaux* who had asked people in five countries—France, West Germany, Italy, Great Britain and the United States—what advances would be of the greatest benefit to the human race between now and the year 2000. In every one of these countries, the overwhelming majority (91 per cent in France, 79 per cent in the United States) gave priority to *la guérison du cancer*. Closely following in second place was the abolition of warfare; sixth on the list was prolongation of life to one hundred years, and last was space travel *sans danger*.[1] Undoubtedly the conquest of cancer would head the list in a similar survey carried out almost anywhere in the world (except in those areas where cancer, for good reasons, is relatively rare). Every director of a cancer research institute, every cancer scientist, is acutely aware of it, and the burden of personal responsibility sometimes becomes exceedingly heavy.

Cancer is not one disease. The term is used generically for many diseases (a hundred, two hundred, or more, according to the criteria applied to their classification) that are in many respects quite dissimilar yet have certain features in common. This lack of precision, in fact, pervades the entire subject, a point which is well expressed in one of the latest publications of the National Cancer Institute: "In 1806, a committee of eminent physicians posed important questions regarding such fundamental problems as an exact definition of cancer, identification of precancerous conditions, if any, and proof that cancer is either a contagious or hereditary disease. The fact that many of these questions are not completely

---

[1] Obviously, the advance that would be of the very greatest benefit to the human race between now and the year 2000 would be to find means for the effective and equitable control of world population; but this proposition was not included in the questionnaire.

answered today, more than a century and a half later, serves to underscore the magnitude and the complexity of the cancer problem."[2] The phrase "the cancer problem" is in itself inadequate. We are much nearer the truth if we look at cancer, in the words of Dr. Francis J. C. Roe, as "a galaxy of problems."

Most scientists (not all, by any means) seem to agree that cancer essentially involves disease of individual cells. For example, cancer of the kidney is not a disease of the kidney *in toto* but a condition in which cells in the kidney have become cancerous and have proceeded to multiply; if all of these cancerous cells are removed or destroyed, the kidney (hopefully) will continue to exist and function more or less like any other healthy kidney, depending on how much healthy tissue remains after therapy is completed. At the outset, therefore, we need to inquire briefly into the nature of the normal cell, and the nature of the malignant cell.

The Normal Cell

About forty years ago, the cell—the fundamental unit of all living things—was a mystery, but a relatively simple mystery. Biology textbooks presented diagrams of what was termed an "ideal" cell, shaped like a somewhat compressed sphere; and, as a unit should, it looked neat and functional. It had a skin, or membrane, which kept its contents from oozing out but permitted nutrients to ooze in; its most prominent feature was a spherical nucleus inclosing a tangle of chromosomes; and surrounding the nucleus was the cytoplasm, permeated by granules, globules, and vacuoles of assorted sizes. One readily accepted the fact that thirty trillion of these sturdy little objects—spherical, polygonal, scale-like, star-shaped,

[2] *Progress Against Cancer*, 1967.

elongated, cuboid, according to necessity—assembled themselves to form tissues, which in turn formed organs, organ systems, and a bony framework, all of which ultimately combined harmoniously to form the total human organism.

With improvements in the means of viewing and investigating the cell, an immense amount of information has accumulated in the past thirty years about its anatomy; about its elaborate systems of membranes, rough, smooth, inner, outer; about its chemistry; about its aggregation of boat-shaped structures, granules, coils, tubules, stacked discs, helixes; and about a thousand other matters. But little has been fully resolved, and the cell almost daily becomes more complex and more mysterious, a baffling micro-universe. If you take a very fine needle and lightly prick this page so that the impression is invisible you will have a mark that is two or three times the size of a liver cell, whose diameter is about one fiftieth of an inch. If you allow the tip of the point of the needle to penetrate the paper and go no further, you will have a hole roughly the size of the human egg cell, about one tenth of a millimeter in diameter and just visible to somebody with good eyesight. Some white blood cells are considerably smaller—only one three-hundredth of a millimeter in diameter. Within these absurdly tiny things occur the diverse activities that are recognized as life; and occasionally within these tiny things some event occurs that results in the catastrophe of cancer. The untrained human mind cannot possibly project itself into such an ultra-Lilliputian landscape, just as it cannot project itself into the radio-astronomer's universes beyond our universe. The image has to be transformed: we mentally magnify the cell to, say, the size of a ping-pong ball, and on this scale we would all be rather more than a mile high.

Similarly, to aid in visualizing it, we can describe the cell as consisting of two sacs or compartments, one inside the other.[3]

[3] It is worth bearing in mind that this is purely a concept of the human intellect. The cell would never describe itself in this way; just as we would rarely describe ourselves as consisting of two sacs, the thoracic (the chest) and the abdominal, plus various attachments above, below, and to the side.

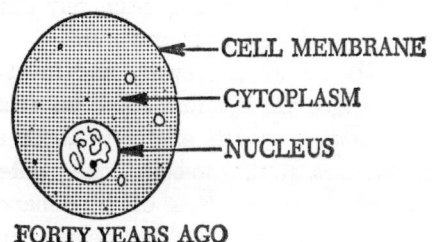
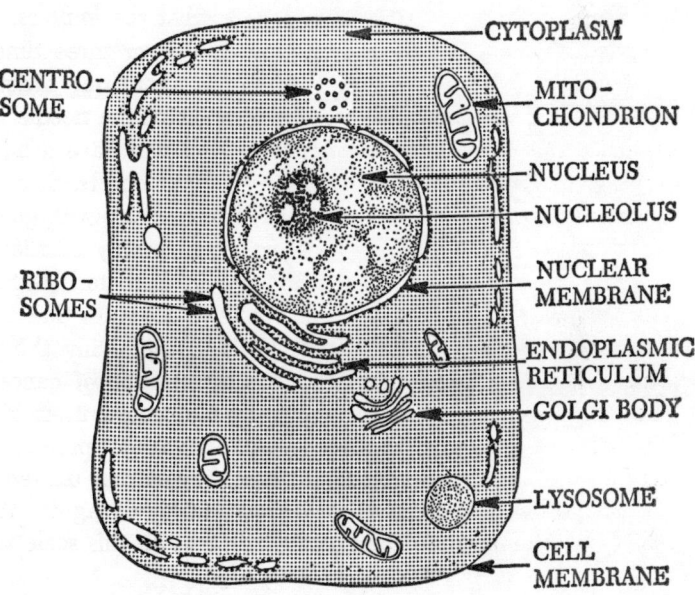

The cell: forty years ago and today

A GALAXY OF PROBLEMS

The inner sac, called the nuclear membrane, surrounds and encloses the nucleus, which contains the hereditary material. The outer sac, called the plasma membrane, encloses the cytoplasm, a translucent substance containing numerous particles of different kinds.

Until recently it was customary to define the cytoplasm as a clear viscous fluid and leave it at that, but the electron microscope has shown that it contains an elaborate system of membranes called the endoplasmic reticulum (which simply means the network within the plasma), that extends from, and is continuous with, the nuclear membranes inside the cell and the plasma membrane on the outside. Thus, the cell is provided with a kind of internal skeleton, bathed by the cytoplasmic fluid. Inhabiting the cytoplasm are a variety of structures, or organelles: sausage-shaped mitochondria, of which there may be a thousand or more—the furnaces or powerhouses of the cell; a lesser number of Golgi bodies, which look like stacks of folded membrane; ribosomes, small spheres which line some parts of the endoplasmic reticulum. Close to the nuclear membrane is a small particle called the centriole, made up of nine double rods arranged in a circle, forming a barrel or cylinder, held together by two belts, or girdles. It is actually a part of the nuclear apparatus.

The nucleus, as far as we know at present, contains nothing much more than the hereditary material, in the form of the chromosomes, plus one or two small granular bodies called the nucleolus, or nucleoli.

This arrangement, whereby the contents of the nucleus occupy a separate compartment, is the same in all cells, the only exceptions being bacteria which have the chromosomal material distributed throughout the cytoplasm or only loosely assembled in a "nuclear area" without any enclosing membrane. (Viruses, which are non-cellular organisms, are simply a strand of nuclear material surrounded by an overcoat or shell of protein—they contain nothing resembling the cytoplasm.) Otherwise, plants, insects, animals of every kind, follow a similar cellular pattern and are even constructed of the same substances, a principle that has been expressed in admirably lucid terms by the French microbiologist, André Lwoff: "When the living world is considered at the cellular level, one discovers unity. *Unity of plan:* each cell possesses a nucleus embedded in protoplasm. *Unity of function:* the metabolism is essentially the same in each cell. *Unity of composition:* the main macromolecules of all living beings are composed of the same small molecules. For, in order to build the immense diversity of the living systems, nature has made use of a strictly limited number of building blocks. . . . Each macromolecule is endowed with a specific function. The machine is built for doing precisely what it does. We may admire it, but we should not lose our heads. If the living system did not perform its task, it would not exist."

The duplex design of the cell (again, as viewed by the human intellect) enables it to play a double role. Firstly, it carries out its functions as a unit in the total organism. If it is a liver cell, it carries out liver functions; if it is a skin cell, it carries out skin functions. But in addition, when it is called upon to do so, it fulfills the responsibility of passing on life to a new generation of cells.

The cytoplasm and its organelles within the plasma membrane constitute, in a sense, a miniature factory—infinitely more efficient than any man-made factory. Here the cell manufactures new parts to replace those that are worn out, refines and assembles its multitudes of proteins, converts food into the energy that enables the processes of life to take place. The plasma membrane itself does far more than merely hold the cell together. It selectively permits the entry of molecules needed by the cell, and the exit of waste products, as well as those products made by the cell for use by other cells, such as hormones. It is flexible enough to provide certain cells with an amoeba-like mobility; it facilitates communication between cells; it acts as a sort of launching pad for antibodies (and as a receptor for invading organisms); and, because it has a peculiar "stickiness," which may be mechanical or electrical, it enables cells to adhere tightly to each other in the formation of tissues.

The nucleus, so conspicuously set apart in its own sac, is the regulatory center of the cell, controlling growth, development, and division. Remove the nucleus from the cell with microneedles and the cell will gradually die; replace the nucleus with the nucleus from another cell of the same kind—a nuclear transplant—and the cell, if all goes well, may continue to live.

Control, we believe, is effected through the chromosomes, which have inherited from their cellular predecessors instructions about how this cell must conduct itself. The information will be passed on, again via the chromosomes, to succeeding generations of cells. But it is important to realize that the chromosomes we see in microphotographs are in a dense, compressed form which is only assumed when cell division begins. During most of their existence, in the stage known as interphase, they are difficult to perceive, even when special stains are used, and are most probably spread throughout the nucleus in a tangle of fine, extended threads. This is their normal condition. This is how they carry out their tasks up to the point, in human cells, where cellular events require them to assemble as twenty-three pairs of separate entities.

The precise structure of chromosomes, therefore, is still a mystery. The precise nature and extent of their activities is equally a mystery. We know that they are composed of nucleic acids and various proteins, and it is generally agreed that the molecules of DNA (deoxyribonucleic acid)—which have the ability to duplicate themselves with unvarying precision—are the ultimate units of heredity.

Cells multiply at different rates. In the liver the interval may be as long as a year and a half. Some cells—nerve cells are the best example—never divide after they are formed, and cannot be replaced if they die. The blood cells work exceedingly hard and, as a result, wear out rapidly, so they must be constantly replaced. The same is true of other cells which of necessity are used up at a high rate in the course of our daily life, such as the skin cells, the cells lining the intestinal tract, and the male reproductive cells.

The process of cell division is so spectacular that we sometimes overlook the fact that the greater part of the cell's existence is spent in interphase, performing its general duties and making the necessary preparations for reproducing itself. Nuclear material must be manufactured so that two sets of chromosomes will be available. The various organelles in the cytoplasm must be duplicated (although how and when this is accomplished is unknown). A cell may go from division to division in as brief a period as eighteen hours, but more than seventeen hours will be passed in interphase and less than an hour in division. Then, in a dramatic succession of stages (called prophase, metaphase, anaphase, telophase) the membrane of the nucleus slowly disappears, the tangled threads of chromosomes become visible, split longitudinally, arrange themselves across the cell's equator, and by means of a remarkable cellular mechanism called the spindle, or the mitotic apparatus, the two sets of chromosomes are pulled to opposite ends of the cell. Nuclear membranes now appear around each set of chromosomes, which reassume their form as a tangle of slender threads; the cell is pinched into two parts, each containing its own nucleus; and two cells now exist where only one existed before. The performance is fascinating and awe-inspiring, and no scientific explanation can adequately account for it. "When I look at a dividing cell," wrote the English geneticist William Bateson, "I feel as an astronomer might do if he beheld the formation of a double star: that an original act of creation is taking place before me." The cells of every living thing have been created in the same way.

A human life begins with the meeting and fusing of a maternal germ cell, an ovum, and a paternal germ cell, a sperm. Both, at the time fertilization takes place, have undergone a process called meiosis (from the Greek, to make smaller) whereby the number of chromosomes possessed by each is reduced to half, from 46 to 23. *The fertilized cell* thus has a normal complement of chromosomes, 46, or 23 pairs, half of which come from the female parent, half from the male. Without meiosis, of course, the fertilized cell would have 92 chromosomes, an impermissible state of affairs since it would bring about the extinction of the species in a few generations.

The fertilized cell with its 23 pairs of chromosomes now proceeds to undergo division. Its chromosomes carry all the information necessary for the development and functioning of a particular human being, and the fertilized cell is consequently said to be "totipotent"—that is, capable of giving rise to every kind of cell required by the mature organism.

But one of the most striking features of cell division is that each time division takes place the daughter cells receive a complement of chromosomes precisely identical to those of the cell from which they have just originated, and therefore *every* cell in the entire organism can be considered to contain all the information required for the development and functioning of a mature human being. This is evident because the mature human being—the end product of the original fertilized cell—possesses the germ cells which (combined with the appropriate germ cell of the opposite sex) will enable the entire sequence to begin all over again. One can at this point paraphrase Samuel Butler and suggest that just as a hen is an egg's way of producing another egg, a man is the way sperm cells make more sperm cells, an idea that has a certain validity since the mature sperm cell by itself is incapable of reproducing itself by division.

Fairly early in the embryonic history of the organism, though, the dividing cells cease to be openly totipotent. They begin to specialize, in order to produce the different kinds of cells required by the body—nerve cells, muscle cells, skin cells, connective tissue cells, and so on, all in an almost infinite number of forms. This process is called differentiation, and it is of profound interest to biologists and cancerologists. It implies, among other things, that much of the information carried by the chromosomes is superfluous in specialized cells and is consequently suppressed. Furthermore, once specialization has begun the change is irreversible—a skin cell or a muscle cell cannot turn itself around and go back to the carefree and uncommitted life of a totipotent cell: its destiny has been decided. Yet the chromosomes in all the differentiated cells still carry (as far as we know) the full complement of genetic information, including the information about *suppressing* whatever is superfluous in any particular kind of cell.

Finally, we reach the most fascinating and the most formidable of all the problems in cellular biology: integration, the process whereby all parts and elements combine to form a complete organism. A human being, or a fish, or a mouse, comes to life not as an assemblage of cells, or of tissues, or of organs, but as a *whole*. How do the cells communicate to achieve this unity? How is development controlled? How is growth halted? If the skin is damaged, new skin cells will soon replace those that have been destroyed, but the manufacture of new cells will stop immediately the damage is repaired: what mechanism controls the cells so that they duplicate the original skin structure? How is it that the total organism exhibits such harmony: everything made to a certain size, everything working in a certain way, everything occurring in a certain order?

The answer to all these questions is quite simple: We do not know.

The Malignant Cell

The normal cell is competent, integrated, and (wherever necessary) industrious and purposeful. Its maladjusted counterpart, the malignant or cancerous cell, is anarchic, purposeless, and only too likely to become a threat to the existence of the organism in which it arises. In the words of Ronald W. Raven, by ending the organism's life it ends its own life, and it is unable to justify or modify its activities to avoid final self-destruction.

A malignant tumor can be defined as a discernible accumu-

A GALAXY OF PROBLEMS

lation of malignant cells (from the Latin: *tumor*, a swelling, from which we also derive *tumulus*, a mound, and even *tomb*). Some of the chief characteristics of malignant cells can be tabulated here briefly:

> They multiply—sometimes rapidly, sometimes slowly—in an uncontrolled manner.
> In the course of this unrestrained multiplication they invade and destroy adjoining normal tissue.
> They may escape from the site where the malignancy originated and spread within the organism, establishing new colonies of lawless and invasive cells. These colonies, or secondary growths, are called metastases.

It is the invasiveness, resulting in the destruction of healthy cells and tissues, that makes the malignant cells a deadly threat to the organism (whether this happens to be a plant, a mouse, or a man). On the other hand, the organism often tolerates without serious ill-effects so-called "benign" tumors that remain localized and non-invasive. Whether a tumor is actually malignant is a matter for the pathologist;[4] if the tumor is in an early stage, diagnosis may be difficult, for the differences between normal and cancerous cells may be small and extremely hard to discern even by an expert.

One of the basic principles of biology, enunciated in the middle of the last century by Rudolf Virchow, is that cells arise only from cells: *Omnis cellula e cellula*.[5] Normal and malignant cells alike are subject to this law. Thus, at some

---

[4] In a broad sense, a pathologist is a physician specializing in the nature, causes and development of disease. He is also concerned with the various physiological changes that arise as the result of disease. *Pathology* is really a portmanteau term: it covers many disciplines and sub-specialties. Among them are *anatomical pathology*, which deals with both the broad and microscopic study of organs and tissues; *clinical pathology*, which deals with aspects of chemistry, bacteriology, virology, immunology, etc., in relation to the diagnosis and treatment of disease, in individual human patients and in the community at large; *comparative pathology*, which deals with diseases of animals particularly in relation or in comparison to similar diseases in human beings; *plant pathology;* and so on.

[5] Virchow's statement appeared in 1855. An English biologist, Martin Barry (1802–1855) had expressed the same idea fifteen years earlier.

stage in their history, malignant cells must have "arisen" from normal predecessors: there is no other way in which they could come into existence. Here we are close to the heart of the problem. How and why do normal cells become cancerous, breaking away from the organism's control mechanisms? We have not learned what really occurs within the cell in the process of transformation, but we do know some of the agents which bear responsibility, in whole or in part, for initiating the change. There are numerous chemical substances which are known to be carcinogenic: many of them are listed in later chapters. Carcinogenic substances may be found in foodstuffs; in the atmosphere, as pollutants; in tobacco smoke; in materials that affect the skin. Some may be manufactured within the body itself. Ionizing radiation, as from X-rays (or nuclear explosions) can transform the cell; so, in excess, will ultra-violet radiation—thus implicating the life-giving sun. There are a few forms of cancer that are known to be hereditary—a distressing tumor of the retina of the eye, found in young children, called retinoblastoma, and a condition characterized by multiple intestinal tumors, usually appearing between the ages of fifteen and twenty-five, called familial polyposis coli. And there are, of course, viruses, known to cause a variety of animal tumors but not yet directly implicated in human cancer.

Theoretically, from what has been established about cell growth, a single malignant cell is capable of initiating a tumor that will ultimately be lethal; and, in fact, this was demonstrated as long ago as 1936 by Dr. Jacob Furth of New York, who transplanted a cell taken from a cancerous mouse into a healthy mouse, with the result that the healthy mouse developed cancer. The experiment has proven of value recently in providing new ideas about the treatment of human leukemia; for calculations have shown that one leukemic cell, doubling every four days, will produce a condition of acute leukemia (in which the patient has approximately a trillion leukemic cells) in 164 days—a little more than five months. Killing 99.9 per cent, or even 99.9999 per cent of the diseased cells is not enough to *cure* leukemia. There must be a total kill, down to

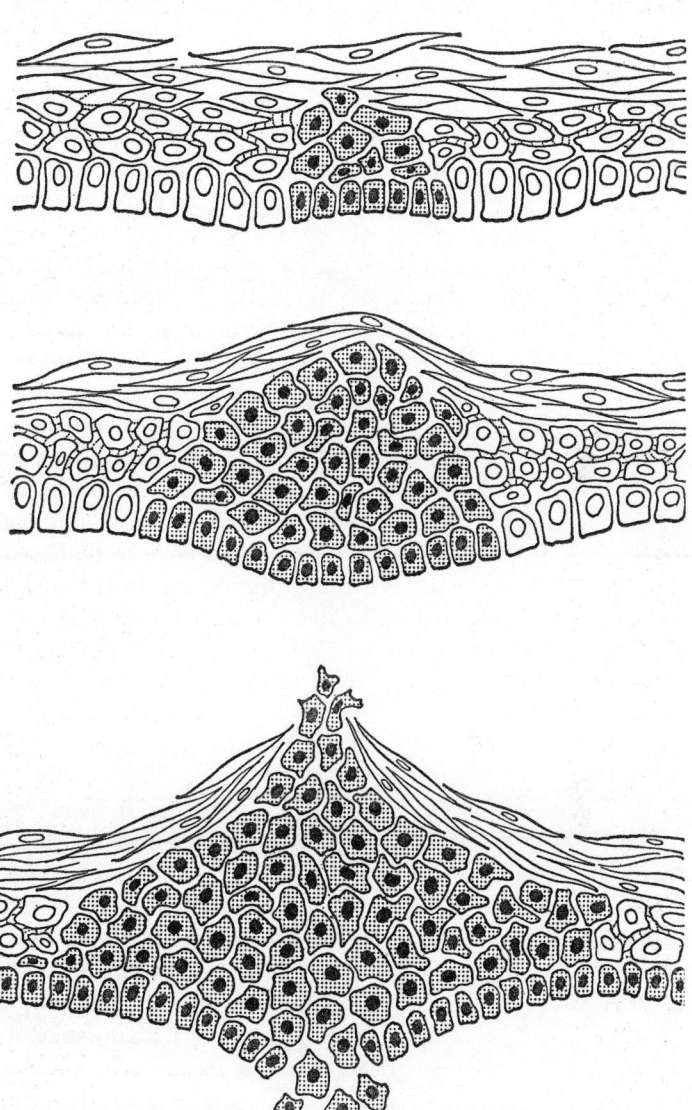

Stages in the development of cancer cells in epithelial tissue

the last malignant cell, otherwise the disease reestablishes itself, a condition seen in leukemia too often.

It is generally believed that, in some way, the stage is set for a malignancy to develop by a series of virtually imperceptible changes within the organism, affecting a fairly considerable population of cells in a particular organ, or at a particular site—a kidney, for example, or a patch of skin. The transformation would manifest itself gradually, rather than in a single jump, over a great many cell generations, each new generation becoming increasingly abnormal and probably more vigorous, until a condition is reached in which some cells are recognizably malignant. The old, popular concept of a ferocious cancer cell coming into existence spontaneously—out of nowhere, so to speak—and proceeding to multiply at an enormous rate is somewhat erroneous, like so many old, popular concepts. "There is no all-or-none difference between normal cells and cancer," writes Professor Michael B. Shimkin in his excellent handbook, *Science and Cancer*,[6] "but rather a series of transformations from the temporary, benign hyperplastic masses, to benign tumors that remain localized and non-invasive, through dependent neoplasms that can continue to grow and invade only if certain hormonal or other conditions of the host are met, to cancers with varying degrees of normal appearance and normal functions, to the relatively completely independent anaplastic cancer without any recognizable normal functions."[7]

Since cancer often behaves in a quite unpredictable way, it is possible for the change to occur abruptly, in just a few steps; but no matter how malignant the cells are from the outset, they must still go through the process of division in order to

[6] Public Health Service Publication No. 1162; U. S. Department of Health, Education, and Welfare, 1964.
[7] *Hyperplastic masses* refers to the enlargement, in size or bulk, of tissues or organs, resulting from an abnormal increase of the number of cells. This kind of enlargement, or overgrowth, is non-malignant. *Anaplasia* is the reversion of cells to a more primitive or embryonic form, with greatly increased reproductive activity. In this condition the cells are immature, have no specific function, multiply rapidly and without purpose, and are therefore considered to be malignant.

increase their numbers, and they are rarely able to increase any faster than some of the more active cells of the body, such as those lining the intestines, or the bone marrow cells. Certainly, no tumor grows as fast as the unborn child in its nine months of uterine life.

Other factors play a part in the rate at which malignant cells multiply. Since they are anarchic, they divide haphazardly, eventually producing a population of cells not only unlike normal cells but also unlike each other. A mixed population provides the tumor with certain advantages. Whereas normal cells are held in check by the body's control mechanisms, the malignant cells are delinquents to the extent that they have escaped partly or wholly from responsibility to the organism; and those cells that are most aggressively malignant, and can reproduce most rapidly, in due course become dominant. The result is that the cancer becomes increasingly malignant and its growth is more implacable.

How long is the interval between the first cellular changes and the appearance of a recognizable cancer? The answer, like everything else relating to this disease, is that it is widely variable and is complicated by factors we understand imperfectly and factors we do not understand at all.

It is usual to turn to the laboratory mouse for data on this matter, but despite its many scientific virtues the laboratory mouse is rather remote from us as a species, and its responses cannot be assumed to provide a reliable pattern for human responses. Nevertheless, it is worth reporting that the mouse, exposed to a cancer-inducing substance, may develop recognizable tumors in less than three months or, in other instances, the tumors may not become apparent for upwards of two years—that is to say, until the animals have almost lived out their lives.

When we turn to human beings we find that the latent interval of various forms of the disease is to some extent dependent on age. In adults the interval is generally quite long. Skin cancer following heavy irradiation may not occur for fifty years, and about the same length of time is required for the induction of cancer as a result of chronic exposure to arsenic-containing dust. The length of time to which a human being is exposed to a carcinogen is also a factor; thus, at all levels of cigarette smoking the risk of cancer development increases with age and the length of exposure. The young smoker rarely develops lung cancer: it is a disease, essentially, of the elderly, heavy smoker. In Britain today, Dr. Richard Doll has pointed out, lung cancer can now be expected to kill one in every twelve males born, and it is responsible for 12 per cent of all male deaths between the ages of forty-five and sixty-four years.

Some interesting statistics have been gathered by Dr. J. Q. Matthias, of the Royal Marsden Hospital, London, dealing with cancers alleged to have resulted from physical injuries. While Dr. Matthias concludes that a physical injury to healthy tissue is unlikely to be a primary cause of cancer, he believes that an injury may act as a co-carcinogen[8] in tissues that have already been exposed to a carcinogen. Even with this reservation a few of the latent periods he cites are surprisingly long. Skin cancer in the scar of burns may occur after twenty-three to forty-five years; following ulcerated gunshot wounds, tumors may occur after forty-one years, and after open knife wounds in thirteen years. Exceptions, of course, are inevitable. "There are also well-documented cases," Dr. Matthias writes, "with much shorter latent periods, such as the girl reported by Lambert (1964) who developed a malignant neoplasm in the frontal region (the forehead) 5 days after being hit by a tennis ball, the carcinoma of the tongue occurring 5 months after injury (Wirth, 1963), and a male patient (Lendrum, 1948) who was found to have a malignant tumor 4 months after a blow on the breast." The probability in these cases is that the injury drew attention to the disorder, or activated a tumor that was already present.

When we look at the malignancies of children we find problems of an entirely different order, related to the inescapable fact that it is the destiny of children to go through a lengthy process of growth. They grow at a prodigious rate *in utero;*

---

[8] A co-carcinogen is an agent that may not itself be carcinogenic, but combines with a carcinogen to hasten or to enhance its effects.

they grow at an almost equally prodigious rate for the first three years after birth; they continue to shoot up until they have passed through adolescence. Rapid growth implies the rapid multiplication of cells; and if, during this time, some abnormal cells arise they will almost inevitably participate in the general proliferation and perhaps span the gap from a benign abnormality to outright malignancy in a few brief cell generations. For this reason, cancer is exceedingly serious when it occurs in childhood. Its most common forms are the leukemias and lymphomas (which are also found in adults), but as we descend the age scale we find certain forms that occur as a rule only in young children. These include cancers of the central nervous system, called neuroblastomas; cancers of the kidney, variously called nephroblastomas, embryomas, or Wilms' tumor; cancer of the retina of the eye, retinoblastoma; liver cancer, hepatoblastoma. Technically they are described as originating in embryonic tissue: they may arise while the embryo is being formed, or soon after birth in tissue that is still immature, with the distressing result that the cancer is already evident when the child is born, or makes an appearance in the first two or three years of a child's life. The chances of developing cancer lessen as children pass through puberty into young adulthood: the incidence of leukemia, for example, in the age group 15–34 is half that of children under fifteen, while lymphosarcoma drops to one-twentieth. In the following two decades, between thirty-five and fifty-four, leukemia again doubles itself, and we also see the rise of the typical malignancies of late middle age—breast, lung, uterus, colon and rectum, and so on—all of which may have been latent throughout the preceding twenty years.

The chromosomes have been shown to be responsible for the general welfare and conduct of the cell, and it might seem reasonable to argue that the lengthy tragedy of cancer begins with a molecular disaster in the nucleus of the cell: an assault upon the chromosomes, accidental or deliberate, initiating the sequence of events that will result in the ultimate destruction of the entire cellular edifice. The accident might be a random X-ray, or an encounter with a chemical carcinogen. The deliberate attack might come from a virus.

Ever since chromosomes were seen by the microscope, scientists have been looking hopefully for a relationship between cancer and chromosomal changes, for signs that would warn that cancer was on its way. As far back as 1889, a German-American pathologist, Edwin Klebs,[9] observed that tumor cells often had unusual numbers of chromosomes: some had too few, some had too many. A few years later another German investigator, D. Hansemann, suggested that where any large numbers of abnormally dividing cells were seen in a tissue, this might indicate that a malignancy was present; he suggested, further, that the malignancy itself might be caused by abnormal division. In 1912, still another German, Theodor Boveri (famous for the definitive explanation of how spermatazoa and ova originate) came up with a Chromosome Theory of Cancer, which postulated that cancer is the outcome of cells acquiring abnormal numbers of chromosomes through abnormal division.

The chromosomes as they are seen in metaphase (the most favorable stage of division for this purpose) can be photographed and then arranged systematically in pairs and in descending order of size. This is known as a karyotype (from the Greek, *karyon*, a nut or nucleus) and it is in effect a presentation of the chromosome characteristics of any particular individual or of any particular cell line.

A karyotype of a normal human cell will show two sex chromosomes and 22 pairs of chromosomes that have been distinguished by number and divided into seven sub-groups designated by letters from A to G. Thus, if a researcher in, say, California suggests that an abnormal E-16 might be the basic reason for the uncontrolled cell division found in cancer, scientists all over the world will know where to look, with the reservation that identifying individual chromosomes is immensely difficult, even for experts. The five largest pairs, which

---

[9] Klebs was born in Prussia in 1834. In 1896 he became professor of pathology at Rush Medical College, Chicago.

make up groups A and B, and a few of the smaller pairs, called acrocentrics (groups D and G, joined at the top and looking like wishbones) can usually be recognized without too much trouble. Others—more than half of the total—are less easy to distinguish: the variations in size are minute.

Several pathological conditions in human beings have been linked to chromosomal abnormalities. Down's syndrome,[10] or mongolism, is marked by mental retardation, slanting eyes with prominent epicanthic (Mongoloid) folds of the upper eyelids, and a great many physical deformities. It is caused by an extra chromosome-21—that is, there are three of these chromosomes instead of two, a condition called trisomy. Klinefelter's syndrome, affecting males and marked by eunuchoidism (absence of sexual characteristics) and excessive development of the breasts, which sometimes secrete milk, is another defect resulting from trisomy. Turner's syndrome, a form of dwarfism, is due to the lack of the X chromosome. Trisomy D, which results in malformation of children and their early death, is trisomy of one of the D group of chromosomes, number 13, 14 or 15; while Trisomy E, also a cause of malformation and early death, is a trisomy of one of the E group, either number 17 or 18. The *cri du chat* syndrome of infants, marked by congenital defects and a curious cry like a cat's mew, is due to the absence of a short arm of one of the number 5 chromosomes.

Unlike these disorders, where the addition or loss of a single chromosome leads to widespread injury, cancer is usually typified by cells carrying chromosomes that are wildly abnormal in numbers and structure. Instead of 46, there may be 70, 80, or even hundreds of chromosomes; in one case, tumor cells were found to contain more than a thousand. With a single notable exception these abnormalities seem to be utterly random: there is no pattern which is specific for a particular malignancy, and a tumor will often contain cells with different numbers of chromosomes as well as cells that appear to be

---

[10] A syndrome is a group of signs and symptoms occurring together and characterizing a particular disease.

quite normal. The exception is a form of leukemia called chronic myloid leukemia,[11] and some findings about it which were announced in 1960 have aroused a great deal of speculation. A majority of patients suffering from this form of leukemia have an abnormal chromosome (identified as chromosome-21) which has been seen in all phases of the disease in blood and bone marrow cells and seems to have some relationship to the patient's survival time. Called the Philadelphia chromosome, or Ph^1 (after the city where it was discovered, not because it occurs there more frequently than anywhere else) it is the only chromosomal abnormality which, so far, has been found consistently in cancer cells.

What is the precise significance of this discovery? Nobody can say. The experts are divided. The Ph^1 chromosome may be the cause of this specific form of leukemia, or it may be one of the results of the disease. In broader terms, chromosomal abnormalities may lead to cancer, or cancer may lead to chromosomal abnormalities. To add to the puzzle, children with Down's syndrome (mongolism), possessing an extra chromosome-21, are thirty to fifty times more likely to develop leukemia than the general population, while patients with Turner's syndrome (dwarfism, due to lack of one of the sex chromosomes) have, mysteriously, a higher incidence of ovarian cancer.

Under the microscope the cancer cell often looks somewhat larger than the normal cell, with a more prominent nucleus. If it is seen in the process of dividing there is usually evidence of chromosomal abnormalities, and sometimes the normal pattern is completely changed—three or four daughter cells may be produced instead of two as in normal division.

But a great deal more occurs in the malignant cell than chromosomal disorders. About forty years ago, the German physiologist Otto Warburg (who was born in 1883) advanced a theory that cancer was the result of a fault in the cell's

[11] Also termed myelocytic, myelogenous and granulocytic leukemia.

metabolism[12] due to the inability of the cell to make normal use of oxygen because of an injury to its respiratory system which, in turn, was due to an enzyme defect. Warburg received the 1931 Nobel Prize in Physiology and Medicine for discoveries relating to the respiratory enzyme, and his theory attracted wide attention and an enormous amount of controversy, leading to wild charges and countercharges and astonishing bitterness. Today, Warburg is out of favor, but research continues into the role of enzymes in cancer, a subject of such monumental complexity that those engaged in it seem to occupy a principality of their own in the kingdom of biology, some distance from a similar principality occupied by the high priests of immunology.

More recently, the mitochondria—those sausage-cucumber-boat-shaped organelles in the cytoplasm, considered to be the cellular powerhouses—have come under scrutiny, following the unexpected announcement in 1962 that they almost certainly contain DNA. This is perplexing indeed. Why should the mitochondria, bustling around the cell *outside* the nucleus, possess DNA, the stuff of life, the double helix of all existence, which until now was assumed to be unique to the chromosomes? There is discussion, too, of the origin of these organelles (and the unknown way they replicate), and it has been suggested that early in evolutionary history they were parasites —or, more accurately, *symbionts*—not unlike the earliest forms of bacteria, which took up residence in primitive cells and actually helped, in the words of Dr. E. H. Mercer, to create the efficient cell as we now know it. This concept might explain their possession of DNA: they brought it into the cell with them. And it might also imply that any defects in the

---

[12] Metabolism can be defined as the aggregate of the chemical changes taking place in the cell necessary to maintain life. It can be regarded as a dual process. *Anabolism* consists of using energy to build food molecules into the complex amino acids and proteins of protoplasm. *Catabolism* consists of breaking down and oxidizing the constituents of protoplasm, which results in the release of energy for vital purposes. However, *protoplasm* is now infrequently used by biologists. It is a portmanteau term for the material which comprises the essential substance of the whole cell.

mitochondria themselves could have a bearing on a cell becoming malignant.

Carcinoma *in situ*, a tumor arising in one place and remaining there without signs that it is invading other tissue, is a threat to the individual that can be met by decisive action: the tumor, at an appropriate time, is removed by the surgeon or destroyed by the radiologist; and that—if the tumor's status was actually benign—should be the end of the matter. It is above all the *invasiveness* of cancer, malignant cells scattering out of the surgeon's reach, that is the real threat, establishing colonies of malignant cells far from the site of the original malignancy. How and why cancerous cells acquire the ability to invade adjoining tissue and travel through the body is, therefore, a problem of the utmost importance: if it could be solved, if the invasive cells could be eliminated by some means, we should have cause for rejoicing.

Normal tissues, we know, are orderly. The cells grow at different rates; they specialize in order to carry out different duties, and the outcome is unified and harmonious—the cells produce a particular kind of tissue with absolute precision and then stop growing. The mucous membranes of the intestinal tract, for example, go through a process of continuous replacement, but the new cells faithfully maintain the form and structure of the tissue or organ of which they form part, so that no change is evident. The cornea of the eye, too, has an extremely high replacement rate: here it is easy to see how precisely the cells obey whatever forces control them.

Still another characteristic of cells is their specificity: kind clings to kind. If individual kidney and liver cells are mixed together, they immediately proceed to un-mix—the kidney cells seek out fellow kidney cells, the liver cells turn to fellow liver cells.

Cancerous cells do not obey these rules. They have lost any familial urge; they have lost the compulsion to arrange themselves in an orderly way and to comply with the rules governing form and structure; they go as they please.

Some brilliant work has been done on these phenomena in the past decade, notably by two British scientists, Professor E. J. Ambrose and Professor Michael Abercrombie. Ambrose has shown, with some extraordinary stereo-microphotographs, how cells move on a glass surface: "It can be seen that the cell membranes are in continuous activity. Ruffles form on the leading edge of the cell, which travel backwards towards the nucleus. . . . The cell is able to migrate across the glass by forming intermittent contacts. The movement is rather similar to that of the earthworm, except that only single cells are involved. . . . When the ruffled membrane of a migrating fibroplast makes contact with another cell, adhesion generally takes place. This adhesion arrests the movement of the cell for two reasons. Firstly, the adhesion between the two membranes holds up the forward movement of the membrane. In addition, the ruffling activity is switched off. The locomotory mechanism of the cell is therefore brought to a halt."

The process whereby the cells switch themselves off has been called by Professor Abercrombie *contact inhibition of movement*. The term implies that once the cells have made contact with each other they obey some signal and thus are inhibited from any further movement: they adhere to each other, and in this way they proceed to assemble orderly tissue. Furthermore, the surface of the cellular membrane is so constructed that permanent adhesion occurs only between cells of the same type.

Malignant cells ignore the signals. They are indifferent to contact inhibition. When they encounter each other, instead of halting and forming orderly interlocking groups, their movement continues and the cells pile up on top of each other, forming a structureless mass. Because they do not adhere tightly to each other, individual cells can break away from the tumor and go on to invade adjoining tissue, competing greedily with normal cells for available food supplies; and, again, because of their lack of "stickiness" they can be dislodged from a tumor and carried by the bloodstream or the lymph to distant parts of the body. Most of these loose vagrant cells are destroyed; but a number will inevitably survive,

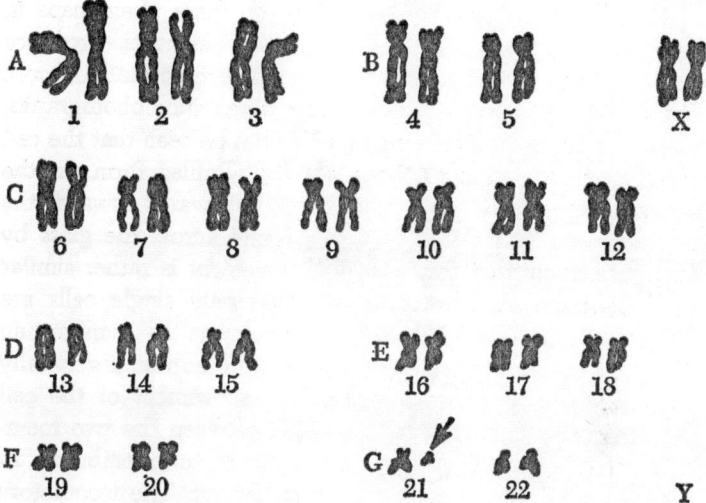

Karyotype (arrow indicates Philadelphia chromosome)

A GALAXY OF PROBLEMS

trapped in lymph glands and in connective tissue, spreading to the liver or the lungs or the brain. Sometimes in the course of weeks, sometimes gradually over many years, new malignant colonies are established, and the condition of disseminated cancer is reached.

What can be done about these cells that are indifferent to the laws that regulate contact inhibition? What can be done about cells with defective membranes, defective organelles, defective enzymes, defective chromosomes; about cells that trespass, about cells that spend a quarter of a century preparing to become malignant? These are some of the basic problems which face the research scientist. He is—at the opposite end of the scale—like the astronomer peering through his telescope at some enormous upheaval taking place in the outer reaches of the universe, powerless to influence it in the slightest degree.

But man's ingenuity is boundless, and he may find a way to become master of the infinitely small catastrophes, the cellular upheavals, that threaten all living things.

3

World Around Us

FOUR

Of People and Places

One of the most dramatic episodes in the history of medicine took place, with no fanfares and with few spectators, in the parish of St. James', London, on Friday, September 8, 1854. Superficially it appears unconnected with the search for the cause and cure of cancer: it arose out of an outbreak of cholera, and its central character was a physician named John Snow who was then forty-one years old and who was to die only four years later. Snow achieved a measure of fame as the first English doctor to specialize in the use of anesthetics (particularly chloroform, which he administered to Queen Victoria in childbirth) and also as the inventor of a pulmotor for the resuscitation of asphyxiated newborn children; but he is best remembered, and by some scientists revered, for his part in the events of 1854.

Cholera is caused by a bacterium called *vibrio cholerae* or —from its very distinctive shape—*vibrio comma*, discovered by Robert Koch in 1883. The source of infection is usually a water supply that has been contaminated by sewage, and from this focus the microorganism can be spread by contaminated foodstuffs, by flies, by its victims, and by passive carriers. Even today it is far more lethal in the underdeveloped areas of Southeast Asia than the sum of all forms of cancer; it has been prevalent for centuries in India, notably in the great jungle wilderness—the Sundarbans—of the Ganges River delta; and as recently as 1965 the World Health Organization announced that one form, El Tor cholera, had invaded new areas, spreading northward and westward to Afghanistan, Nepal, Iran, and the USSR.

There had been a series of fearful cholera epidemics in Europe, and also in America, in the first part of the nineteenth century. Thus, the epidemic which suddenly erupted in London in the middle of August, 1854, must have aroused the utmost terror. John Snow, who had been appointed secretary of a Cholera Inquiry Committee, has left a superb account of what happened. "The most terrible outbreak of cholera which ever occurred in this kingdom, is probably that which took place in Broad Street, Golden Square, and the adjoining streets, a few weeks ago. Within two hundred and fifty yards of the spot where Cambridge Street joins Broad Street, there were upwards of five hundred fatal attacks in ten days. The mortality in this limited area probably equals any that was ever caused in this country, even by the plague; and it was much more sudden, as the greater number of cases terminated in a few hours. The mortality would undoubtedly have been much greater had it not been for the flight of the population. . . . As soon as I became acquainted with the situation and extent of this irruption of cholera, I suspected some contamination of the water of the much frequented street-pump in Broad Street. . . . On proceeding to the spot I found nearly all the deaths had taken place within a short distance of the pump. . . . There were sixty-one instances in which I was informed that the deceased persons used to drink the water from Broad Street, either constantly or occasionally. . . . I had an interview with the Board of Guardians of St. James's parish, on the evening of Thursday, 7th September, and represented the above circumstances to them. In consequence of what I said, the handle of the pump was removed on the following day."

Snow's conduct in this epidemic was remarkable for several reasons. He did not spend time looking for a causative agent. True, he examined the water, finding at first "little impurity in it of an organic nature," then on a later examination finding "small white flocculent particles" that he surmised rendered the water impure. *Vibrio comma,* even if he had found it by microscopic examination, would have meant nothing to him. But his immediate and most significant activity was assembling the evidence which clearly established that the pump was the source of the cholera. Once this was known the next step was simple (although any observer of the medical scene must remain astonished that this simple step was in fact taken, that there was no vehement opposition to an act manifestly infringing on the rights of the individual). The handle of the pump was removed on Friday, September 8—a day that should be celebrated in a suitable manner every year by all epidemiologists;[1] even the most freedom-loving, the most addicted of pump-water drinkers could not pump themselves a glass of Broad Street pump water; and the cholera epidemic thereupon subsided, having killed only 530 men, women, and children, although—if it had continued—it might easily have killed ten times that number.[2]

The method is capable of extension to cancer in certain forms. For example, nobody knows precisely what happens to cells in the human bronchial tree when cigarette smoke is inhaled. But there is every probability that cigarette smoking is *at least* partly responsible for the present-day pandemic of lung cancer. In the United States lung cancer is the leading cause of male cancer deaths: 44,000 men died of the disease in 1967, as well as some 8,000 women—about 140 deaths a day, considerably higher than the cholera mortality in the vicinity of Broad Street. In England, 40 per cent of all cancers of men

[1] There is no satisfactory *contemporary* definition of this term, as the reader will find in the next few pages.
[2] An outbreak in Hamburg in 1892 caused 17,000 cases of cholera in two months, of whom 8,605 died. Altona, a neighboring city using the same tainted water from the River Elbe, was saved because the water supply included a sand filter which effectively held back *vibrio comma,* a preventive measure inspired by Robert Koch himself.

are lung cancer, and the same pattern is becoming evident wherever cigarettes have shown the way to perfect pleasure (*It is exquisite*, as Oscar Wilde said of smoking, *and it leaves one unsatisfied. What more can one want?*) even in equatorial Africa and far-off Borneo. There is really no need for research costing untold millions of dollars into the carcinogenic fractions contained in cigarette smoke and their fate in the cytoplasm. Snow's method is applicable. Unfortunately for everybody concerned, it is difficult in this particular case to remove the pump-handle.

Most dictionaries are unimpressed by epidemiology, taking it merely at its face value as, medical science dealing with epidemics (Webster) or, the science of epidemics and epidemic diseases (Stedman). But an epidemic is considered to be an outbreak of a specific disease, affecting an unusually large number of individuals at the same time and in the same general area; and, more particularly, an outbreak of this kind is by its nature infectious. Since cancer does not occur as an outbreak affecting numerous people simultaneously, and since it is not (as far as we know) infectious, there seems to be little point in discussing the epidemiology of cancer. It would appear to be a branch of medicine that by definition is nonexistent. The truth is, the epidemiology of cancer not only exists: it is alive and well, and contributing perhaps more to our knowledge of the disease than any other kind of investigation.

What may have occurred, indeed, is that the epidemiologists found themselves riding a very spirited horse; instead of merely pursuing epidemics they took off for broader pastures and larger game, so that it is impossible to provide a really concise definition of the full range of their current activities. The science of epidemiology now inquires into all the aspects of the occurrence of disease, the distribution of disease in time and space, the pattern of disease within a community. It accumulates and analyzes the statistics of disease; it is concerned with the geographical variations of disease; it deals with the relationship of the environment to disease; and it can often suggest the means whereby a disease may be controlled or, better still, prevented. Epidemiologists have been described as the detectives of public health; and engraved on the heart of every epidemiologist are the magic words *John Snow, Broad Street Pump*. There, in 1854, was the perfect model, the perfect case.

"We are impressed by the probability," said Professor Sir Alexander Haddow in an address before the Crown Prince in Tokyo in 1966, "that a much higher proportion of human cancer than we had even recently suspected—perhaps amounting to as much as 80 per cent—may be due to environmental causes." This estimate, in the opinion of many scientists, may be too conservative, and in private conversations recently a few scientists have speculated that perhaps all cancer (with the exception of a few hereditary forms) may arise from the environment, and even these hereditary forms may be found to have their origin in the environment—wholly or in part—if one traces them back far enough. Clearly, the term environment in this context has a broad scope. It includes virtually everything, except the individual himself: the air he breathes, the ground he walks upon, the sunlight that sustains him, the food he eats, his religious faith, even the spouse who shares his bed (or, more accurately, the spouse who shares *her* bed). All, all, in some way contribute to the incidence of cancer: an utterly dismaying finding in most respects, for it seems to imply (to adapt the words of Noel Coward) that life is just one damned carcinogen after another—there is no escape, there is no umbrella which will keep us dry in this endless downpour of cancer-producing substances and situations.[3]

The epidemiology of cancer has a long and honorable history. More than two hundred years before Percival Pott described cancer of the scrotum in young chimney sweeps, a German physician and scientist, Agricola (who lived from

[3] An encouraging note, perhaps, is the discovery that certain chemicals (anthracene, phenanthrene and pyrene) act as anti-carcinogens. Laboratory animals treated with these substances show resistance to carcinogenic chemicals.

1494 to 1555 and whose name was Latinized from Georg Bauer), described a strange condition he had found in miners, called *Bergkrankheit,* or mountain disease.[4] The same disease was described only ten years later by that remarkable Renaissance figure, Philippus Aureolus Theophrastus Bombastus Paracelsus von Hohenheim (whom Sir William Osler dubbed "the Luther of medicine"). In 1879, two German pathologists, F. H. Hürting and W. Hess, recognized that this condition—which is still common among men working in the same mines at Schneeberg (Germany) and Joachimsthal (now called Jachymow, in Czechoslovakia)—was cancer of the lung. Later still, these mines were found to be rich in radioactive ores —they supplied, in fact, the pitchblende from which Madame Curie extracted her radium. Here, then, is an epidemiological highlight: an occupational cancer that has been occurring in the same localities for at least five centuries, almost certainly due to radiation, and responsible until recently for fifty times more lung cancer deaths than occurred in the general population. Over the past few years this ratio has changed: the consumption of tobacco has increased the incidence of lung cancer to the point—as one observer has noted—where many heavy smokers are in much the same state as if they had spent their lives inhaling radioactive gas in the Erz Gebirge mines.

Atomic radiation has been under epidemiological suspicion ever since 1909, when doctors found that repeated exposure to X-rays (discovered fourteen years earlier by Röntgen) caused dermatitis. This condition was often followed by the growth of warts which were likely to become malignant. A memorial erected in 1936 in Hamburg was inscribed with the names of 110 scientists and technicians who died as a result of injuries caused by X-rays in early experiments: the number has now risen to about 200. After 1930, as scientists learned more about the dangers of rays of various kinds, the incidence

---

[4] Agricola is known as the father of mineralogy. The description of *Bergkrankheit* occurs in his chief work, published a year after his death, *De Re Metallica,* which was translated from the Latin into English in 1912 by a mining engineer who was to become the thirty-first President of the United States, Herbert C. Hoover. Assisting in the translation was his wife, Lou H. Hoover.

of cancer due to radiation subsided, and then rose again during World War II chiefly as the result of exposure to radiation produced by the atomic bombs exploded over Hiroshima and Nagasaki. These ghastly incidents have alerted every intelligent human being to the cancer-inducing potentialities of high doses of radiation; but a certain amount of sensationalism has clouded the subject and it is worth quoting an expert on radiobiology, Professor Peter Alexander: "A very important *quantitative* difference must be borne in mind between the long-term hazards such as cancer-induction (and induction of mutations) and the immediate effects such as radiation sickness. Cancer or leukemia does not appear in every individual. Radiation merely increases the likelihood of their occurrence. Thus, the incidence of leukemia was doubled among the 18,000 Japanese who were between 1,500 and 2,000 yards from the Hiroshima bomb and who survived. Seven of the 18,000 have since died of leukemia. On the basis of the normal incidence in Japan one would have expected to find three cases among these people even without the bomb. For any one irradiated individual it is not possible to say if this leukemia was due to radiation or to spontaneous factors which we know nothing about at present; the evidence that radiation does induce leukemia is that statistically the incidence of leukemia is greater in an irradiated group."[5]

We owe much of our knowledge of the effects of radiation on the human organism to a group of young women who had the misfortune to work with radium during World War I, and it could be argued that they, too, deserve to have their names inscribed on some memorial. Dr. J. T. Boyd, an associate of Dr. Richard Doll at the British Medical Research Council, told me the story during an interview in London.

The research began in the United States, where medical

[5] *Atomic Radiation and Life*. Penguin Books, 2nd Edition, 1965. Authorities appear to disagree about the number of leukemia victims in Japan: a figure given in a study by Brill, Tomonaga and Heyssel indicates a tenfold increase in the incidence of leukemia.

authorities first recognized that something strange was happening. The young women, now officially called luminizers, were employed to paint the dials of clocks and military instruments with luminous paint containing radioactive substances—either radium or mesothorium. The process was new. Nothing was known of its hazards. The girls were on piece work, and they found that they could apply the paint to the dials more effectively and speedily if they first licked the applicator brush, twirled it between the lips to form a fine point, dipped the brush in the paint, painted a figure or two, then again put the brush up to the mouth to reshape the point. In the process, of course, they licked off any radium or mesothorium on the brush, and this was absorbed by the body through the lips and tongue.

"In the middle 20s and early 30s," Dr. Boyd said, "it became evident that things were going wrong with these girls. First, they were developing an intractable osteomyelitis (that is, inflammation of the marrow and the adjoining bone and cartilage). Then, some time later, many of them developed bone tumors. The reason was that once radium enters the body it behaves very much like calcium—it makes its way to the bones and is more or less permanently fixed to them." Radium, in other words, is bone-seeking, but, unlike calcium, once trapped it proceeds to destroy the bone and gradually produces cellular changes that lead to cancer. Another obvious danger is to the white blood cells in the bone marrow: if these are irradiated by radioactive deposits the result may be leukemia. The larger doses cause death within a few years through anemia and hemorrhages; smaller doses take effect over longer periods of from twenty to twenty-five years, and it is in these cases that cancer is most likely to arise.

In one small factory in New Jersey where luminizing was carried out during World War I, more than forty girls developed bone cancer through ingesting luminous paint. Many cases must have occurred in England, but these appear to have escaped official attention. However, another group of victims now came on the scene: people who had been given medicines containing radioactive substances—"radium water," which was guaranteed to cure everything and anything—and some who even had these deadly substances injected intravenously. Salesmen in shoe stores were cheerfully X-raying their customer's feet to help in fitting shoes, at the same time absorbing enormous doses themselves. Doctors were exposing their patients to X-rays for purposes of diagnosis—particularly pregnant women in order to see what was going on in the uterus, at the same time exposing themselves and their nurses to irradiation; dentists were almost audibly crackling with their accumulated radioactivity. There was a general belief that X-rays in one form or another could point the way to universal well-being.

But it was the luminizers who were the focus of Dr. Boyd's investigations. "By the beginning of World War II," Dr. Boyd said, "we were able to establish some protection standards of permissible levels of radioactivity, mostly from the basic knowledge derived from this so-called natural experiment—the effects upon the American girls in World War I. It was realized that there would be a considerable expansion of the industry, to provide instrument dials for aircraft, for the Navy, and so on; and the Ministry of Labour laid down regulations governing working conditions which included regular examinations by one of the Ministry's doctors. In 1941 the use of brushes was prohibited, and the workers used pens or other applicators which did not need to be licked."

Then, in the late 50s there were second thoughts about these girls. It was certain that at least some of them must have ingested radium in minute amounts, despite the stringent regulations applied to the industry. Radium remains active for a very long time (its half-life is 1,580 years) and even the smallest doses, once they have lodged in the bones, can be located by instruments and measured. It seemed worthwhile to examine the World War II luminizers, if possible, for two reasons: first, to ascertain whether they had developed what are known technically as "undesirable sequelae"—that is, whether cancerous or pre-cancerous conditions had appeared; and, second, to obtain data about the effects of low levels of radiation on human beings over a period of twenty years or more.

"That is what we are now doing," Dr. Boyd said. "We have now traced a group of seven hundred women who spent at least two years working as luminizers during the last war, and we've collected a lot of data. It wasn't easy tracking them all down. In the war years they were in their teens or early twenties; now most of them are married, they've changed their names and their residences, they've moved all over the country. When we find them we ask them to come to a center in the south or north of England—whichever involves the least amount of traveling—for measurement of the radium they're carrying, if any; and we shall be following their histories indefinitely into the future. So far we haven't found any bone tumors. But the group is close to the period when the signs will be coming up, if they're going to produce anything dramatic. We've done various kinds of studies of the girls who show a measurable amount of radium: we've looked at the chromosome patterns, and these suggest that there might be some relationship between even a low body burden of radium, such as these girls are carrying, and chromosome damage. What this means remains to be seen. There are so far no clinical findings to relate to the chromosome findings."

A detective story of a special kind: searching all over the United Kingdom for these girls who are now married, settled, the mothers of families. Something similar has been done in the United States, and (one hopes) in all the other countries that had a need for hand-painted luminous instrument dials in order to conduct a world war—Germany, France, Italy, the USSR, Japan. "Our approach is an epidemiological one," Dr. Boyd said. "Essentially it's a question of finding cases with a particular disease, digging into their history to see what's different from the history of people who don't have the disease. That, in a way, is what Snow did with cholera in the last century, in the Broad Street pump episode. He was able to halt the epidemic, long before the organism that causes cholera was discovered."

As for these radioactive young women: "For the present," Dr. Boyd said, "we are very careful not to alarm them."

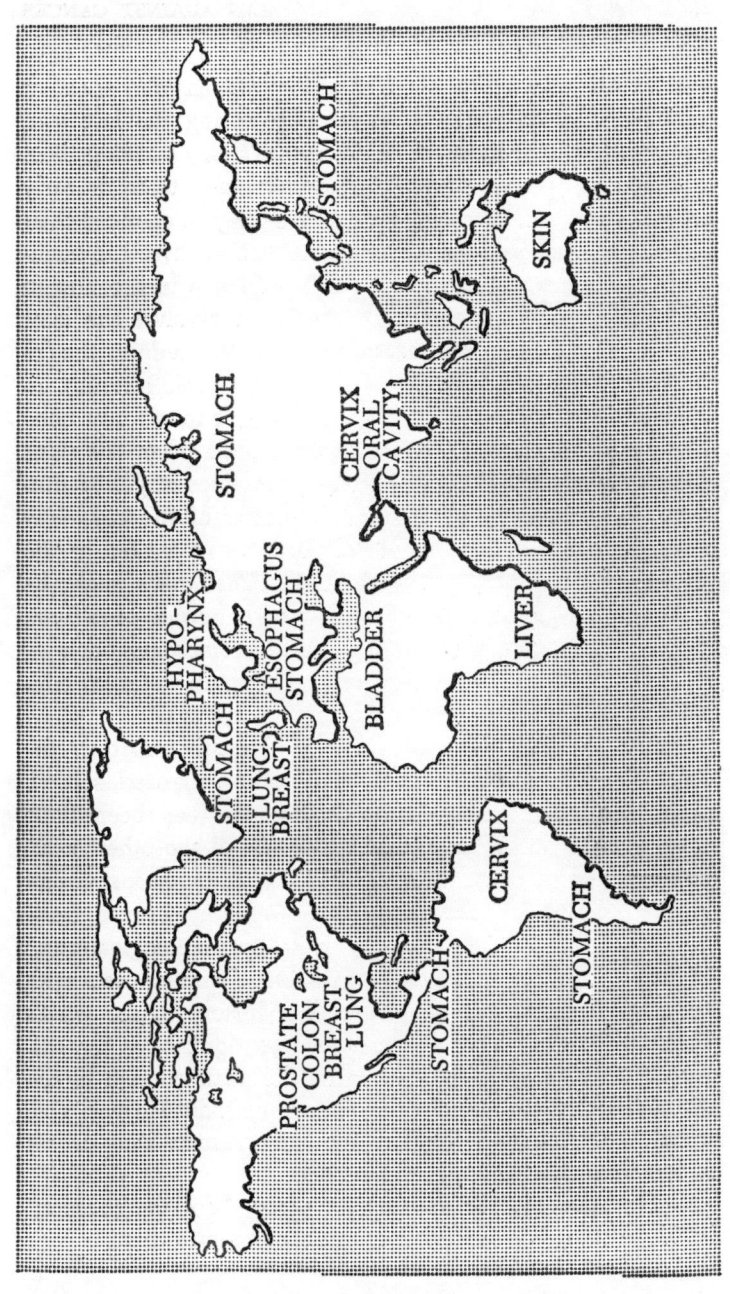

The epidemiologist looks out on a strange and puzzling world. Displayed on a sheet of paper as, say, in Mercator's projection, a cancer map of the world seems to make no sense whatever.

In the center of this map we can place the United States. Of two dozen countries (omitting the USSR and China) it ranks fourteenth in the scale of death rates from cancer. It has the third highest leukemia death rate, a median incidence of cancer of the breast, uterus, lung, prostate, and the lowest incidence of stomach cancer. To the north, Canada has a fairly high incidence of oral, breast, colon and rectum cancer, and leukemia. In South America, cancer of the cervix and of the stomach are high. In Iceland, half of all cancers in men are of the digestive organs, particularly the stomach. In Ireland, skin and oral cancers are high, with ten times more cancer of the lip than in England, sixty miles away. In England, lung cancer is the second highest in the world: the leader is Scotland, which also has the second highest total cancer death rate for men.

The puzzle continues across the English Channel. France has the highest oral cancer death rate for men, almost the lowest for women. Belgium is high in colon and rectum cancer, lung, stomach, uterus, leukemia. Germany has a high rate of stomach cancer; Austria has the highest rate in the world of male cancers, the third highest rate of female cancers. To the north, Norway and Sweden are third and second, respectively, in prostate cancer. To the south, Italy has a fairly low incidence of most forms of cancer except oral and stomach cancer in men, uterine cancer in women. Portugal has a proud place—the lowest cancer incidence of all countries in the world. Israel, for men, is the next lowest, but it has the world's highest incidence of leukemia for both men and women.

Egypt is high in bladder cancer; across equatorial Africa there is a high rate of liver cancer and cancer of the esophagus. Russia apparently has a high rate of stomach cancer and is now troubled by a rise in lung cancer; China (with no statistics to support the assumption) is high in cancer of the liver, of the back of the mouth, of the penis. Japan, which suffers severely from cancerophobia—a widespread obsessive terror of cancer—actually has a fairly low incidence of the disease: it is nineteenth in total male cancers, twenty-third in total female cancers, but both sexes have the second highest rate in the world of stomach cancer. Australia has the second highest skin cancer for males, the highest for females. In New Zealand, males and females hold third place in skin cancer, but the males have second place in leukemia while females are thirteenth.

From mountains of statistics that appear to be equally haphazard the epidemiologist attempts to extract reason and meaning. Why should the women of Chile have the highest general cancer rate in the world—more cancer of the uterus and of the stomach than any other women, and at the same time almost the lowest rate of skin cancer, colon and rectum cancer, and leukemia? Why should Danish women have the highest breast cancer rate, South African men the highest incidence of cancer of the skin and of the prostate? If he could provide the answers to these questions, and to all the other questions that arise simply from looking at a world cancer map, the epidemiologist might be well on the way to taking the first steps in a program for preventing the disease (but not for curing it, a totally different matter).

Clearly, the environment—the total environment, the sum of all the elements surrounding the individual human being—plays a significant part in the induction of cancer. Otherwise one would expect the different forms of the disease to appear in a more or less uniform manner in all communities throughout the world. But this is not so. Countries that are geographically adjacent may confront the epidemiologist with startlingly different statistics, like Ireland with its high skin cancer rate and England with a comparatively low rate—a difference that is reversed in the rates of lung cancer, breast cancer and cancer of the uterus, all of which occur more frequently in England. The differences may manifest themselves in even more circumscribed conditions. Dr. Mavis Gilmour, a surgical specialist at Kingston Public Hospital in Jamaica (West Indies), has reported that she rarely sees a cancer of the breast among the large Chinese population on Jamaica but in her practice she sees at least two new breast cancers every week among the Negro, mixed blood, and white populations. Something of the same kind may be happening in Fiji, where there are two distinct populations, the native Fijians, and Indians who arrived in the islands between 1880 and 1916 to work on the sugar plantations. Many years ago a local doctor announced that cancer of the cervix was more frequent among the Indian women than among the Fijian women; and recently studies were begun to try to learn (a) if this is indeed so, and (b) whether any local factors can be found to account for the different cancer incidence. There are excellent reasons why epidemiologists should travel to the fragrant West Indies or to the balmy Fiji Islands to pursue their studies; but a similar state of affairs may be found in any big city with mixed populations, in Europe or in the United States.

More than thirty years ago a scientist named W. Cramer put forward a theory that has succeeded in establishing itself in what may be called the folk lore of cancer. "There appears to be a general law," he stated, "that when in a given population the incidence of cancer in one particular organ is markedly increased as compared with another population, there is then a compensating decrease in the incidence of cancers in a number of other organs. As a result, the incidence of cancer in different populations, whether of the same sex or not, may represent a very different distribution over the various organs or tissues, but the sum total—the total incidence of cancer—remains on an even level."

What one perceives through this thicket of words is the proposition that in a given community there will be a certain pre-ordained amount of cancer, fixed and invariable, and at any particular time the different kinds of cancer will always add up to the specified amount (an idea that corresponds to the steady-state theory of the universe). If the aggregate of male cancer drops for any reason, the specified amount will be made up by an increase of cancer among females. If there are fewer cancers of the breast, the general law will accommodate an adjustment whereby somehow or other there will be more uterine or skin cancers. An increase of cancer of the kidney may result in a corresponding decrease in cancer of the liver or of the brain or of the thyroid.

The thought underlying this argument is that human cancer is governed by genetic factors; and people who are destined by their genes to develop cancer will do so willy-nilly. In any community there will be a specific number of these gene-doomed people: each of them, sooner or later—unless death from some other cause overtakes them—must encounter a carcinogen that will trigger cancer. There is no way out. The form of cancer may vary; but the total number of deaths from cancer (like the total number of people in the community with red hair) is immutable.

Theories of this kind are pernicious because they are demonstrably false yet statistics can be assembled to support them, and they will in consequence be accepted by many people, often with distressing results. It can be shown, for example, that in two widely separated countries the cancer death rate per million may be approximately the same, yet the *forms* of cancer in each country may have a totally different incidence, thus supporting the theory. But the argument collapses when one considers, say, the tremendous increase of lung cancer in Britain without any corresponding decrease of other cancers, or the increase in virtually all forms of cancer in Japan which has accompanied the growth of that nation's industries. A few— very few—cancers are known to be inheritable; a few—very few—forms of cancer afflict people of certain physical types. Otherwise there is little to support the theory of an unvarying pool of cancer, the Wagnerian concept that a specific number of us are condemned by our genes, long before we are born, to die of this disease in one form or another.

Nevertheless, anybody who spends a little time brooding over the statistics of cancer must be struck by their unexpected constancy. From year to year the figures for each form of cancer show remarkably little variation. There are several exceptions. Lung cancer, of course, shoots up like a rocket on any chart of cancer deaths over the past quarter of a century: it has more or less replaced tuberculosis as the pestilence of our time. Stomach cancer, at least in the United States and Britain, has declined. Taking a period of fifteen years or more, one sees an increase of, say, urogenital malignancies, a decrease in, say, oral malignancies. But the yearly figures often show little variation. Here, for example, are United States cancer figures, assembled by the American Cancer Society, for the age group 55–74. The first figure is the actual mortality in 1963, the second figure is the actual mortality in 1965.

MALES
Lung: 25,546–26,935   Colon & rectum: 11,012–11,423
Stomach: 6,429–6,051   Prostate: 7,101–5,827   Pancreas: 5,355–5,427

FEMALES
Breast: 11,932–12,632   Colon & rectum: 10,599–10,729
Uterus: 6,862–6,721   Ovary: 4,599–4,770

One can select examples that are even more striking. Here are a few statistics of cancer in Ireland. The first figure is the actual mortality in 1960, the second figure is the actual mortality in 1961.

MALES
Pharynx: 27–27   Pancreas: 120–122   Prostate: 218–221
Kidney: 30–30   Bladder: 68–75   Bone: 49–46   Leukemia: 88–82

FEMALES
Pancreas: 110–112   Breast: 355–373   Uterus: 95–92
Ovary: 87–87   Kidney: 22–21   Bone: 26–28   Leukemia: 48–50

By the finer standards of epidemiology, which insist upon the most exhaustive processing of all available evidence, these examples are insufficient to prove anything. They have been selected simply to illustrate a phenomenon that so far has not been explained: the mathematical regularity with which certain forms of cancer occur. One rarely sees extreme fluctuations, as in the infectious diseases where something like an influenza epidemic may send that particular statistic sky-high. Here there are 5,355 cases of cancer of the pancreas one year, 5,427 cases of cancer of the pancreas two years later—almost the same number. Or, in another country, there are 218 cases of cancer of the pancreas one year, 221 cases of cancer of the pancreas the following year. This, one has to say for the present, is the way Nature operates—a conclusion that is scientifically inadequate.

FIVE

More of People and Places

We exist, according to some authorities, in an environment composed chiefly of carcinogens. Sometimes it would appear more appropriate to say that a handful of us miraculously manage to survive in this seething ocean of carcinogens, for as soon as one begins to catalogue everything that might initiate a malignancy the impression grows that the only way one can evade cancer is to stop breathing (polluted air may be a co-carcinogen), stop eating (certain foods may be carcinogenic, many foods may contain traces of carcinogens) and never to venture out of doors (because of the viruses which sooner or later may be proved to be the cause of all the trouble).

The environment does not really deserve its bad name. It is not quite as hostile as the experts say it is. Some of the environmental carcinogens are substances most of us have never heard of and are not likely to encounter, such as isonicotinic acid hydrazide, or pyrrolizidine alkaloids derived from Senecio plants, or nuts from the cycad palm (relatively harmless except that they contain a substance called cycasin which may be transformed into a carcinogen in the intestines of rats and *possibly* of man). Then there are substances that are part of our everyday lives such as photographic film, which may initiate a cancer when it is sewn under the skin of experimental animals; and plastic sponges, which may initiate a cancer if a surgeon leaves them inside the body after an operation, in the course of plastic surgery or reconstruction surgery; and common sawdust, which is believed to have caused cancer of the nasal passages among cabinet workers in England. The Scots and Welsh have a peril all of their own in the bracken that grows on their hillsides: there is evidence that this vicious plant has caused tumors in sheep ("that curse of the hill farmers," it was called by the normally mild-mannered London *Times*).

Arsenic is a well-known carcinogen, apart from its other disagreeable properties; but few of us use it to excess unless we are farmers who utilize it in pesticides and sheep-dips. Vineyard workers in the Moselle valley have contracted lung cancer presumably as a result of inhaling arsenic spray; but it more often causes a pre-invasive variety of cancer called Bowen's disease. Asbestos causes, principally, lung cancer and mesothelioma (a cancer arising from the coverings of the lungs and the linings of the chest wall and abdominal cavity). A number of metals are carcinogenic: nickel, iron, beryllium, chromium, lead, zinc, copper and cobalt; but, again, it is only fair to point out that few of us absorb large amounts of these substances. Various oils, such as turpentine oil, orange oil, eucalyptus oil, have been found to enhance the induction of tumors in experimental animals; anthracene, obtained from green oil which in turn is derived from coal tar, has the distinction of being listed as a highly potent carcinogen by some authorities and as an anti-carcinogen by the National Cancer Institute at Bethesda, Maryland. "The possibilities of contaminating food with carcinogenic chemicals," say Ronald W. Raven and F. J. C. Roe, "are endless. Carcinogens in plastic wrappers, or in the lining of cans, can get into food by elution (a process of washing out). Printer's ink and dyes used in labelling may find their way into food unless precautions are taken; and accidental contamination may occur during storage and transportation." By and large, few of these environmental carcinogens pose an immediate threat to the general population. There are some carcinogenic substances, dealt with in more detail elsewhere in this book, that are unquestionably suspect, to say the least; but there is little reason in the normal conditions of daily life to go in fear of anything listed so far. Where any serious hazard is believed to exist, more often than not action has been initiated by government authorities to reduce or isolate the danger. One example is the very great care taken in industrial plants where radiation may be at a dangerous level; another is the banning of a carcinogenic substance called butter yellow, once used to color margarine. An *exception,* of course, is the permissiveness shown by virtually all governments toward tobacco in general and cigarettes in particular.

But the cancer scientist continues to regard the environment with suspicion, and rightly so. It is constantly providing him with sinister surprises.

Standing on the window sill of Dr. Francis J. C. Roe's office in the Chester Beatty Research Institute in London is a rather dusty and unattractive plant, about two and a half feet high, with numerous branches curving upward like the arms of a candelabra. "This," Dr. Roe told me with a certain proprietary pride, "is called *Euphorbia tirucalli.* It's a common hedgerow in South Africa. During World War II, when the Japanese overran Malaya and cut off rubber supplies, natives in South Africa attempted to collect latex from a related plant, *Euphorbia ingens,* in the hope that it could be used as a substitute for rubber." With a sharp blade, Dr. Roe made a tiny incision in the stem, and a thin white line of latex immediately oozed out. He went on, "If you were to rub that latex in your eye, you would have the most severe conjunctivitis which could proceed to blindness. If you were to put it on your skin it would produce blisters. We've tested it on the skin of mice: if it's applied after a very small dose of a chemical carcinogen, tumors are produced. It's an irritant which promotes the development of cancer; and, in fact, it's the second most potent co-carcinogen ever discovered. We found it after Dr. J. S. Fawcett, a biochemist at the London Hospital, told us about his part in the efforts to produce a rubber substitute from *Euphorbia ingens*. There are about twelve hundred species of Euphorbiaceae and most of them are latex producers, including some that are common weeds in England and America. Many of them produce a latex that is irritant, but none so irritant as that of *Euphorbia tirucalli*. So here we have a group of plants that may grow freely in gardens and produce secretions that are extremely irritant in a way that is of some significance in the induction of cancer. Most flattering to me is the fact that in Heidelberg there is now a whole department working on the chemical nature of this latex." Other members of the Euphorbiaceae yield castor oil and croton oil (known to promote tumors); one yields cassava, or manioc, a staple food throughout the tropics; *Euphorbia pilulifera* is used in asthma, angina pectoris, and for colds in the head; *Euphorbia resinifera* was once widely used as an emetic and cathartic but is now used only in veterinary medicine.

The African is beset by many problems, besides the latex of the Euphorbiaceae. Immediately north of the equator, the Bantus living on the slopes of Mount Kenya seem to be highly susceptible to cancer in several forms: liver cancer, cancer of the esophagus (the food passage from the back of the mouth to the stomach), and cancer of the nasopharynx (the air passages leading from the nose to the back of the throat). The natural history of this tumor of the nasal passages was described to me by Dr. Jan Stjernswärd, a young scientist who works with George and Eva Klein at the Karolinska Institutet. When I met him he was preparing to leave Sweden to spend a year with the famous surgeon Peter Clifford in Nairobi; and we talked about his future work in his home (on what was once a royal estate) at Trångsunds Gård, about twenty kilometers from Stockholm.

Nasopharyngeal cancer (or cancer of the epipharynx, or postnasal space cancer) occurs most commonly among the poorer people of China. The Chinese and Malays in Singapore suffer from it; in Taiwan it is the leading form of cancer among men, while in Hong Kong it is the second most prevalent form of cancer among both men and women. The cause may have something to do with poor living conditions, overcrowding, lack of ventilation, fumes from communal stoves, burning wood, charcoal, tobacco, and soot from kerosene lamps. In addition, Ronald W. Raven has suggested that a causative carcinogen may be produced by smoking opium.

In Kenya, the highest incidence is among the Kikuyu who live above 2,000 feet, where the rainfall is heavy. Members of the same tribe living in low-lying coastal districts are virtually free of the disease. One theory—unproven so far—is that in the cold, rainy mountain areas the Kikuyu men prefer to remain in their huts where they can build a good fire, relax with tobacco or snuff, and stay dry, while their wives take care of household and agricultural duties out of doors. The huts, constructed of mud and wattle surmounted by grass thatch, have no chimney and no door: one enters by crawling in on all fours—an architectural feature that effectively keeps fumes and smoke in, and keeps fresh air out. The fire is built on the soil floor in the center of the hut and is kept going with any kind of fuel that happens to be available: wood from eucalyptus or acacia trees, or dried cattle dung. Scientists who have examined soot deposited on the walls of the huts and in the soil of the floor have found ample amounts of 3,4-benzpyrene and other aromatic hydrocarbons—a discovery that must have been fully anticipated.

The result of this way of life for the men is that they are assured of plenty of rest, but they also contract a number of diseases, of which nasopharyngeal or postnasal space cancer is the most serious. On the other hand, their wives—driven out to attend to their duties in the open air and thus given little opportunity to inhale the cloud of carcinogenic material inside the huts—are rarely afflicted by this tumor. The tragedy is that the risk could be removed almost completely by relatively simple changes in living conditions. Once the tumor has established itself, according to Dr. Stjernswärd, it is usually inoperable and can only be treated by radiotherapy; and the unhappy fact must be reported that African patients cannot enter the hospitals in Johannesburg or Cairo where radiotherapy units are available, simply because they are Africans. (*Note:* Shortly before this book went to press, the author visited Kenya and met a team of Swedish radiologists installing a radiotherapy unit in Kenyatta National Hospital, Nairobi. This, the only unit of its kind between Salisbury, Southern Rhodesia, and Cairo, was a gift from the Swedish people to the people of East Africa.)

Cancer is inevitably the subject of endless superstitions, and one of the first was started by Hippocrates when he named the disease after that timorous crustacean, the crab, whose name in Greek is *karkinos*. Ever since, the creature has evoked fear not as a symbol (Hippocrates is said to have thought that cancer of the breast had a crab-like appearance) but as an evil force in itself, capable of inflicting the disease upon its victims, although the crab has rarely been known to do more than nip an unsuspecting toe in shallow water. It is a remarkably interesting animal biologically; the hermit and fiddler crabs are delightful to watch; the larger kinds are excellent to eat and easy to prepare; and there is absolutely no justification for associating the crab with the malady most alarming to mankind. The danger is that this association tends to be melodramatic, and it thereby harms the patient and hinders the physician. Smoking cigarettes causes cancer; heavy irradiation causes cancer; viruses cause cancer in animals; crabs have never been shown to cause a single cancer, and in the opinion of many people the use of the crab as a symbol is meaningless and a source of alarm, and it should be discontinued.

Not quite as ancient is the superstition that just as there are haunted houses, there are also houses which in some mysterious manner affect their inhabitants so that these unhappy people unfailingly develop cancer and thus die a horrible death. "Cancer houses" have been known for centuries, and the superstition has been expanded to include entire streets where deaths from cancer occur constantly. *One does not* walk those dark streets at night, one dare not abide in those accursed houses, for there the crab lies in wait.

Clearly, this is all quite absurd, and it has been proven beyond a shadow of a doubt to be absurd. In 1932 and 1933 two French scientists, A. Lumiére and P. Vigne, published accounts of their research into the subject: *Existe-t-il des maisons à cancer?* and subsequently *Statistiques et maisons à cancer*, proving that deaths from cancer in so-called cancer houses in several different communities fitted into the pattern of pure chance. In other words, careful scientific investigation demonstrated that this superstition, like most superstitions, was sheer nonsense.

"Cancer research," said the late Charles Oberling, in *The Riddle of Cancer*, a classic of cancer literature, "is one of the most entrancing chapters of contemporary science, one of the most forceful witnesses of the power of invention, of the tenacity and acuity of the human mind."[1] What deserves to be added to this statement is that cancer research, because it is always exploring unknown territory, is a cause of endless intellectual unrest. Established facts are unexpectedly shown to be nonfacts. Silly old superstitions are shown to be not quite so silly, after all; and this is the case with the "nonsensical superstition" of cancer houses.

The matter is referred to briefly by Dr. Richard Doll in a recent monograph.[2] Discussing local factors that may have significance in the etiology (or cause) of cancer, he says, "The suggestion that the occurrence of cancer may be related to the *character of the soil* or of the *water supply* (Dr. Doll's italics) has been made frequently, but the evidence to support it is extremely weak. In Britain, gastric cancer tends to be commoner in areas where the water is soft, and it may be relevant that patients with gastric cancer show unusually little evidence of calcification in the abdominal aorta. More impres-

[1] Translated by William H. Woglom, M.D., Yale University Press, revised edition, 1952.
[2] "Prevention of Cancer: Pointers from Epidemiology," by Dr. Richard Doll, O.B.E., D.Sc., M.D., F.R.C.P.S., F.R.S. The Rock Carling Fellowship Lecture, 1967, published by The Nuffield Provincial Hospitals Trust.

sive but equally incomprehensible observations have been made by Stocks and his colleagues on garden soils."

These "incomprehensible observations" are in a report by P. Stocks and R. I. Davies published in the *British Journal of Cancer* in 1964, entitled prosaically, *Zinc and copper contents of soils associated with the incidence of cancer of the stomach and other organs*. Stocks' study consisted of taking samples of soil from the gardens of houses in which there had been deaths from one of eight different types of cancer. These were then compared with similar samples of soil taken from the gardens of houses in which there had been deaths from causes other than cancer. In both sets of samples, sex, age, and district of residence were matched as closely as possible, and altogether more than 750 samples were examined in twelve districts in North Wales, Cheshire, and Devonshire.

The results justify Doll's term *incomprehensible*. "In each district," he writes, "the average zinc content of the soil was found to be greater when death had been due to gastric cancer and the subject had lived in the house for more than fifteen years. Less consistent differences were found in relation to the chromium content of the soil, and no differences were found for the other six elements examined (cobalt, titanium, vanadium, nickel, lead, and iron). . . . These observations are particularly striking because they are specific for one type of cancer (gastric cancer), and the differences appear only when the houses were inhabited by the subjects for more than ten years."

No hypothesis, Dr. Doll remarks in conclusion, has been formulated to explain these observations. Studies similar to Dr. Stocks', in other countries with a high incidence of gastric cancer (such as Finland, Japan, and the USSR) might help to clarify the matter. For the time being, "cancer houses" remain as one of the unresolved mysteries of cancer research, shadowy and just a little disturbing.

Another highly-colored superstition, reminiscent of Baron Munchausen, is the belief that husbands and wives may pass cancer on to each other in the process of sexual intercourse, the husband contracting penile cancer from the wife's uterine cancer, and vice versa. Oberling refers to it, in a phrase that lingers in the mind, as *cancer à deux;* and demolishes it by pointing out that one must beware of deducing, from a few coincidences of dubious authenticity, that cancer is contagious. "If cancer really were contagious," he says (in an earlier passage), "it might be expected to attack frequently nurses, surgeons, and pathologists, all of whom come into contact with it without taking any special precautions. But it is no more common among them than among the members of any other profession, nor does it spread through the patient's family as may tuberculosis and other truly infectious diseases."[3]

But here once again cancer research springs a surprise, and what seems to be a ridiculous superstition turns out to have an element of truth in it, for there is one quite extraordinary example of *cancer à deux,* among animals; while among human beings there is evidence that the process works at least in one direction, and untold numbers of husbands bear some measure of responsibility for initiating malignancies in untold numbers of wives.

Every type of cancer affecting man can also be found in animals; but different kinds of cancer occur in different proportions in various species and each seems to have its own particular spectrum of tumors. "In experimental work," Dr. H. Hamperl told me, in his *Pathologisches Institut* in the Univer-

[3] In a strict sense, *contagion* is transmission of a disease by personal contact with someone suffering from that disease (from the Latin: *contactus*, to touch together). Diseases such as mumps, measles, chickenpox and influenza are contagious. *Infection* is invasion of body tissue by disease-producing organisms. Many diseases caused by infections are not contagious. Typhus, one of the most devastating infectious diseases in the history of mankind, requires an intermediary, the louse, to transmit the disease. The same is true of malaria: the infectious agent, the malaria plasmodium, can only be transmitted by the Anopheles mosquito after going through a complex biological cycle in the stomach of the mosquito. Thus, a person suffering from typhus, or malaria, or a similar disease, cannot pass that disease on to another person by direct contact.

sity of Bonn, "you can easily produce a tumor in an animal which is prone to develop this kind of tumor even without your intervention. But if the animal has no natural disposition to develop a certain tumor you may have to use an enormous carcinogenic dose to *force* that tumor to arise." There are good reasons for research into the cancers of animals, apart from immediate economic reasons such as the control of cancer in livestock and poultry. Dr. William I. J. Beveridge (Professor of Comparative Medicine at Cambridge, and a special consultant to the World Health Organization) stated the case briefly and clearly: "The basic idea of comparative medicine is that we will benefit from studying the spontaneously occurring diseases of animals, using them as experimental models for the investigation of human problems. The two most important areas of research are the cardiovascular diseases and cancer. . . . If we only knew why some cancers are common and others are uncommon in different species, we would be very much further along the road to understanding the fundamental factors that produce cancer."

The dog is more susceptible to cancer than any other domesticated animal. One explanation, applicable also to the domestic cat, is that it is kept as a family pet, and it is more likely to live out its full life span than animals bred for food purposes. "Animals that are killed for meat," Dr. Beveridge explained, "are killed quite young. Those that are used for production of milk or eggs are killed as soon as they become unproductive. So we have really very few old animals in the farm world, except dogs and cats." In addition, the dog, like man, has benefited from advances in nutrition and medicine: the life span of both has been extended. But both, as a result, are increasingly subject to diseases associated with old age.

Leukemia is not common among dogs (but very common in cats and cattle). Nor do dogs have a high incidence of lung cancer (although the rate, mysteriously, seems to be increasing). Cancer of the gastro-intestinal tract is infrequent, but dogs may have tumors of the thyroid, spleen, liver, vagina and ovary. They have a high rate of oral cancer, including oral melanoma (an extremely malignant cancer arising in pigment cells), and they also have high rates of lymphomas, skin cancer, cancer of the testis, and cancer of the mammary gland (a type of cancer, curiously enough, that is practically unknown in cows). A report by two experts on the subject[4] indicates that some forms of cancer occur more frequently in certain breeds. Osteosarcoma (a bone cancer) is most frequent in large dogs, particularly Great Danes and St. Bernards; brain and certain skin tumors in boxers and Boston terriers; melanomas[5] in highly pigmented breeds such as cocker spaniels and Scotch terriers.

But the dog is subject to one form of cancer that represents, in the words of Prier and Brodey, "a unique biological phenomenon": a transmissible venereal sarcoma—that is, a cancer of the genital organs which is transmitted from one animal to another in the act of sexual intercourse. If the cancer is present in the female, the male will acquire it as a result of coitus; the tumor can then be transmitted by the male to other females.

Transmissible venereal sarcoma is another of the puzzles of cancer, almost in the same way that the duckbilled platypus is a puzzle of zoology. It was the first malignant tumor to be transplanted experimentally, from dog to dog—a laboratory triumph that occurred nearly a century ago, in 1876, and marked the beginning of research in tumor transplantation. The tumor affects dogs only: transmission, according to Prier and Brodey, "apparently is by direct transplantation of tumor cells on to the mucosa [the mucous membranes]. It is difficult to classify the tumor as either benign or malignant. Usually it regresses but occasionally metastasizes [spreads] to regional nodes and rarely to distant sites." Another singularity of the

[4] *Canine Neoplasia: A Prototype for Human Cancer Study*, by J. E. Prier, Associate Professor of Virology, School of Veterinary Medicine, University of Pennsylvania, and R. S. Brodey, Associate Professor of Medicine, College of Veterinary Medicine, University of California, 1963.

[5] Malignant melanoma is a form of cancer arising from pigment cells. It may occur in the skin of any part of the body, or in the mucous membranes. In human beings it arises most often on the hands or feet, and it may spread rapidly to such organs as the lungs, the liver, and the brain.

tumor is that when it regresses—whether it was originally acquired by sexual intercourse or in the laboratory—the dog then seems to become resistant to any further transplants. This induced resistance does not occur with any other tumor (except certain papillomas)[6] and it might be described as a form of inoculation against a particular kind of cancer. Duplicating this process in human cancer is the immunologist's golden dream, and a curiosity of cancerology has therefore acquired, in the eyes of some investigators, considerable general importance.

Cancer à deux has not been observed directly in human beings. But it is possible that we come close to it in one form of cancer, and that in certain circumstances one human being may play a part in inducing cancer in another human being.

The uterus is a pear-shaped organ normally about the size of a clenched fist. The broader part of the pear, at the top, is called the fundus, and attached to it are the appendages of the uterus—the Fallopian tubes and the ovaries. The large, main portion is the body of the uterus, or corpus uteri. The elongated lower part, opening into the vagina, is the cervix of the uterus.[7]

The types of cancer affecting these three areas of the uterus are quite distinct. Cancer of the cervix is the most common, and it is this kind that can more readily be detected by the well-known Pap smear technique. The disease, if discovered at an early stage, can then be treated before it becomes invasive. In the United States about 44,000 women develop uter-

[6] *Papilla* means a nipple. Papillomas are small, benign, nipple-like growths such as warts and various polyps. A papilloma that becomes cancerous is called a papillocarcinoma.

[7] *Cervix* means neck. It is the name given to the lower part of the front of the neck, and to various other *necklike* structures in the body, such as the cervix of the bladder. To avoid confusion, consequently, the cervix of the uterus is often referred to by its full name, as the uterine cervix or as the cervix uteri. Similarly, *cervical*, derived from cervix, means pertaining to the neck, as in cervical vertebrae (the seven vertebrae of the neck), cervical nerves, and so on; but in this case the term *cervical cancer* is generally taken to mean cancer of the cervix uteri.

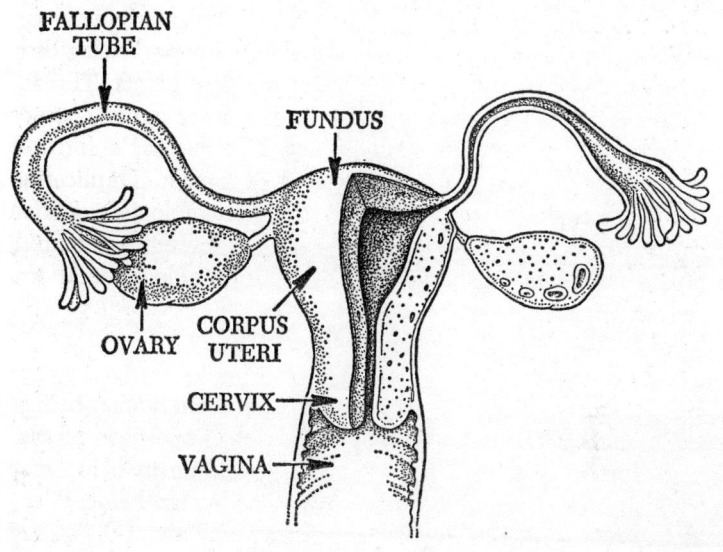

The uterus and its appendages

ine cancer each year; and 14,000 women died of it in 1966. The mortality in different age groups is significant: age 15–34: 486. 35–54: 4,052. 55–74: 6,271. 75 and over: 2,572. The incidence of cancer of the uterus rises sharply from the age of 30 or 35, and this rise is largely due to cancer of the cervix uteri. Cancer of the corpus uteri—the body of the uterus—usually occurs later, reaching its peak in women who are 65–70 years of age.

An enormous amount of information has been gathered about cervical cancer, and it is possible to extract a number of key points and present them almost in the manner of Euclidean propositions, leading to a conclusion that is almost unavoidable:

> Surveys in Scandinavia have shown that prostitutes have a rate of cervical cancer six times higher than that of the general population.
> The disease is almost unknown in nuns.
> The disease is rare in virgins.
> It occurs less frequently among women who have been married once than among women who have been married twice or more.
> It occurs more frequently in women who begin to have regular sexual intercourse before the age of twenty than in women whose sexual activity starts later.
> It is more frequent in women who have sexual intercourse with a number of partners.
> It occurs more frequently in women of lower socioeconomic groups.
> It occurs less frequently when the sheath type of contraceptive is used by the male partner.
> The lowest incidence is found among Jewish women. The disease is almost unknown in Israel.
> Jewish women in Israel almost never marry outside their faith.
> Jewish males are circumcised soon after they are born.
> The incidence of cancer of the cervix is also low among Moslem women whose husbands are circumcised.
> It is less common in circumcised African tribes than in those tribes that do not circumcise.

Cancer of the penis is extremely rare among men who are circumcised early in life.

The interpretation of these findings is relatively simple (in the opinion of some scientists, possibly *too* simple). Presented in this manner, the evidence strongly suggests that the vital factor in cancer of the cervix uteri is whether or not the male partner is circumcised. Thus, women who do not take part in sexual intercourse—nuns and virgins—are almost totally free of risk. Prostitutes, who accept numerous men indiscriminately, are high risks. Jewish women and certain Moslem women, married to circumcised males, are low risks.

Circumcision has been practiced among the Jews since the exodus from Egypt, when God commanded Joshua to make sharp knives and "circumcise the children of Israel" (Joshua V, ii); but the rite goes back even earlier, to the ancient Egyptians, Ethiopians and Copts. In the prehistoric cemetery of Naga-adder, north of Luxor, dating back to 5000 B.C., all the male corpses were found to be circumcised.[8] But circumcision is not merely a sectarian relic. The reasons for carrying it out are medically substantial. Quite often the prepuce, or foreskin, fits too tightly over the glans penis, causing a painful and dangerous condition called phimosis (from the Greek, *phimos*, a muzzle). More important as far as cervical cancer is concerned is that under the prepuce is a secretory gland, called the glandula preputialis or Tyson's gland, which produces a fatty substance known as smegma (also from the Greek, meaning an unguent). Circumcision allows this secretion to be washed away without difficulty, since there is no prepuce; but in uncircumcised males the smegma may accumulate under the prepuce, and it may then be deposited in the vagina of the female during sexual intercourse. Smegma has been very strongly implicated in cancer of the penis; and there are good reasons to believe that the in-

---

[8] This remarkable observation comes from Castiglioni's very valuable *History of Medicine*. It is nevertheless a little difficult for a reader to believe that the soft tissues of prehistoric corpses, even embalmed, would remain so well preserved after seven thousand years as to permit of such a broad and positive statement.

duction period of the disease falls within the first ten years of life. Thus, among certain groups who normally carry out circumcision at puberty, the operation may come too late. Phimosis, resulting from tightness of the prepuce, adds to the problem of washing away the smegma; and this condition has been found in more than 40 per cent of cases of cancer of the penis.

It would be erroneous to assume that smegma is directly responsible for all cancer of the cervix uteri. Medical opinion at the present time seems to be that smegma is best considered to be a promoting agent, causing cancer when it is in association with some other agent which is still unidentified. Nevertheless, smegma is implicated in cervical cancer just as it is in penile cancer; and it makes the concept of *cancer à deux* something more than a foolish old superstition.

In these terms, the situation is not hopeless. A well-known epidemiologist, during a conversation in New York, said confidently, "Keep in mind John Snow and the Broad Street pump. If you don't drink contaminated water you won't get cholera. If you don't allow smegma to contaminate these particular tissues you won't get these cancers. I could eliminate all cancer of the cervix and all cancer of the penis, if I were given absolute power, by issuing a single decree: every male in the world must be circumcised."

Other epidemiologists, with whom I discussed this statement, deplored its dramatic tone but generally agreed with its sense. A symposium arranged by the International Union Against Cancer in Mexico, in February, 1964, expressed similar opinions in more guarded terms: "The most promising method (of preventing the disease or reducing its incidence) is to raise the standard of general hygiene. This can best be achieved by education, concentrated perhaps on the schoolchild and the mother, and by provision of satisfactory washing facilities. In some areas where carcinoma of the cervix is particularly common, circumcision of males should be considered. Where carcinoma of the penis is also common, routine circumcision of male infants born in hospitals might be a valuable measure."

There remains to be added, as a sort of footnote, the problem of cancer of the breast; and here we seem to return to the discouraging theory of Cramer, that there is an unvarying pool of cancer and where one type decreases another type will inevitably increase. Those women who suffer least from cancer of the cervix, nuns and unmarried women, have a much higher incidence of breast cancer than the general population, and the women of Israel have the third highest incidence in the world. On the other hand, Chile—which has the highest incidence in the world of uterine cancer—has almost the world's lowest breast cancer rate, surpassed only by Japan where, again, the extremely low rate of breast cancer is accompanied by a high rate of uterine cancer.[9] For this strange relationship the epidemiologists have no satisfactory explanation. A popular theory is that women who have numerous children and breast feed them for a fairly long time are less susceptible to cancer of the breast; but this, like so many other theories, is under investigation and remains to be proven.

[9] Denmark adds to the epidemiological confusion, with the world's highest rate of breast cancer and the second highest rate of uterine cancer.

SIX

Visit to a Sub-Continent

It is inevitable that each country should be most concerned with its own predominant forms of cancer, or those forms which have received most public attention. In the United States and in the United Kingdom the preoccupation is with lung cancer (and perhaps cancer of the prostate) among men, and breast and uterine cancer among women; colon and rectum cancer, for unexplained reasons has not affected the national consciousness in either country, although it is a leading cause of death. Halfway around the world, in Japan, the overwhelming concern is with cancer of the stomach. "Every Japanese," a novelist in Tokyo assured me, "is worried about it. I am worried about it. My wife is worried about it." This man had a gourmet's passion for certain mushrooms, and he might have been distressed to learn that some investigators believe that cancer of the stomach in Japan may be related to toxins produced by various kinds of fungi. It may also be related to emotional stress, which seems to afflict all Japanese, novelists and non-novelists alike.

In India the national concern is entirely different. The observer—particularly if he is actually there and not dependent upon that country's sparse statistics—sees an unusual spectrum of cancers; but what is of outstanding interest is that nearly all of them can be related directly to the environment, to the conditions of life governing huge masses of people. One can quite easily isolate and identify these epidemiological forces, and their range is astonishing: from the cultural and social habits of various groups, to local politics. It is not often that we can think of politics as a cancer promoter, but here the relationship is clear, inescapable, and disturbing.

"The disease cancer existed in the world among all kinds of multicellular living organisms even before the human being came into existence. Dreadful nature of the disease was observed many years before Christ. But just after World War II it was felt that some types of cancer had begun increasing in incidence and it has become the second greatest killer of man. So vigorous work began throughout the world to control this fell disease. Scientists of all disciplines—medical and nonmedical, the benevolent people of the Society, and the people connected with publicity works, have come forward to work from a common platform. So unlike other diseases, the cancer problem is not a problem of only medical and para-medical people in the field. So cancer societies were established in different advanced countries like U.S.A., U.K., U.S.S.R., France, Scandinavian countries & Latin American countries. India also did not lag behind. A band of workers started the Indian Cancer Society in May 1951."

This racy account of how the Indian Cancer Society came into existence, by an official of the society, is of interest among other things for one curious statement: that cancer has become the second greatest killer of man. It is perfectly true of many Western countries including, of course, the United States, where people connected with publicity works are constantly stressing the melancholy fact; but it is definitely not true of India, for reasons which serve to illuminate the entire field of cancer research.

Nothing prepares the visitor for his first encounter with

India. Whatever he has read, whatever he has heard, whatever his imagination has conjured up, seems totally unrelated to the facts of Indian life. He arrives filled with sympathy and admiration for the mother of civilization, the fountainhead of art and philosophy; but his admiration quickly turns to alarm. He is put up, perhaps, at a splendid hotel in Bombay, in surroundings of solemn elegance; at breakfast, lunch, or dinner he is served whatever his heart desires by bearded waiters in turbans and skin-tight trousers whose fathers may have graced the pages of E. M. Forster; everything is immaculate; an army of zealous servants is constantly at work polishing floors, tables, the woodwork in the vaulted corridors; but at night, when he looks down from the windows of his airconditioned bedroom, he sees the sidewalks below crowded with skeletal figures who have no other place to sleep. They reside there, on the streets, and in Bombay alone they number more than 40,000. During the day the visitor is reluctant to walk out of his elegant hotel, for the beggars descend on him like flies, thrusting their twisted limbs and their maimed babies at him—the babies are maimed by the parents, or by specialists in the art of baby-maiming, for greater appeal to the visitor's charity. Across the road from the hotel, on the shore of the fabled Arabian Sea, is a great ornamental arch, the Gateway to India, which he read about and dreamed about in his youth; but he can hardly reach it—the beggars bar his way, and the arch itself is teeming with beggars. He goes out to the villages, and he is reluctant to take photographs of the villagers and their dusty, broken-down surroundings—it would be an offense to these people with their pinched, beautiful faces and their beautiful children with the too-bright eyes. Wherever he moves in the city he is conscious of the *crowds* of people, the press of bodies; and in due course he begins to find some explanation of the Indian scene in the available statistics of India. Here, in a million and a quarter square miles (about one-third the area of the United States) are approximately—nobody knows precisely—five hundred million Indians. "As a matter of fact," said one Indian scientist during an interview, "part of the trouble with India today is that we are trying to find ways to *increase* the population rather than decrease it. Every man, every family, wants sons. Daughters are quite good, but sons are the important thing; so the people go on having children." So the people go on having children, and within fifteen years there may very well be seven hundred million Indians, and by the end of the century more than a billion. Of the five hundred million now alive, a handful, relatively, are wealthy —some so wealthy that their gold is piled brick upon brick in long walls and there is said to be more than enough of it to pay off all of India's debts. ("We must have a French Revolution," cried a harassed middle-aged business man to me in New Delhi: "We must send all these filthy rich people to the guillotine. That is the only way to solve our problems.") Roughly five hundred thousand Indians form the middle class, living in conditions that might be called tolerable. The rest live for the most part in unimaginable poverty: hungry, ill-housed, hopeless, facing the permanent threat of drought and famine. Starvation is a reality for these human beings. Today there is starvation in the State of Bihar. Tomorrow there can be starvation anywhere in the Republic of India.

It is almost impossible to believe that conditions were ever worse than they are now. Yet in the first decade of this century, the life expectancy of Indian men was 22.6 years, of Indian women a few months more. Between 1941 and 1950, life expectancy had risen to 32.5 for men, a few months *less* for women. By 1960 the figure had again risen; in the cities men could expect to live 41.9 years, women 40.6. In rural areas men gained an additional 4 years, women an additional 6 years. For comparison, the average length of life in the United States was 47.3 years at the beginning of the century, 63 years in 1940, 68.2 in 1950, and 70.2 in 1965.

Since cancer *generally* attacks man in the latter part of his fourth decade and the years that follow, one might reasonably assume that it is far less of a scourge in India than it is in more fortunate lands; and the statistics tend to confirm this assumption. The greatest hazard to the Indian comes from the infections and diseases of birth and early infancy: about one-third of India's children die before they reach the age of five. If he survives the first few years of childhood, the Indian is then menaced by the classic diseases of poverty and malnutrition: tuberculosis; infective and parasitic diseases such as cholera, dysentery, typhoid fever; respiratory diseases such as influenza, pneumonia and bronchitis; disorders of the gastrointestinal tract; heart disease; and—ranging from eighth to tenth among the leading causes of death—cancer. The average Indian simply does not live long enough to develop cancer as it is known in the West. He does his best, however, within the limited span of his life to develop cancers which are virtually unknown and nonexistent in the West, and the cancer pattern of the Republic of India is therefore grimly fascinating.

Some two hours after my arrival in India I was driven out to the home of Dr. Vasant Ramji Khanolkar for an interview. Dr. Khanolkar is one of India's most distinguished scientists. He is Director of the Indian Cancer Research Centre (which should not be confused with the Indian Cancer Society); he was Vice-Chancellor of the University of Bombay for three years, and President of the International Union Against Cancer from 1958 to 1962.

The house, or as the driver of the car preferred to call it, the villa, is in Sion, on the outskirts of Bombay. It stands on the edge of a dirt road surrounded by shade trees, and it looks not at all unlike a modest house on the outskirts of a small Southern town in the United States. A swarm of youngsters came running up to inspect the car and its occupants, kicking up a cloud of dust. The evening air was very warm, very humid, and charged with a peculiarly Indian odor, sweet and peppery.

Inside, Dr. Khanolkar awaited us in a white robe and sandals. Through an open doorway the ladies of the house could be seen talking quietly to each other; occasionally, during the interview, they brought us refreshments—a dish of honey cakes, bottles of cola. A large slow-moving ceiling fan had to be switched off because its rumble affected the tape recorder, and the interview was carried on in somewhat trying circumstances: the interviewee perfectly calm and collected, but the interviewer almost overwhelmed by his first experience of Indian heat.

Dr. Khanolkar is of medium height, spare, lithe, very alert. One would have guessed that he was in his early sixties. He was actually seventy-one, he told me to my surprise, and he had worked in New York for a year with one of the legendary figures of cancer research, Dr. James Ewing. "I was a pathologist originally," Dr. Khanolkar said with a smile. "Then some madness drove me to specialize in cancer."

I was led to protest. "It's hardly madness. I've found that all the people I've met who are engaged in cancer research are very extraordinary people indeed. I'm drawn towards them. They're doing something that's of great importance, and they care about it tremendously. You don't find cancer researchers who leave their office at 5:30 every evening."

"Yes," Dr. Khanolkar said. "Cancer goes on, you see." It did not stop, he implied, at 5:30 in the evening.

We went on to discuss the purpose of my visit, which was to learn whatever I could about cancer and the status of cancer research in India. Dr. Khanolkar meditated for a few moments. "It is a little difficult to tell you. The country is so big—five hundred million people, after all—and the level of development is so varied. But one can say this much: formerly it was thought that cancer was a disease of civilization. According to the Europeans, however, there was no civilization east of Suez. So there was no cancer east of Suez." He laughed. "But we started work here, and we found there was almost the same total amount of cancer in India as in Europe and America. The great difference is in the localities, the body sites of the cancers. And, besides, there are different types of cancer in different communities. For example, we have a very strange thing here in Bombay. There are two communities among many others: the Hindus—I am a Hindu—and the Parsis, who are supposed to have come originally from Persia.[1] The inter-

---

[1] These were followers of the Zoroastrian or ancient Persian religion who fled from Persia in the seventh and eighth centuries to escape Mohammedan persecution and settled mainly in the Bombay area.

esting thing is that the men who came from Persia took the women here and drove the local men out. These women were Hindus, and after all these years they still dress like Hindu women and have kept up many Hindu customs. Now, what is remarkable from a cancer point of view is that the most common cancer in Hindu women is a uterine cancer. But with the Parsi women the most common cancer is of the breast. But this is unusual. You see, we are like experimental animals. We have different populations living close together; they don't intermarry, but they intermingle. Environmentally, their conditions appear to be the same. What is so interesting is that we find some cancers more common in certain groups of people than in other groups living in almost identical circumstances. Among the Gujarati men—most of the business people in Bombay are Gujaratis—cancer of the back of the throat, the upper part of the pharynx, is relatively common. But it's very rare in Gujarati women, and found very infrequently in other communities."

Dr. Khanolkar went on to discuss some of India's medical problems. "India is, in a sense, divided into two parts," he explained: "The urban and the rural populations. If you consider the matter of collecting health statistics, for example, you will find that in the urban part—say in Bombay and Calcutta—we are doing as well as Europe or the United States. In the rural areas, however, the health statistics are not at all reliable because there are not enough doctors. We *train* the doctors to go and work in the rural areas, but they are reluctant to do it because they are not given enough facilities. You see, if I go to work in a village, I want a school for my children, I want other facilities: but often these do not exist.

"Nevertheless, it is obvious that an improvement is taking place. Look at cholera. Everybody talks of cholera in India. Bombay doesn't have it. I have only seen one case of cholera in thirty years in Bombay. Plague: the home of plague was Bombay City. But all that is changing. The improvement in our economy, in the living habits of the people, in the environmental conditions—all these things, and many others, make a lot of difference. Take another example: leprosy. At one time it was highly prevalent in India. Today it is rare. In Bombay City you have hardly any leprosy."

"Isn't it kept under control today by drugs?"

Dr. Khanolkar said, "We now know that leprosy is transmissible—although people in Europe and America sometimes write all sorts of things without knowing enough about it—by direct skin contact. The disease is acquired in childhood, but it manifests itself after fifteen or sixteen years. I was in charge of the committee of the Leprosy Institute, and I did a lot of work myself on the manner in which leprosy is transmitted. What happens is that when our women go to sleep they like to keep the child close to them. The child is naked; the woman has only one sari which does not cover the upper part of her body completely, so during the critical years of childhood skin contact between mother and child is very intimate and the microorganisms—if they are present—will be passed on. In Bombay this habit is now changing; very few women sleep with the child like that. And as a result the incidence of the disease is becoming much less."

"Does the population accept the findings of the pathologist? If you go to these people in Bombay and say, This is how leprosy appears to be passed from one person to another, do they listen to you?"

"It all depends who is talking to them," Dr. Khanolkar said. "If you approach them like a man who is going to give a lecture, it is useless. But we have a number of social workers who are very close to them. Women, especially, are our best social workers; and they look after the children not just for leprosy or cancer but for all health matters, and the people feel the social worker is one of themselves. So, when she tells them *Don't do this,* they listen to her."

"If these social workers went around and told the people about the dangers of smoking cigarettes, do you think they would have any better results than we've achieved in America with all the millions of dollars we've spent?"

Dr. Khanolkar laughed. "Well, the point is, Indians don't smoke cigarettes. They have these things called bidis, rather like small cigarettes, and they take just a few puffs and throw the bidi away."

"You have a low incidence of lung cancer, then?"

"Yes. We had relatively little lung cancer in India. But now it seems to be increasing, and we don't know what it is due to. At least, we are seeing more."

At the Indian Cancer Research Center there are about a hundred workers (not all of them senior scientists, Dr. Khanolkar pointed out) engaged in an impressively wide range of specialized research. I asked whether there were any lines of research which the Indian scientists had found particularly promising and were exploring more extensively than researchers in other countries.

"It is rather difficult to say," Dr. Khanolkar replied, "because we take ideas from them, they take ideas from us. I don't think we can stay in a sort of isolation, doing only certain kinds of studies and not other kinds."

"Will your health services be able to expand sufficiently in the next twenty years to take care of your growing population? And are they training the men and women at Tata Memorial Hospital to carry on with cancer research?"

"Let me answer you in this way," Dr. Khanolkar said. "In Bombay there are, let us say, four medical colleges. Each one takes about 150 students a year. So, quite a number of doctors are being produced. Some of them will specialize in cancer, and these are very valuable people. But as far as my own work is concerned, I deal mostly with non-medical people—the physicist, the chemist, the biologist. In any case, a medical man can make ten times as much money by practicing medicine than doing research."

"That's true almost everywhere," I said. "It's a complaint I heard expressed with great bitterness in several European countries, some of them very prosperous, where cancer researchers with the highest qualifications get little help from their government. America seems to be the one country which provides adequate funds for research."

Dr. Khanolkar commented, "I may be wrong, but in my opinion the disposal of funds in America is not very intellectual, not very wise. They have lots of money, but I don't think they spend it to the best advantage." He did not enlarge on this point, but we went on to discuss in broad terms some of the problems faced by the scientist who is forced to rely upon government support. One of these problems he denounced as "most pernicious." He said, "The financial year starts on April 1, and we cannot carry any funds over from one year to the next. Now, if I have, say, 20,000 rupees, I know that if it is not spent it will be taken away from me, and also the grant will be cut down for next year. So one goes out and spends it, very often not in the most productive manner."

It is a problem that is not exclusively Indian. Bureaucracies all over the world tend to mimic each other.

At Dr. Khanolkar's suggestion, a friend, T. R. Ramachandran, obtained for me a package of bidis (spelled *beedies* on the package itself, and *biris* in Webster). The bidi, called "a smoke for the common man," is quite unlike the cigarette smoked by the common man in Western countries. It is about two inches long and consists usually of a rectangular piece of a greenish-white leaf with the thick spongy consistency of blotting paper, wrapped very cunningly around a few grains of tobacco which have been sun-dried and cured. There is a hint of the romance and mystery of the East here, for the leaf comes from a species of ebony tree (*Diospyros melanoxylon*) called by the Indians temburni. The bidi is tapered like a long, thin cone. At the broad end the leaf is neatly tucked in so that the tobacco grains cannot fall out, while the narrow end is tied with a fine red thread and flattened by pressing. It is the narrow end that the Indian characteristically holds between his incisor teeth; the broad end is lit. Because of the dryness of the tobacco and the temburni leaf the bidi is quickly consumed, lasting only a minute or so; but there are various ways of shielding it so that the smoke lasts a little longer. One way is to hold the bidi in the cupped hand; another is to invert it so that the lighted end is inside the mouth—a trick which is accomplished by a flick of the lower lip and is performed in certain parts of India—for example, Vijayawada in Andhra Pradesh—by boys no more than eight years old. As a consequence, these are the only places in the world where eight year old boys have been found to be suffering from cancer of the roof of the mouth.

Of the fifty known kinds of tobacco only two are grown at present in India, and they serve a dual purpose, being used not only for smoking in the bidi but also for chewing. The betel chew is as prevalent throughout India and other areas of Southeast Asia as chewing gum is throughout the United States; perhaps more so. As you fly into Bombay the air hostess may pass around what appear to be candies wrapped in glassine. The glassine is actually a sort of envelope, less than an inch square, containing a few dried scraps of betel nut, betel leaf, tobacco, slaked stone or shell lime, spiced with cardamon (the seeds of an Indian herb), cloves, aniseed, and other substances; and this mixture—with the addition of saliva—forms a long-lasting quid. If you are a lonely Indian male and go to what is known loosely as a place of entertainment, you may find that the courtesans will pass around a slightly more interesting version of the betel chew, spiked with aphrodisiacs: in this way the ladies make sure that they will have an adequate number of patrons for the night. You can buy the unspiked betel chew from vendors squatting on the hot sidewalks, or it can be prepared by one's loving wife, or mother, in the home. An important distinction must be made: the betel *nut* is the fruit of the areca or betel palm (*Areca catechu*), whereas the betel *leaf* is the leaf of the betel vine, a climbing species of pepper. "The betel leaf gives you a red mouth," a scientist explained to me: "Here, in some parts of India, the women keep the chew in their mouth while they sleep, for the cosmetic effect, as Western women use lipstick." The betel nut, on the other hand, stains the teeth black; and one stain, presumably, enhances the other.

The varying roles of the bidi, the betel chew, and other carcinogens, were discussed during a series of interviews in the Indian Cancer Research Center, which is attached to the Tata Memorial Hospital in Parel, Bombay, rather as the Sloan-Kettering Institute is attached to Memorial and James Ewing Hospitals in New York. The first of these interviews was with one of Dr. Khanolkar's senior scientists, Dr. (Mrs.) Satyavati M. Sirsat,[2] Chief of the Ultrastructure Section.

At the outset of the conversation, in a small cramped cubicle of an office leading to her laboratory (almost exactly like the offices of most scientists everywhere) I asked Dr. Sirsat for an account of how the Indian Cancer Research Center came into existence; in particular, I wanted to know more about the part played in its establishment and growth by Dr. Khanolkar.

"When the laboratories of the Tata Memorial Hospital were started," said Dr. Sirsat, "they were headed by Dr. Khanolkar, who was already well known in the field of general pathology, and cancer pathology too. Gradually he collected a group of young people—as we all were then—who studied for their degrees with him. In the late 40s he sent some of us overseas to be trained in techniques of tissue culture, electron microscopy, medical genetics, medical biochemistry, and so on. Then the government of India decided to upgrade a few departments; this was one of them; and that is how, in 1952, we started the Indian Cancer Research Center, with a nucleus of people who had been trained outside this country. For example, my field was electron microscopy: I began at the Chester Beatty Research Institute in London; then I went to Sloan-Kettering in New York, the National Cancer Institute in Bethesda, Maryland, and eventually to the Cancer Research Institute in Paris."

Dr. Sirsat had given me an impressive document consisting of about a dozen large, closely typed pages summarizing the program of work at the Center. One project, listed under the general heading, *Testing of Carcinogens in Relation to Cancer*

---

[2] This particularly Indian form of address is used by Dr. (Mrs.) Sirsat to avoid confusion with her husband who, also, is a doctor engaged in research. Since he did not take part in this interview, she is referred to in a style more familiar to Western readers.

Etiology, was entitled Chinar Tar and Kangri Cancer. Dr. Sirsat explained what this was all about.

"Quite a few years ago," she said, "it became apparent that compared to the rest of India there was a much greater incidence of a certain kind of skin cancer—*abdominal* skin cancer—in Kashmir. It was then discovered that the incidence of this skin cancer could be correlated to a custom of these people in Kashmir: that is, when the weather is very cold they carry around a wicker basket known as a kangri which is attached to the front of the body. Into the kangri they put a sort of vessel which is filled with live coal; and in order to keep the coal burning they add a lot of chinar leaves.[3] This tree has a rather broad leaf like the maple. Many workers wondered whether the leaves might have something to do with the high incidence of cancer of the skin of the abdomen, and what we have done here is to isolate the chinar tar and test it on the skin of various strains of mice. We have found that there definitely seems to be some kind of change produced by the tar."[4]

I asked Dr. Sirsat whether the information about chinar tar had been passed on to the people in Kashmir who used the kangri and chinar leaves. She replied, "It has been published in scientific journals. One does not quite make a point of bringing it up at governmental levels or public health levels so early in the schedule. . . . Now, another problem we have in India is oral cancer. This, definitely, is one of our major health problems."

I had been told that there were estimated to be more than two million Indians suffering from this disease.

Dr. Sirsat said, "Not from oral cancer itself, but from a precancerous condition, which we are studying very intensively

[3] The chinar—also, chenar—is the Oriental plane tree. (Merriam-Webster)

[4] Some authorities consider that a major cause of this cancer may be infra-red radiation from the burning materials carried in the kangri. A similar condition believed to lead to cancer is called erythema *ab igne,* or erythema *caloricum* (meaning redness and inflammation of the skin caused by fire or heat); this occurs on the shins of bakers and stokers exposed to radiant heat from ovens and furnaces.

in relation to oral cancer. This condition is called submucous fibrosis, and the name describes exactly what happens in the oral mucosa (the tissues lining the mouth). A person develops fibrosis (a hardening into a fibrous-like texture) of the mucous membranes of the mouth, and he is then very uncomfortable: he cannot eat hot food, and he cannot open his mouth because of the fibrous bands. Not uncommonly there is an associated cancer. Studies with animals have shown that the eating of chilies can produce the same kind of tissue changes that we see in oral submucous fibrosis. The chili, *Capsicum frutescens*, and the Guinea pepper, *Capsicum annum*, are the chief sources of cayenne or red pepper. They are ground up and used as a seasoning in most types of India food."

"The inclusion of chilies in the food may produce this precancerous condition?"

"In relation to other factors," Dr. Sirsat answered, "like malnutrition, Vitamin B deficiency, and possibly a certain susceptibility or sensitivity."

This raised a question I had always found puzzling. "The seasoning passes through various parts of the gastrointestinal tract where there may be equally sensitive mucosa. Why, then, does it seem to affect only the mouth?"

Dr. Sirsat replied, "We don't know whether it does or does not affect other mucosa in the gastrointestinal tract. But in some parts of India where they do eat more chilies, for example Andhra Pradesh, there is a slightly higher incidence of stomach cancer."

"How long has this been under investigation?"

"For about ten years now," Dr. Sirsat said. "In the early days we just called it a collagen[5] disorder, and left it at that. But recently the World Health Organization has become very interested in it and we are working in collaboration with the Royal Dental College in Denmark, which is extremely active in research on oral pathology."

"Does oral submucous fibrosis occur in Denmark?"

"Not at all. That is a most fascinating thing about this dis-

---

[5] Collagen, from the Greek *kolla*, glue, is a protein which is the chief constituent of the connective tissues and the bones.

ease: it is highly endemic to India, and the only other country that has reported it is Thailand, where they also eat a lot of chilies. Now we are preparing to carry out a very full survey of the other chili-eating countries—Mexico, and some parts of China, if that is possible."

I said, "If your deductions are right it should be possible to take steps to correct this situation. You have to persuade people to stop eating chilies, or to neutralize the irritant in some way, just as you have to persuade them to stop smoking in order to reduce the possibility of lung cancer. I suppose this is really outside the scientist's terms of reference: it's really up to the people themselves to decide whether they want to avoid contracting these diseases."

"Here again I would repeat," said Dr. Sirsat firmly, "that to convince the lay population that they face the danger of cancer is extremely difficult when all you can do is present statistics and laboratory experiments which are completely remote from the everyday life of the average person. As a worker in this field for many years I feel that one has to be very careful about telling people what they should or should not do. . . . Now, whenever we collect data on submucous fibrosis we always go closely into the other habits of the individual, besides eating chilies; that is, his habits regarding the chewing of tobacco and the chewing of *pan*, which is a mixture of tobacco, lime, various spices, and the leaf of the piper betel. This is known as the betel chew, and the tobacco and the lime are the two substances we believe cause trouble. The lime—shell lime, calcium hydroxide paste—is first spread on the leaf; then tobacco, catechu, betel nut and the various spices are added. This mixture is extremely irritant. We have now studied it in some detail, and we find that in conjunction with vitamin deficiency and protein deficiency it can cause a great deal of tissue damage to the oral mucosa of experimental animals."

In a room on one of the upper floors of the Indian Cancer Research Center, overlooking the roofs of the Tata Memorial Hospital, I spoke to Dr. L. D. Sanghvi, head of the Division of Cancer Epidemiology and Statistics, a voluble and exceedingly cheerful man. He was not really an epidemiologist, he explained to me: "My training was in human genetics at Columbia University in New York. But before that I took a Master's degree at Bombay University in pure mathematics. The bulk of my work here at the cancer institute is now concerned with a variety of genetic problems relating to our populations. For instance, the castes in this region have a greatly variable distribution of genes, blood groups, hemoglobin variants, and so on; and we have some interesting basic differences between the castes and the tribes.

"We have a two-fold classification," Dr. Sanghvi continued. "One is linguistic. Our States are based on linguistic groups. The second classification, which runs across the first, is based on religion—Hindu, Moslem, Christian, and so on. The Hindus comprise almost 75 per cent; Moslems are now 13 per cent; and 7 per cent of the population—that is, almost thirty million —are tribals: animistic populations who are outside the fold of the castes and outside the fold of the village economy. They live in the forests, remote from civilization (and remote even from the land revenue tax). Genetically, these thirty million people are very different from the rest of the Indian people. Now, the Hindu society is basically divided into a caste hierarchy: the Brahmans, the highest or priestly class; the Kshatriyas or warriors; the Vaisyas, who are farmers and merchants; and the untouchables who can be divided roughly into two kinds—the untouchable workers, and the lowest of the untouchables, the Harijans, a name which was given to them by Ghandi and means Children of God. Each one of these groups is itself a genetic group, so that for a geneticist this is an experimental laboratory."

He went on to discuss a subject on which he has done considerable research—the very high incidence of oral cancer in India. Several years earlier, in 1963, a group of epidemiologists and pathologists from Ceylon, Denmark, India, South Africa and the Soviet Union, meeting under the auspices of the World Health Organization in New Delhi, had reported that oral cancer accounted for about 40 per cent of all cancer cases in India, compared to less than 5 per cent in other countries. This was believed to be due (in the words of the report) "to the habit of chewing a mixture of tobacco and lime"—the betel chew described by Dr. (Mrs.) Sirsat. A high incidence of oral cancer was also reported from Central Asian districts of the USSR, where people chew "nass," an unappetizing mixture of tobacco, ashes, slaked lime and cottonseed oil.

Chewing, however, was not the only factor in oral cancer. Smoking the bidi—"the smoke for the common man"—played a part, too; and long before the New Delhi conference, Dr. Sanghvi published a report[6] which surveyed both habits—chewing the betel and smoking the bidi—among nearly fifteen hundred patients attending the Indian Cancer Research Center. The results were remarkable.

> The habit of *chewing* was found to be associated with cancer of the mucous membranes and other parts of the mouth, including the front of the tongue and the palate (the roof of the mouth).
> The combination of *chewing the betel* and *smoking the bidi* was associated with cancer of the base of the tongue, and of the lower part of the pharynx.
> *Smoking the bidi* was associated with cancer of the oropharynx (the part of the pharynx continuous with the mouth), cancer of the tonsils and to a lesser extent cancer of the esophagus.

Thus, as a result of varying habits, different cancers seemed to be induced in different parts of the same general area; and this curious variation was observed in entire communities. The Gujarati Hindus, who are accustomed to smoking hand-made bidis, have a greater prevalence of cancer of the base of the tongue than the Deccani Hindus, who prefer to chew the betel and therefore have a greater prevalence of cancer of the inner lining of the cheek.

[6] *Smoking and Chewing of Tobacco in Relation to Cancer of the Upper Respiratory Tract.* L. D. Sanghvi, K. C. M. Rao, and V. R. Khanolkar, Indian Cancer Research Center, Parel, Bombay. *The British Medical Journal*, May, 1955.

These findings raised a question which, in another form, I had asked Dr. (Mrs.) Sirsat earlier. "Dr. Sanghvi, have you any explanation for the fact that smoking the bidi, in India, produces cancer of the mouth (or, to be more accurate, the back of the mouth); whereas in Western countries the smoking of cigarettes causes cancer of the lung?"

"We discussed this very question in our paper more than ten years ago," Dr. Sanghvi replied, "and it was also discussed in an editorial in the British Medical Journal. I wish I could answer it today. My own concept is that it is possible that the populations of Western countries have a different tissue susceptibility, and perhaps that is why they get more lung cancer; while our oral cancer is due to a racial susceptibility of the oral tissue, enhanced by the use of spices, and so on."

The editors of the British Medical Journal had come up with another explanation, equally imprecise: "Instead of postulating racial differences in tissue susceptibility to account for the appearance of cancer of the upper alimentary tract among Hindus who smoke and cancer of the bronchi among Europeans who smoke, the possibility may be considered that the physical state and dispersal within the upper respiratory and alimentary tracts of the smoke particles from the bidis may differ from that of cigarettes of American and European type. To suggest that this is so is in fact no more than to suggest that bidis resemble in their effects cigars rather than cigarettes."

At the conclusion of our talk I told Dr. Sanghvi, "I am greatly enlightened, and at the same time greatly puzzled." He beamed. It was a state of mind, he seemed to think, that was not at all uncommon among workers in this particular field.

Beatriz M. Braganca was abroad when Dr. Khanolkar started the Indian Cancer Research Center. She had gone expecting to stay away for two years; instead she stayed for eight years, studying biochemistry in Canada, the United States and Europe. When she returned to India in 1954 she joined the Center, which was just embarking on its many programs. "I was given this room," she explained to me, "without any facilities, with only bench space and a few test tubes some other person had left behind, and I was told to develop an enzyme chemistry department. So I gradually acquired some equipment which would enable me to go ahead with what I wanted to do, because I was full of ideas and very enthusiastic. And it was just right."

It was just right, indeed, for some unique and intensive research on the properties of cobra venom. "I felt that this was an interesting problem to work on because in India we have access to this material, more so than people in most other countries. It is not so easy to get venom abroad, particularly cobra venom, but we can get it here. And it is somehow characteristic of India—I suppose that is one reason it attracted me."

Dr. Braganca, a tall and remarkably dignified woman, spoke with great fluency. She wore a white laboratory coat over a silk sari, a detail which is of no scientific significance whatever, but has remained in my memory, and the interview opened with a feeble jest which was perhaps unavoidable in the circumstances. I said, "I expected, when I arrived here, to see cobras in the streets."

"Oh, no!" Dr. Braganca exclaimed. "We use them for better purposes."

"You have a cobra farm near here?"

"There used to be a farm nearby in the Haffkine Institute," Dr. Braganca said, "but they are no longer breeding cobras. It is rather difficult in the city. The cobras are highly sensitive to any type of vibration, from street traffic or from trains; so, since the cobras will not breed under city conditions, the cobra farm turned out to be not very successful. Now they have people who go into the jungle to get cobras; these people sell the cobras to the Institute, and the Institute milks the venom."

"Is the venom of the cobra different from the venom of other poisonous snakes?"

"Yes," Dr. Braganca said. "The lethal action of the cobra is due to a very potent neurotoxin (a poison that acts on the nervous system). The venom of Russell's viper (another very dangerous snake, common in India and Southeast Asia) causes death by acting on the blood, and other snakes have venom that acts in still other ways."

I asked Dr. Braganca to explain what led to her use of cobra venom. She said, "I have been working on it for the last ten years. We were interested in characterizing and purifying these particular neurotoxins. Various chemical studies had been made of cobra venom in the past, but I felt we could go deeper into the subject with the more modern methods of protein chemistry now available to us. I also wanted to study the biochemical mechanism of this neurotoxin—that is, how it works. This is absolutely unknown. Nobody knows what changes it induces to bring about its effects."

The process followed by Dr. Braganca and her fellow workers was to put crude cobra venom—untreated venom taken directly from the snake—through a process known as agar electrophoresis. This separated the crude venom into a series of bands, or fractions, of different proteins. Seven fractions separated out and were identified alphabetically: A, B, C+D, E, F, G, and H. In some preparations C+D appeared to be one rather vague band; in other tests C+D separated into two distinct bands.

The next step was to learn if these components of crude venom were equally poisonous. This was done by establishing the minimum lethal dose (or, more conveniently, the MLD) for each of the seven protein fractions. The MLD, as defined by Dr. Braganca, is the smallest amount of a substance, in milligrams (thousandth parts of a gram), required to cause the death of a mouse weighing 20 to 25 grams within eighteen hours, when injected subcutaneously.

The results, like the results of so many tests of this kind, were unexpected.

First, the MLD of crude venom, direct from the cobra, was established as 17—that is, 17 milligrams were required to kill a mouse.

The scientists then found that the MLD of fraction F was 6. In other words, *it was almost three times as toxic as crude venom.* Fraction H, with an MLD of 12, was also more potent than crude venom.

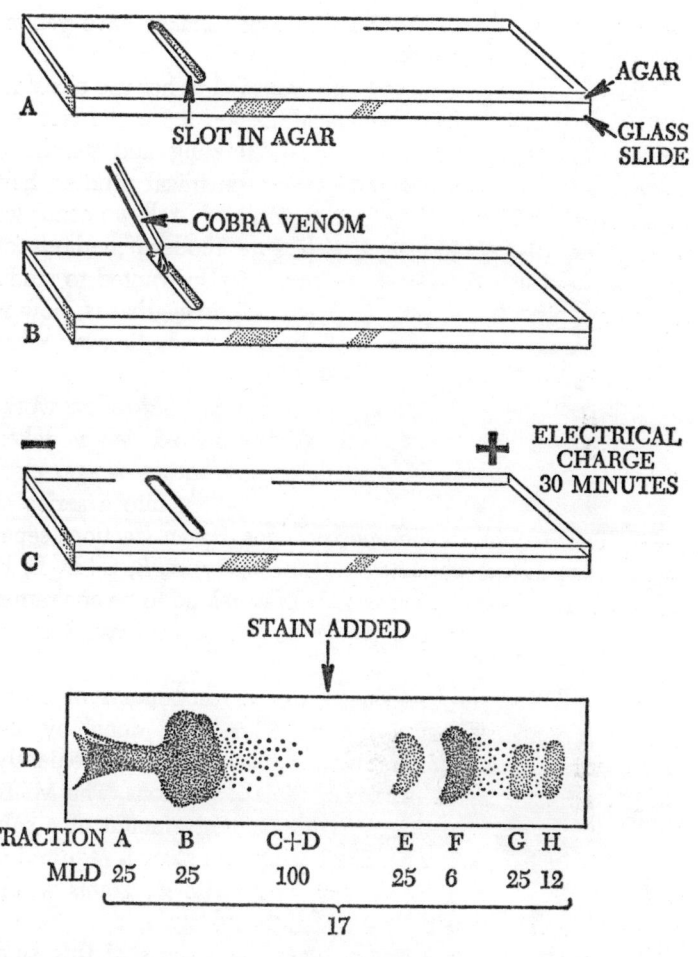

Agar electrophoresis

On the other hand, fractions A, B, E and G were less potent than crude venom: they were remarkably alike, each having an MLD of 25. Most surprising of all was the discovery that the combined fraction, C+D, was virtually non-poisonous, with an MLD of 100.

Thus, two of the substances which make up cobra venom were found to be *more toxic* than the whole venom; of the rest, four were markedly *less toxic*, and one was so inert, relatively, that the scientists immediately asked what it was doing in the venom. There was also the larger question: why, in the deadliest of all snake venoms, should only two of the seven components be highly poisonous? The explanation seems to be that in some way still not understood the non-toxic substances enhance the action of the toxic substances. In scientific terms, the overall toxicity appears to be the resultant of the multiplicity of components. But this curious state of affairs enabled Dr. Braganca and her co-workers to start an important new line of investigation.

"There are a considerable number of isolated reports in the literature," Dr. Braganca explained, "which say that cobra venom has an effect on cancer tissue, that it causes regression of tumors. Some are clinical reports. Others are from work on animals. However, the trouble with all this earlier work is that it was carried out with the crude venom, which contains the highly potent neurotoxin. Consequently one could not study the effect—the beneficial effect if any—because it was simply impossible to inject large doses of venom. But since we were now able to extract the toxic part of the venom I decided to see if the rest of the material—the fraction with low toxicity—could be used on tumors. We had some work on experimental tumors going on here, so I tested it on one type, the Yoshida sarcoma [a standard form of cancer used in laboratory experiments]. I found that the non-toxic fraction of the cobra venom did have a delaying effect on the growth of the tumor." Then, in collaboration with Professor E. J. Ambrose of the Chester Beatty Research Institute, Dr. Braganca proceeded to work on a different problem. Many substances which attack tumors will also attack certain kinds of healthy cells, and as a result the substances will do more harm than good. "So," Dr. Braganca said, "we decided it would be interesting to see what effect the non-toxic fraction of cobra venom would have on cells of various types. What we hoped to find was a reasonable differentiation—that is to say, it would not be unexpected if the substance attacked normal cells, but if it destroyed *a much higher proportion* of tumor cells then it might prove to be useful in chemotherapy."

"Had you given this substance a name by this time?"

Dr. Braganca said, "Yes. It was called B6, because that is the position where it appeared in our method of preparation. The results of our tests were extremely interesting because we found that B6 had a very wide differential. If one part of B6 is required to destroy tumor cells like the Yoshida sarcoma cell, ten times more is required to destroy healthy bone marrow cells, about fifteen times more to destroy healthy lymphocytes, and red blood cells are not destroyed at all. In other words, it was found to be considerably more destructive to tumor cells—at least with the particular tumor we used. In fact, several animals have been cured of Yoshida sarcoma tumors, so we consider that our preliminary work has been quite encouraging."

This was reminiscent of the work done earlier on the rauolfia compounds, used so widely in tranquilizers and other drugs. These compounds originated in India, and had been known for many centuries in Indian folklore.

"Oh, yes," Dr. Braganca said. "They are as old as Sanskrit literature."

"Does cobra venom have a similar history?"

"It was used in the therapy of cancer, but not successfully," Dr. Braganca said. "In the old literature of India there are many descriptions of cancer, and cobra venom was one of the many things the people tried as a remedy. The technique of milking the cobra is quite ancient. Primitive people knew how to do it. There are also stories that the cobra venom was used to cure leprosy; and whether this is scientifically true I do not know. But cobra venom has many enzymes whose properties we still have to discover, and it has one great advantage. You can prepare enzymes from animal tissues and from plant tissues and from bacterial systems. With all these, however, you have to go through several operations before you can get the material in solution. But cobra venom, and other snake venoms, are all completely soluble in water, so it is perfectly simple to obtain a solution. Today in India cobra venom is very costly. It is being exported to many European countries as well as to the United States. They purify the enzymes and then they sell them back to us. It is my idea that in the course of my work we should ourselves explore the purification of these enzymes because there is so much that might be done with them for cancer research and for other purposes."

The story of cobra venom does not end here. Nearly six months after this interview, a scientist at the University of Miami described experiments with a "non-poisonous factor" of cobra venom which may open up new avenues of research in organ transplants. Human trials were not yet possible, but the substance had greatly prolonged the survival time of pig kidneys transplanted to dogs. In time, the scientists at the Indian Cancer Research Center may find ways of utilizing cobra venom in a direct attack upon human tumors; while the scientists in Florida and elsewhere may find ways to use the venom to aid in the transplantation of organs from animals to human beings. It was indeed, as Dr. Braganca had assured me, a most interesting and versatile substance.

A Postscript on Politics and Epidemiology

When I visited the World Health Organization in Geneva I was advised that I should make every effort, when I reached India, to call on officials at the World Health Organization Regional Office for Southeast Asia, which occupies a handsome building erected by the Government of India in New Delhi.

There, I was told, I would be able to learn all about the fight against cancer not only in India itself but in Afghanistan, Burma, Ceylon, Indonesia, the Maldive Islands, Mongolia, Nepal, and Thailand. Letters were sent off on my behalf; I was assured that the World Health Organization in New Delhi would welcome me with open arms and place itself fully at my disposal; and I was deeply grateful (and still am) for the help and encouragement I received from those hardworking gentlemen in their gleaming new Swiss palace.

Accordingly, when I completed my interviews at Tata Memorial Hospital, a telegram was sent to the officers at World Health House advising them that I was now about to leave Bombay, and that I would call upon them as soon as possible after I arrived in New Delhi. This I did; and I was met at the entrance of the WHO building by a young man whom we can call Mr. Brown, of the public relations department.

Mr. Brown was greatly agitated. "Didn't you receive my letter?"

"No."

"Didn't you receive a telegram from me?"

"No."

"I'm terribly sorry. There has been some awful mix-up. I am afraid you're wasting your time coming here."

"Oh? Why?"

"I understand you are collecting material about cancer research. We have nothing to do with cancer research in Southeast Asia."

"But in Geneva they told me—"

"It's all most unfortunate. I sent you a letter and then a telegram, explaining the situation and urging you not to come. But communications in India—" Mr. Brown shrugged his shoulders. He led me into his office and showed me the last annual report of the Regional Director, a large volume of 235 pages describing in detail the activities of the Regional Office for Southeast Asia. The account of activities in the field of cancer appeared on page 47 and occupied exactly five lines, merely stating that some research on oral tumors was being done at Agra, and a

WHO epidemiologist had visited various places in India, Ceylon, and Afghanistan.

"We are principally concerned with the communicable diseases," Mr. Brown explained, full of apologies: "Tuberculosis, malaria, smallpox, cholera, plague, and so on. We have limited funds and limited personnel. We couldn't possibly do anything in depth about cancer. And, besides, cancer in Southeast Asia is not a tremendously serious problem, except, of course, for those people who happen to get it."

Misunderstandings of this kind occur. There is nothing one can do about them. One has to accept them as a natural hazard. Later we learned that at the very time Mr. Brown was apologizing for WHO's lack of activity in the field of cancer an important WHO conference on new aspects of cancer in Southeast Asia was being held at Agra University, about a hundred and fifty miles from New Delhi. Nobody had bothered to inform Mr. Brown about this conference, presumably because it might be considered bad form to let one's right hand know what one's left hand is doing.

Throughout the underdeveloped parts of the world a number of hotels of almost unbelievable splendor have recently been built. These effectively insulate the visitor from anything unpleasant in that particular area. New Delhi itself is not wholly underdeveloped, but the hotel in which I was staying gave the impression that India was a land flowing with milk and honey. Some of the most elegant human beings I have ever seen strolled through the vast foyer; dozens of bellboys struggled with mountains of expensive luggage; aristocratic ladies of stunning beauty, swathed in glorious saris—possibly the most beautiful of all garments—hurried to the elevators like heroines of Indian fairy tales hurrying to the arms of heroic Indian princes.

Outside, late in the afternoon, I sat drinking tea beside the swimming pool with a man who had just resigned from the World Health Organization and was returning to Europe. He was from one of the Scandinavian countries, and we can call him Jensen. The scene was very peaceful: some pretty girls were splashing about in the pool, a number of huge jackdaws were hopping from table to table gulping down any scraps of food they could find; a couple of wealthy Indians were abusing a cringing waiter who had forgotten to bring them an ashtray.

Jensen said, "I can't wait to get home."

"Have you been here long?"

"Too long." He laughed bitterly. He said, "I came out here three years ago. Young, you know. Full of ideals. Wanting to do something—*anything*, anything to help. The people here don't want your help. They despise you for wanting to help them. They resent WHO being here, they're doing everything they can to get rid of WHO."

"Who exactly are *they?*"

"The Indians," Jensen said.

"*All* Indians?"

"All Indians. They feel it's an insult, a blow to their pride, having a lot of foreigners come here advising them to boil their water, sterilize their food, build sewers, and so on. We tell them they should get early treatment for syphilis, and they say who the hell do we think we are, ordering them to do this and do that. After all, they were civilized when we were still painting our bodies blue.— Do you know what's going to happen in this country? Next year or the year after or the year after that?"

"What?"

"The population is increasing at the rate of twelve and a half million a year. That's like adding the entire population of Tokyo to India, every twelve months. And there's no food for these new Indians. There's no housing for them, no sanitary facilities. We are going to see in India the worst famine, followed by the worst epidemics of cholera, plague, and all the rest, that the world has ever seen."

"You're very pessimistic."

"I don't think so. You know, the stocks of surplus grain in the United States are running low. The USSR is running low, too. How are the Indians going to feed themselves?"

"They have plans for increasing food production—"

"It's impossible. They can't catch up with the population increase."

The two wealthy Indians at the nearby table told the waiter, "The service here is so disgraceful, we refuse to pay our bill." They pushed their chairs back and prepared to leave. The waiter pleaded with them; if they did not pay, he would have to pay for them. They were greatly amused.

Jensen said, "We had a conference here three years ago about oral cancer. Did you hear about it?"

"Yes, I've heard about it."

"I mean," Jensen said, "did you hear about the outcry?"

"No."

"We were violently attacked by a lot of politicians. They said we were abusing our position, we were insulting them. Nobody in the world, they said, knows what causes cancer; and here we were saying that cancer of the mouth was caused by chewing the betel. They said we were trying to rob the Indians of their one pleasure." He added angrily, "Do you know why the politicians *really* attacked us?"

"Why?"

"Because most Indians are lucky if they get a full meal once in three days. Chewing the betel does one very specific thing: it allays the pangs of hunger. So if the Indians listened to the cancer experts and stopped chewing the betel to avoid getting cancer of the mouth, there would be a lot of Indians feeling very, very hungry; and hungry people are apt to cause trouble. The politicians aren't anxious for that kind of trouble, so they call us a bunch of rogues and liars and want us to get the hell out of here."

It was a depressing conversation, after the stimulating interviews in Bombay. I said, "I'm sure that isn't the attitude of the Government."

Jensen said sourly, "I wish you were right."

We have to hope that in some way a major catastrophe will be averted in India, that despite the handicaps of undeveloped resources, of ignorance and superstition, of staggering population growth and hopelessly inadequate social services, *somehow* India will survive, and not only survive but become stable and self-sufficient. There is a possibility, according to observers like Chester Bowles, that in the next few years an agricultural revolution will take place, with a dramatic increase in foodgrain production, enabling the Indians for the first time in modern history to feed themselves. The act of survival itself might be the prelude to a succession of miraculous acts, for theoretically, a reasonably efficient Indian agriculture could feed the whole of Southeast Asia; theoretically, Indian industry could leapfrog into the atomic age and overtake Japanese industry, which lacks room for growth; theoretically, India with its tradition of intellectual brilliance, its outstanding mathematicians and physicists and philosophers, might become one of the world's leading nations, active and prosperous. It is a possibility. History makes a habit of tipping the balance in unexpected ways.

If so, Dr. V. R. Khanolkar's policy of selecting scientists like Dr. (Mrs.) Sirsat and Dr. Sanghvi and Dr. Braganca and ensuring that they received the best training available, in India and abroad, will be applauded for its remarkable wisdom and foresight. The Indian is already living longer, and like Western man he will soon be faced with the inevitable consequences of longevity: a steep rise in deaths from the two major degenerative diseases, heart disease and cancer. Instead of being eighth or tenth, cancer may become one of the leading causes of death; and for three quarters of a billion people, or more, the programs of Dr. Khanolkar and his fellow workers will have profound significance.

4

Burkitt and Others

SEVEN

The Implications of Mr. Burkitt

A legend has existed for many years that *The New York Times* keeps in its composing room a front page with headlines in 60-point Gothic Black—one inch high—CURE FOR CANCER FOUND. A few explanatory lines have to be dropped in—who discovered the cure, when, where, how, and so on; otherwise the page is ready for instant use. Legends of this kind are harmless; they are mildly colorful, providing science with a kind of folklore; and consequently one accepts them for what they are and does not scrutinize them too closely.

On Thursday, December 15, 1966, one of London's leading newspapers, the *Evening Standard*, appeared with huge headlines running right across its front page:

> **A WORLD AUTHORITY TALKING**
> **IN LONDON TODAY . . .**
> **'REAL REVOLUTION IN MEDICINE'**
> **CANCER CURE—NEW HOPE**

The last four words were printed in 60-point Gothic Black— one inch high. The wind, it seemed, had been taken out of *The New York Times*' sails: but *The New York Times* the following morning paid little attention to the whole matter, presumably on the grounds that CANCER CURE—NEW HOPE is a far cry from CURE FOR CANCER FOUND.

The world authority quoted by the *Evening Standard* was Professor Sir Alexander Haddow, Director of the Chester Beatty Research Institute in London, and past President of the International Union Against Cancer. He had spoken at a press conference in St. James's Palace, announcing a National Cancer Day in Britain to be celebrated the following September which, by permission of the Queen, would culminate in a race meeting at Ascot with some of the best horses in the country competing for prize money totaling £26,000 (about $65,000).

Professor Sir Alexander Haddow is, of course, one of the most distinguished cancer scientists in the world. As Director of the renowned Chester Beatty Research Institute he is intimately in touch with the entire field of cancer research. His authority is indisputable. What he has to say merits the utmost respect; and what he said on December 15, 1966, resulting in those gigantic headlines, was that in the past year or two medical scientists had "for the first time applied chemical treatments which can completely cure two types of cancer in a proportion of cases." He added (the text is taken from *The Times* of London), "The first is Burkitt's lymphoma, a form of the disease which mainly strikes African children and in which the rate of success has been about 16 per cent. The second is choriocarcinoma, a tumor which sometimes follows pregnancy and in which the rate of success is about 80 per cent. In neither case does the chemical treatment have to start early in the history of the disease for it to be successful. This gives us tremendous hope for the future."

Choriocarcinoma is a strange, highly malignant type of cancer which arises from the placenta either during or soon after pregnancy. Until recently it had been considered to be relatively rare: the frequency in Europe and America is given variously as 1:10,000 to 1:30,000 pregnancies, but it is now known to occur in Asia and the Middle East more often than had been suspected. In terms of the world's population, according to an expert on choriocarcinoma, Dr. K. D. Bagshawe, it may possibly be one of the more common tumors of early adult life.

Press conferences are not ideally suited for the dissemination of precise scientific information. Misunderstanding and misinterpretation of what actually was said are only too likely. The treatment of both Burkitt's lymphoma and choriocarcinoma by means of drugs had been going on, in fact, with considerable success for rather more than a year or two before the news was announced in those gigantic headlines. Burkitt had been using methotrexate, of course, since 1960; the same drug had been used by Dr. Roy Hertz and Dr. Min Chiu Li of the National Cancer Institute in Bethesda, Maryland, as long ago as 1956 to treat advanced cases of choriocarcinoma, and the results had been impressive: of 110 women who received treatment, 64 per cent (presumably 70) were in complete remission, totally free of the disease more than five years later.

Nevertheless, the inch-high headlines were to some extent justifiable. In two separate forms of the disease, involving substantial numbers of patients, cancer—for the first time—appeared to have been completely cured by means of drugs. It was good news; and the potentialities were even better, for as Sir Alexander remarked, similar forms of treatment could impede the growth of tumors in other types of cancer, giving people many more years of life, even if the cancer was not completely cured. And with a greater knowledge of how the body reacts to its own tumors, "there is no telling," Sir Alexander said, "what great developments we may make."

A less happy note was sounded by several newspapers which, somewhat misguidedly, chose to wave the Union Jack over Sir Alexander's head. "A London doctor," one proclaimed, "has now developed treatment which cures 8 out of 10 cases of choriocarcinoma." "British doctors," proclaimed another, "are now holding out hopes of finding a successful treatment for cancer." A press release, printed by *The Times*, seemed to imply that a certain drug had been developed in Britain whereas it had been developed by associated laboratories in the United States. Cancer research, in every form, is now an international matter, and no country—and certainly no industrial organization—has a clear title to any so-called discovery. This is something for which we should all feel profound gratitude; and it is utterly asinine, even despicable, for any newspaper to attempt to lift a nation's flagging spirits by claiming that "we" have found a cure for this disease, whoever that "we" happens to be.

In the United States nearly a million and a half men, women and children are alive today, five years or more after receiving treatment for cancer. They are considered cured. In Great Britain, there are nearly a million people alive today, cured of cancer. At a guess, some four million people throughout the world have survived after treatment for cancer and are free of the disease.

Most of these four million people were cured of cancer by surgery. A considerable number were cured by radiotherapy. The combination of surgery and radiotherapy also cured a great many people of cancer; and in some cases a combination of surgery, radiotherapy and chemotherapy effected the cure. A small number of people experienced what are known as spontaneous cures: that is, the disease disappeared of its own accord, for no clear reason. And of the total of four million, a pitifully small number—a few hundred women suffering from choriocarcinoma, and perhaps fifty youngsters suffering from Burkitt's lymphoma—were cured by chemotherapy alone. Thus, if we consider the larger picture, what appears to be an outstanding achievement, worthy of inch-high headlines, now appears to be rather disheartening.

Surgery is a cruel necessity. We shrink at the thought of it. Radiation therapy seems less cruel; no flesh is cut, no blood is shed; but living tissue is destroyed, and the quiet dreamlike process, in which nothing of significance seems to happen, can eventually prove to be as painful and as dangerous as surgery. The ideal treatment for all our ills, obviously, is to take a couple of pills with a glass of water every four hours, before or after meals; and man has been singularly successful in finding this kind of cure—but not in all instances quite so simple a procedure—for a number of diseases which not so long ago were always, in varying degrees, calamitous. He has been particularly successful in finding means to treat many infectious diseases: he has learned how to attack them at their source, how to provide immunity against them, how to overcome them when they have invaded the human organism. He is still unable to deal with infections caused by certain viruses which have the ability to modify their form in some unexplained way, such as the influenza viruses: therapy by means of drugs (or by any other means) is ineffective. But, by and large, cancer is the chemotherapist's most prominent failure.

This failure has little to do with lack of funds, or lack of effort, or lack of facilities. Nobody could possibly estimate how much has been spent all over the world since the end of World War II on research into chemical means to cure cancer. Government agencies, private agencies, university laboratories, commercial laboratories, all participate in the work of seeking new anti-cancer drugs. Reference has already been made to the effort supported in the United States by the National Cancer Institute to find new drugs with which to treat cancer. No other country could possibly afford such a program. In ten years, 257,000 materials were tested, at a cost in Federal funds of $257,685,000. Yet the best that the National Cancer Institute could report, at the beginning of 1967, was that "encouraging progress continues to be made in cancer chemotherapy. . . . Exceptionally long remissions in children with acute leukemia have been produced, with survival of five years or longer for more than a hundred children . . . survival of five years or longer of a group of women with choriocarcinoma. . . ." Certain other successes have been achieved, impressive and heartening in themselves but not at all impressive or heartening in terms of the enormity, the virulence, the persistence, of the enemy we seek to overcome.

The ultimate reason is that cancer as a disease is unique. In any infectious disease there is, as a rule, one causative agent—a microorganism specifically related to that particular disease. Here, therefore, the task of research is to find chemical substances which will seek out and destroy the *specific* microorganism responsible for a *specific* infection. Against bacterial diseases, as well as diseases caused by various fungi and protozoa, medical technology has achieved a high degree of success: the research can be conducted quite satisfactorily in the laboratory, for the action of chemicals on these microorganisms *in vitro* (that is, in the test tube or beaker) will be much the same as the action *in vivo*, in the living body. A more perplexing problem is to find means of reaching certain disease-causing viruses which carry on their activities within the cells of the host they have invaded, and here chemotherapy has been less successful. But even if the target is difficult to approach, it is still recognizable: a *specific* microorganism, responsible for a *specific* disease.

A number of unhappy factors complicate the search for anticancer drugs. To begin with, there are no microorganisms known to cause human cancer which can be sought out and destroyed. Theoretically, even if such a microorganism were identified, we would still be faced with the complication that it has to act only once, initiating the cancer: the cancer will then proceed to grow and to spread without any further intervention by the causative agent. We can draw a crude parallel with a rat which has gnawed a hole in the bottom of a sack of sugar: killing the rat will not stop the sugar from flowing out of the sack. The tumor is not dependent upon the agent which brought it into existence, and destroying the agent after the act is not particularly helpful.

In addition, cancer cannot in terms of chemotherapy be considered a single disease. All organs, all tissues, all cells of the body are subject to malignant tumors, which differ in form and structure and in their response to various chemicals. Any anticancer drug, as a consequence, must be capable of seeking out and destroying a particular kind of tumor, in a particular location; it must at the same time avoid acting on healthy tissue, even when exceedingly high dosages are administered. The problem is summed up in the first report in 1962 of an expert committee formed by the World Health Organization to investigate the chemotherapy of cancer:

Tumor chemotherapy is faced with a task of colossal difficulty, since it must learn how to destroy all the cells of each of an enormous number of varieties of tumor and, at the same time, avoid irreparable damage to any of the essential normal tissues, from which tumor tissues differ, in the main, only quantitatively.

In these circumstances the success that has nevertheless been gained in discovering compounds that have a selective effect on some tumors—that may indeed bring about more or less complete regression of some animal and human tumors —must in itself be classed as a great achievement.

It is clear, then, that the present status of cancer chemotherapy is somewhat uncertain. On the one hand, at immense cost of effort and resources, we have acquired a number of drugs which will aid cancer patients, sometimes dramatically, without providing a complete cure for their disease, and we have also achieved complete cures of two rather rare forms of cancer. The score is not enormously impressive. On the other hand, these two complete cures represent such a significant step forward in cancer therapy that they do indeed give tremendous hope (in the words of Professor Sir Alexander Haddow) for the future. They demonstrate, moreover, that the cure of cancer by chemotherapy is not a pipe dream but solid reality, that drugs properly used can eliminate the disease not merely in mice but in human beings.

One remarkable aspect of these two cures is the dosage required to produce the remissions. The first report of the World Health Organization expert committee stated unequivocally: "The dosages used must, in most cases, be very close to the maximum that can be tolerated. It is practically impossible to achieve complete regression of tumors unless doses are used that bring about quite considerable side-effects. Fortunately, these consist mainly in depression of hematopoiesis (the formation of blood), which can be completely restored." This principle was confirmed by Dr. K. D. Bagshawe in relation to the treatment of choriocarcinoma: "Trophoblastic necrosis (destruction of the tissue in which the malignancy forms) can only be achieved by drugs when given in amounts which cause, or at least risk, systemic toxicity (that is, poisoning of the body as a whole). In addition, when given in an ineffective manner, resistance to the drug may develop."[1] Burkitt's treatment (which, of course, may work only in very special circumstances) resulted in what appeared to be complete and permanent cures, in some cases, from a single dose or a single course of treatment.

Dr. Michael B. Shimkin, of Temple University School of Medicine in Philadelphia, who is one of the world's most eminent cancerologists, has applied the term "serendipitous" to those occasions when what seems to be an obscure line of research produces unexpectedly valuable results. He was refering particularly to the curious chain of events which led to the discovery of the aflatoxins, described later in this book, but the term could be applied equally to the very different chain of events which brought Denis Burkitt and Burkitt's lymphoma into world prominence. Serendipity, though, does not simply strike once, like lightning; it seems to attach itself as a personal attribute to certain people; and Mr. Burkitt's contributions to the welfare of his fellow human beings has not been limited to what occurred in Uganda between 1957 and 1962. The implications of his discoveries are considerable; they have led to the most remarkable speculations about the fundamental nature of cancer; and they have led, furthermore, to other discoveries which no scientist in his right mind could possibly have anticipated.

In the course of one of our conversations Mr. Burkitt urged me to speak to Dr. Dennis Wright, of Makerere University College Medical School. "If you want answers to any questions about the pathology[2] of the tumor," Mr. Burkitt said,

[1] "Post-Gestational Choriocarcinoma," K. D. Bagshawe, M.D., M.R.C.P., *The Prevention of Cancer*. Butterworths, London, 1967.

[2] Pathology has been defined earlier as the science dealing with the nature, causes and development of diseases, and the structural and functional changes occurring in the course of a disease. As used here, the emphasis is on the changes arising in tissues and organs as a result of a disease (in this case, Burkitt's lymphoma) and the identification and interpretation of these changes.

"he's your man. In this aspect of the work I look upon him as the world expert."

My talk with Dr. Wright opened with a glance back at the great tumor safari of October, 1961; and Dr. Wright then discussed his part in the story. Once again, what emerges from the narrative is unexpected and revealing.

"Before I went out to Uganda, there had already been an attempt to describe the pathology of the tumor," Dr. Wright said, "but at that time nobody was sure what Burkitt's tumor was, and the pathologist took all the children with jaw tumors and lumped them together in one group; whereas, in fact, all jaw tumors in Africa are not Burkitt's tumor, and all Burkitt's tumors are not jaw tumors.

"When I arrived, as a pretty inexperienced pathologist, I was very puzzled by this. I couldn't understand it. Was Burkitt's tumor a single disease, of one particular type, or did all lymphomas in Africa behave in the same peculiar way? The first thing I did was some histo-chemistry (that is, studies of chemical reactions in the cells making up tissues) and the results of this, by 1962, showed quite clearly that Burkitt's tumor (wherever it arose in the body) was of a single type. Then, a little bit later, we started making special preparations of the tumor and looking at the individual cells; and it became clear that the Burkitt tumor is composed of a particular type of cell that is different from the cells of other types of lymphomas, either in children or in adults, and behaves differently clinically.

"Burkitt's tumor is very common in tropical Africa. The other forms of childhood lymphosarcoma are fairly uncommon. In the ten year period, 1952 to 1963, we had about 550 cases of Burkitt's tumor, and we only had 19 cases of childhood lymphosarcoma. Now: if you go to other parts of the world where the climate is temperate, you find that both diseases are uncommon—childhood lymphosarcoma is an uncommon occurrence and Burkitt's tumor is even less common. Nevertheless, wherever it has been looked for, in London or New York, for example, you find that typical cases of Burkitt's tumor do crop up."

Burkitt's tumor had been connected with equatorial Africa so intimately (it has been called, in fact, African lymphoma) that to find it occurring in other parts of the world—particularly temperate areas—came as a startling surprise. This discovery could only have been made after Dr. Wright succeeded in demonstrating that the Burkitt tumor cell is a separate entity, different from other lymphomas.

I asked him if there had been a history of Burkitt patients in London or New York visiting tropical Africa.

"No," Dr. Wright answered. "The majority of them haven't been abroad. When I was in England in 1964 I reviewed all the childhood lymphomas in the Manchester Tumor Registry and in Great Ormond Street Hospital in London, as well as a few cases in Sheffield and a few in Liverpool. Some of these were absolutely typical cases of Burkitt's lymphoma."

"Is there any explanation for the tumor occurring in such unexpected places?"

"You have to classify diseases according to their cause, or according to what they look like," Dr. Wright explained. "If they look similar, this doesn't necessarily mean they have the same causative agent. So although typical cases of Burkitt's tumor occur outside Africa, say in America and England, they may not be etiologically the same."[3]

"Is it possible for the same disease to have a different etiology?"

"Oh, yes. For example, ordinary skin cancer, squamous cell carcinoma, occurs in Africa as a result of chronic irritation in tropical ulcers of the leg. But it can be caused by X-rays, and it might be caused by arsenic poisoning. In experimental animals it can be caused by viruses. The human body can only react in certain ways to any particular stimulus, and you may get the same final result from a number of different stimuli. The fact that all these cases look like Burkitt's tumor, clinically and pathologically (that is, in their general symptoms and also in laboratory tests), doesn't mean necessarily they have the

---

[3] Etiology is the study of causes, specifically the branch of medicine dealing with the cause of a disease. It is used here in the sense of *the cause or reason for the occurrence of the disease.*

same etiology although, on the other hand, it's possible that they *may* have the same etiology."

"Could viruses be the cause of this disease?"

Dr. Wright said, "A number of viruses have been isolated from Burkitt's tumor. One is herpes simplex. This, though, may be pure chance because herpes simplex occurs everywhere in the mouth and therefore it would be close to jaw tumors.

"We also have a herpes-like virus. In other words, it isn't herpes simplex, but it looks *like* a herpes virus.

"Then T. M. Bell, who is working at Entebbe for the Imperial Cancer Research Fund, has isolated a virus which belongs to a group called reoviruses. He has isolated reovirus type 3 from twenty of seventy-five cases of Burkitt's tumor—over a quarter of the cases; and at the same time he hasn't isolated it from thirty-five controlled cases of other kinds of children's tumors."

"Are these viruses found, say, in Sheffield?"

"Reovirus is known to be world-wide in distribution. Now, if in fact Burkitt's tumor is related to reovirus (of course, all we have so far is in *association,* not an etiological relationship) I think we would then have to postulate a second factor to account for the very high incidence of Burkitt's tumor in tropical Africa and in New Guinea.

"The points *in favor* of reovirus being implicated are (1) it has very frequently been isolated from Burkitt's tumor and has not been isolated from other children's tumors; (2) Professor N. F. Stanley of Perth, Western Australia, has shown that reovirus can be transmitted by mosquitoes; and (3) Professor Stanley has produced lymphomas in mice with reovirus.

"*Against it,* is the fact that it is world-wide in distribution (because this would lead us to expect Burkitt's tumor to occur more commonly all over the world).

"So, to account for the high incidence of Burkitt's tumor in Africa we have two possibilities. The first possibility is that if Burkitt's tumor is due to reovirus *and nothing else,* then the tumor occurs because of the way the African child gets reovirus. The usual way one gets reovirus is by ingesting it (as by swallowing), and normally this wouldn't cause the tumor. But if you got the virus as a result of being bitten by a mosquito, this *might* result in a tumor.

"The other possibility is that in tropical Africa a second virus, or a second *agent* such as malaria, might play a part; so that if you got reovirus plus a second virus, or reovirus plus malaria, you might stand a higher chance of developing the tumor than if you live, say, in Sheffield and you only get the reovirus.

"The thing that has to be borne in mind is that from the records of the past thirty years in the Great Ormond Street Hospital, which covers the eastern part of England, and in the Manchester Children's Tumor Registry which covers an enormous population (in the Midlands and North Country) I've picked up only nine cases of Burkitt's tumor. On occasion, you might have seen that number of children with this disease sitting, in one day, in one ward of our hospital in Kampala. So that although Burkitt's tumor occurs in England and in the United States, there is a very significant difference in the rate we see in tropical Africa."

The three infective agents mentioned by Dr. Wright deserve, at this point, a closer look. They are like the small unnoticed clues in a mystery story which *might* suddenly explode as decisive clues.

Herpes comes from the Greek (*herpein,* to creep, *herpeton,* a snake) and these viruses manifest themselves by creeping, or spreading, from one part to another. The kind mankind knows best is herpes simplex which—in its more harmless aspect—causes fever blisters or cold sores, most frequently around the mouth or the margins of the lips. Occasionally the small moist sores may appear on the skin or mucous membranes of the genital organs; and sometimes they occur on the conjunctiva or on the cornea of the eye, with the danger that they may cause scarring which will impair vision. What is most remarkable about herpes simplex is that it seems to infect human beings soon after birth and then remains dormant in the skin until it erupts (usually quite unexpectedly) as the result of overexposure to sunlight, an upper respiratory infection, or even emotional stress. A girl experiencing an unhappy love affair may find—adding to her woes—that herpes simplex has used this excuse to burst forth in public; a man returning from a skiing vacation may be bronzed and fit but embarrassed by lip sores, the result of herpes simplex responding to excessive ultraviolet radiation at high altitudes. But, generally, herpes simplex stays in hiding, as far as we know in a state of total torpor. When it makes an appearance, drugs cannot affect its course. Drying lotions, such as spirits of camphor or 70 per cent alcohol, may help skin lesions, and recently some success has been reported in chemotherapy of herpes infections of the cornea; but little really can be done (except, perhaps, in the cases cited, to plunge at once into a new love affair, or stay resolutely away from high places) until herpes simplex, obeying some voice we cannot ever hope to hear, decides to go back into its torpor again. One of its relatives is notable for wearing two hats: it may cause either chicken pox, when it is called herpes varicella, or shingles, when it is called herpes zoster.

But herpes simplex is not quite as mild as it seems. It is known to cause the disruption of chromosomes in the nucleus of the cell, and thus may be implicated in carcinogenesis. Furthermore, according to Dr. Etienne de Harven,[4] "the Lucké carcinoma agent can hardly be distinguished from herpes simplex virus." Now, the Lucké virus (which was discovered by Dr. Balduin Lucké of the University of Pennsylvania) causes tumors of the kidney in leopard frogs; and it has been suggested that the Lucké virus, or one of the herpes group very similar to it, may be picked up by mosquitoes which feed on frogs and then transmitted to children, thus initiating the process leading to Burkitt's lymphoma. Another amphibian which has come under suspicion is *Xenopus,* a genus of African toads notable for having no tongue, teeth in the upper jaw, claws on the hind legs and tentacle-like processes on the side of the head. These animals might serve as natural reservoirs

---

[4] *Electron Microscopy of Cancer Cells: A Review.* Etienne de Harven, M.D., *The Medical Clinics of North America,* Vol. 50, No. 3, May 1966. W. B. Saunders Co., Philadelphia & London.

of viruses which are somehow connected with Burkitt's lymphoma, raising new possibilities which were described to me by Dr. M. A. Epstein at the Bland Sutton Institute in London. Dr. Epstein is the leading expert on the *herpes-like virus* found in Burkitt's lymphoma; this virus, in fact, and several additional strains were first found and grown by him in tissue culture and were designated EB_1, EB_2, and so on (E for Epstein, B for Dr. Evelyn Barr, a co-worker).

"This is a synthesis of what many people are thinking," Dr. Epstein said. "First, the virus might be carried to humans by, say, a hypothetical mosquito from an animal reservoir; that's one possibility. Another possibility is that when the virus replicates in these animal reservoirs it might acquire very slightly different properties from what you might call the usual run of the virus, so that when it's carried to a human being it behaves in a slightly different manner and there is a chance of the recipient getting a malignant response. Still another possibility is that the virus may be altered in a similar way when it replicates inside the insect that is carrying it, and we are doing mosquito feeding studies at the present time to see whether we can get any evidence of this. There is also the possibility that the virus isn't altered in any way in the vector which is carrying it, but that it is introduced by the vector[5] into the recipient by an abnormal route. You and I might catch the virus and become infected with it by the oral route, which might be the usual way of picking it up; but the vector might in some cases put the virus directly into the blood stream of the recipient, leading to an abnormal situation."

The reoviruses derive their name not from a place or a person but from an odd combination of words: Respiratory and Enteric Orphans. In the early 1950s, scientists searching for polio viruses came upon a number of viruses which were noteworthy for causing illnesses in man so mild and transient that

[5] A vector is a carrier of the microorganisms of a particular disease (or diseases), picking up the microorganisms from an infected person or animal and transporting them to other individuals, thus spreading the infection. In some cases (as in malaria) the microorganism undergoes vital biological changes in the vector, which are part of its life cycle.

some virologists concluded that these organisms had not, so to speak, found their true *métier* and could be regarded as viruses in search of a disease. Hence, orphans. The original group was known as ECHO (Enteric Cytopathogenic Human Orphan) viruses, and it numbers about thirty; but recently one of these viruses was found to differ from its brothers in certain respects and it became the founder member of a new group, with a new name and a current membership of three. Type 3 reovirus is the kind which has been found in Burkitt's lymphoma.

Malaria is something altogether different. Of all the ills that afflict mankind it is perhaps the most deadly. It kills more people than cancer; it kills more people than heart disease. On a world-wide scale it is said to be responsible for more than half of all the deaths of human beings. It has cast a long shadow on history: some scholars believe that among other catastrophes it contributed largely to the downfall of the ancient Greek empire; but the same claim has been made for other infections, such as typhus.

The agent responsible for malaria is the plasmodium, which has its place among the fifteen thousand species comprising the Protozoa—those microscopic animals that for the most part consist of a single cell but sometimes live in colonies of similar cells. The plasmodia reproduce by forming spores; they are parasitic and have no means of locomotion of their own; and four different types cause malaria in man—*Plasmodium vivax, P. malariae, P. falciparum,* and *P. ovale,* each with a different biological pattern. *P. ovale* is rare; *P. vivax* and *P. malariae* are capable of "hibernating" and may reappear periodically—for five years when the agent is *P. vivax,* and for thirty years when the agent is *P. malariae.* Falciparum malaria is the type most common in the tropics. It has a very high mortality rate; but with early treatment it can be cured by chemotherapy, although there is the possibility of an unpleasant complication known as blackwater fever.

Malaria is carried by mosquitoes of the genus *Anopheles,* which is easily recognized (usually a moment too late) because it appears to be virtually standing on its head while biting its victim. *Culex,* the familiar house mosquito of Europe and the United States, keeps its body parallel to the surface on which it rests while transmitting malaria to birds and filaria (roundworms) to humans. *Aëdes aegypti*, too, keeps its body horizontal while transmitting the viruses of dengue (breakbone fever) and yellow fever.

But *Anopheles* is only one factor in a complex cycle of events. It must first bite a human being who is already suffering from malaria, and ingest blood containing plasmodia which have developed sexual forms. Within the mosquito's stomach these organisms undergo further development, and numerous offspring, known as sporozoites, eventually make their way to the salivary glands of the mosquito, to enter the blood stream of any human being *Anopheles* then encounters and bites. The parasites invade the victim's red blood cells, multiply, consume the cells, and burst out to attack more red blood cells. There is a belief that the simultaneous release into the blood stream of great numbers of parasites, and their poisonous by-products, causes the shivering chill followed by intense fever characteristic of malaria.

In communities where even the most primitive medical facilities exist, the malaria patient is screened from further contact with *Anopheles*, for two excellent reasons. Several mosquitoes may bite him and pick up the infection, thus passing it on to other members of the community. Or, alternatively, he may be bitten again by mosquitoes carrying the plasmodium, thus acquiring more infections in addition to the primary infection. It is quite possible to have two or more infections going simultaneously. Constant infection may build up a fair degree of immunity, but not always; and in many parts of the world this is the real menace of malaria. Human beings, from early childhood on, suffer a virtually uninterrupted series of malarial attacks; the infections may appear to die down, but even a mild illness of a totally different kind—sometimes a psychological disturbance—may precipitate a new attack. At the same time there is continual exposure to new bites and eventually, weakened and exhausted, the malaria victim can offer no further resistance to the disease. One sees photographs of Africans, of the Indians of South America, of the Papuans of

New Guinea—handsome, robust people, with one physiological peculiarity in common: a bulging belly. It usually denotes, not riotous living, but an enlarged spleen resulting from recurrent malarial infection, and it is only too often a harbinger of early death.

The possibility that viruses may be involved in causing human cancer is a commonplace in all discussions of carcinogenesis, so that one is not overcome by surprise when herpes-viruses and reoviruses are found in Burkitt's tumor, even though their role remains unclear. The discovery bolsters the hope that viruses will in due course be found in other human tumors and that a day will arrive when a vaccine will end the threat of cancer in the same way that a vaccine ended the threat of polio.

The malaria plasmodium seems, at first glance, not quite so credible as a leading character in this detective story. It occupies an entirely different niche in the natural history of disease. Nevertheless, some scientists believe that it may play a part of quite unexpected importance both in the induction of certain forms of cancer and in their eventual control.

A reference to malaria occurred when Dennis Wright was talking about adults in Uganda who developed Burkitt's lymphoma.

"We have a population of immigrants," Dr. Wright said, "who come in from the mountains as laborers. They're poor, and if they fall ill in Uganda they usually stay in the hospital until they die. When they die there are no relatives to carry them off, so they're almost certain to come to post-mortem. I was reviewing all the post-mortem cases of Burkitt's lymphoma when I was writing my M.D. thesis, and I noticed that all adults who died of the lymphoma were immigrants. I pointed this out to Denis Burkitt, and we went into it in more detail, in clinical cases (those under treatment) as well as post-mortem cases; and together we published a paper in the *British Medical Journal* pointing out that there was a very high incidence of the tumor in adult immigrants from the highlands."

"Doesn't this underline the possibility that the local children develop some kind of immunity as a result of repeated exposure to the virus, or the infective agent, whatever that happens to be?"

"Yes. The suggestion was best expressed, I think, by Alec Haddow, the director of the East African Virus Research Institute at Entebbe. He postulated that Burkitt's tumor was *an uncommon response to a common infection,* and that all the indigenous people in the lowland areas of Uganda got the virus and developed immunity to it, while a very few unfortunate people developed the tumor. An adult coming in from the highland areas might more easily develop the tumor as a result of never having developed immunity to the virus."

"Is this theory still held?"

"It still fits very well," Dr. Wright said. "The agent might not necessarily be a virus. I think if you believed that malaria was implicated you could still postulate the same theory. The adults who come from the highland areas go down immediately with malaria because they have no immunity to it (malaria doesn't occur in the mountains), whereas our local lowland population has acquired some sort of immunity to malaria fairly early in life."

"Does Burkitt's lymphoma occur with the same frequency in other areas of the world with similar environmental conditions—along the Amazon, for example?"

Dr. Wright answered, "People have looked along the Amazon and haven't found it (which doesn't mean it isn't there). The two places where we know for certain that the tumor occurs are tropical Africa and New Guinea. They have many factors in common. When I was in New Guinea recently I kept wanting to speak to the people in Swahili, and I kept thinking I was back in Africa. They have many disease patterns that are alike; but the one thing that is most striking in both areas is the very high incidence of malaria due to *Plasmodium falciparum.* In South America and Southeast Asia they have different vectors for malaria which result in different forms of the disease."

"The hypothesis, is, then, that the tumor might be caused by two agents—or even more?"

"Yes," Dr. Wright said. "It's possible that you have two agents coming together at one particular time. Or that the host's immune mechanism is altered by malaria (or some other infectious parasite) and then hit by a virus."

The story still remains to be completed. In the most recent developments, as this book goes to press, malaria appears to be even more strongly favored as a possible factor in Burkitt's lymphoma, and the EB virus—now referred to simply as EBV—is perhaps more strongly favored as a co-factor than reovirus type 3. A vast amount of excitement has been generated by the discovery that the EBV found in Burkitt's lymphoma is almost certainly the cause of infectious mononucleosis (better known in Britain as glandular fever)—the outcome of some brilliant work by Drs. W. and G. Henle of Philadelphia. The hope underlying the enormous concentration of energy on Burkitt's lymphoma is that this may well be the first form of cancer to be "cracked"—in other words, to be fully understood by scientists, thus opening the way to our understanding of other forms of cancer such as the leukemias and lymphomas. Put in the most guarded terms, the outlook is good—one even dares to say *very* good.

EIGHT

Stalking Horse

There are today some thirty or forty men and women who constitute a sort of inner cabinet of cancerology. They are scientists of great accomplishment and total dedication; they have immense prestige and, deservedly, considerable power; and they are involved directly or indirectly with virtually every aspect of cancer research all over the world. One can name a few of them more or less at random: Professor Sir Alexander Haddow of the United Kingdom; Dr. Vasant R. Khanolkar of India; Dr. Tomizo Yoshida of Japan; Dr. Otto Mühlbock of the Netherlands; Dr. Pietro Bucalossi of Italy; Professor J. R. Maisin of Belgium; Dr. Victor Ngu of Nigeria; Dr. Isaac Berenblum of Israel; Dr. Hedwig Hamperl of the Federal Republic of Germany; Pr. George Klein of Sweden; Dr. Nikolai N. Blokhin and Dr. L. M. Shabad of the U.S.S.R.; Dr. Pierre Denoix of France; Dr. Ahmed Lotfy Aboul-Nasr of the United Arab Republic; Dr. Prosper Loustalot of Switzerland; Dr. Eduardo Caceres of Peru; Dr. Erkki A. Saxen of Finland. Several names spring to mind when one thinks of the United States and it would be invidious to select just one or two; but in any listing of members of the cancer establishment,

Dr. Joseph Holland Burchenal would most certainly be present. Dr. Burchenal's major field of work (according to a *Who's Who* prepared for the Ninth International Cancer Congress) is cancer chemotherapy, and his qualifications can justifiably be called awesome. He was for more than ten years Chief of the Division of Clinical Chemotherapy at the Sloan-Kettering Institute for Cancer Research, and he is now Vice-President for Clinical Investigation. At the same time he was Chief and then Co-Chief of the Chemotherapy Service at Memorial Hospital and is now Director for Clinical Investigation. More than thirty lines would be required to list the medical and scientific societies of which he is a member and the various committees on which he has served. When I was in Stockholm interviewing Dr. Eva Klein she referred with deep feeling to a conference on Burkitt's lymphoma which she and her husband, Pr. George Klein, attended in Kampala at the invitation of the chairman, Dr. Joseph H. Burchenal. When I was in Geneva a week later, an official of the World Health Organization presented me with a copy of *Chemotherapy of Cancer: First Report of an Expert Committee;* the chairman of this expert committee was Dr. Joseph H. Burchenal. When I was in Tokyo a few weeks later, I met Dr. Burchenal in person: he was chairman of a panel dealing with new developments in the treatment of the leukemias and lymphomas. Acting as chairman on committees such as these always entails a vast amount of work. The reward is not fortune; it is not even fame; it is, one suspects almost entirely intellectual—the satisfaction of helping to bring light to darkness.

In May, 1966, Dr. Burchenal gave the Presidential Address to a meeting of the American Association for Cancer Research in Denver, Colorado. The title of his address was *Geographic Chemotherapy—Burkitt's Tumor as a Stalking Horse for Leukemia,* an unusually romantic title for what was in effect a highly technical survey; and it began, appropriately, with definitions of what the title meant:

Geographic chemotherapy may be defined as the study of

the chemotherapeutic response of similar tumors from different geographic regions. It takes advantage of the differing incidence of certain tumors in various geographic areas, presumably due to environmental or genetic factors: (a) to bring the best chemotherapy available to bear on various sensitive tumors, such as choriocarcinoma or Burkitt's tumor, which constitute a real problem in certain countries, and (b) to determine whether tumors with similar pathological appearance from different regions respond similarly to chemotherapy. If differences are found, this might suggest that environment or genetic factors also affect the response to chemotherapy.

The *Oxford Universal Dictionary* defines "a stalking horse" as "a horse trained to allow a fowler to conceal himself behind it or under its coverings in order to get within easy range of the game without alarming it." Thus the title and its definition are meant to suggest that a careful study of Burkitt's tumor may provide a useful approach to the eventual control of acute leukemia.

The eventual control of acute leukemia has perhaps the highest priority in all cancer research, not merely in terms of budget allocations and laboratory space but in the less tangible terms of heart and mind, for acute leukemia kills mostly those who make the largest claim on our emotions: children between the ages of three and fifteen. In the United States, where the deadly infections of childhood are no longer a major problem, acute leukemia is the leading cause of death of young children, killing some twenty-one hundred each year—more than died of poliomyelitis in the peak year of 1952. Adults are by no means immune: for every child, five adults die of the disease, and the American Cancer Society's latest estimate, for the year 1968, is that nineteen thousand adults and children will contract the disease in one of its forms, and fifteen thousand will die of it.

Surgery is of no help in acute leukemia of childhood; radiation has accomplished little; chemotherapy in general can only stem the disease temporarily. To all intents and purposes leukemia is incurable and it is therefore considered the deadliest of all cancers; yet for the past twenty years some scientists and many publicists have insisted that of all forms of cancer this will be the first for which a practical cure will be found, that a breakthrough is imminent, and that—like polio—it will eventually be brought under control in every civilized part of the world. Mr. Burkitt's stalking horse may in due course help to accomplish that end.

Leukemia comes from the term *Weisses Blut,* white blood, which was first used by the German pathologist Rudolf Virchow in 1845.[1] Virchow was describing a distinctive reaction in which a layer of white blood cells appears in sedimented samples of blood taken from leukemic patients; and the name —perhaps unfortunately, in the opinion of some scientists— has persisted as a sort of historical relic. The circulating blood is not white in leukemia. Certain very severe cases may show a slight milkiness; but quite often the white blood cell count is low, and at least in one form there is such a conspicuous absence of white cells in the circulating blood that the disease is called aleukemic leukemia, or non-white-blood white-blood condition, while yet another form, affecting both red and white cells, is called erythroleukemia, or red-whiteblood condition.

In practice, leukemia is the generic name of a large and complex group of malignant diseases of the blood and the tissues in which the blood cells are produced. There are not only many forms of the disease; the different forms may progress at different rates, which provides one method of classification. In *chronic* leukemias the disease may continue for three to ten years, or even longer, and relatively simple treatment often will enable the patient to live in a state of almost normal health most of the time and perhaps die eventually of an entirely different disease. In *acute* leukemia—the type which most commonly afflicts children—the course of the disease is rapid, lasting from a few weeks (sometimes only a few days)

---

[1] The disease was also described in the same year by John Hughes Bennett, an English physician. The word leukemia itself is derived from *leuko,* white, and *emia,* a suffix denoting a condition of the blood.

after it first manifests itself, to about six months. *Subacute* leukemias may continue for about a year.

A second method of classification is according to the type of cell affected by the disease. The blood, of course, is composed of a fluid portion called the plasma, which makes up about 55 per cent of the total volume, and the so-called formed elements consisting of red blood cells, white blood cells and platelets, which make up about 45 per cent of the total volume. (It might be observed in passing that the *blood plasma* cannot be cancerous, since cancer by definition is primarily a disease of cells that are capable of reproducing themselves; but the plasma, and the lymph, which closely resembles blood plasma, serve to *transport* cancerous cells.)

The red blood cells, or erythrocytes, are formed in the red marrow of the bones, and their chief function is to carry oxygen to all tissues of the body, exchanging it for carbon dioxide. The white blood cells, or leucocytes, are of five different kinds. Three contain numerous small granules which become visible under the microscope when stained with different dyes; and these cells are therefore called granulocytes. The two other kinds of leucocytes appear to lack granules, or the granules are exceedingly fine; and they are called, respectively, lymphocytes and monocytes. There is still considerable difference of opinion about where the various leucocytes are formed, but we cannot be far wrong if we assume that the granular leucocytes, like the red blood cells, originate in the red bone marrow, while the lymphocytes and monocytes are formed in lymphoid tissue, including the lymph nodes, spleen, tonsils, and thymus. The chief function of the leucocytes is protective. They destroy invading bacteria, generally by engulfing them, thus earning the title of phagocytes or eating cells; they are the source of antibodies and other substances which are part of the body's immune system; and, collaborating with the tiny platelets (which seem to have no other function) they assist in the repair of damaged tissue.

Red and white blood cells have some striking differences, related to the kind of work they do. For example, the red blood cells are transported through the body by the normal flow of the blood, and have no power of movement of their own. None is needed, for molecules of the oxygen they carry can seep through the walls of the capillaries without difficulty to supply adjoining tissue cells. On the other hand, most of the leucocytes—while still relying upon the circulating blood for long-distance transport—are able to move in a manner resembling the movement of the amoeba: that is, they thrust a portion of the cell forward, forming a pseudopod or false foot, and the rest of the cell follows. In this way the leucocytes are able to pass through minute gaps in the walls of blood and lymph vessels and enter adjoining tissues to attack hostile bacteria and participate in tissue repair. Furthermore, the leucocytes have a nucleus, which enables them to reproduce by the process of mitosis, the usual method of cell reproduction. The red blood cells in the circulating blood do not have a nucleus and so they cannot reproduce. However, when the red blood cells are being formed in the bone marrow they go through a number of stages in which they possess a nucleus, and this is lost only in the final stage when the red blood cell achieves maturity and is ready to pass into the blood stream: the nucleus disintegrates and is replaced by hemoglobin.

All those factors are of profound importance when any type of blood cells becomes cancerous. Thus, in the rare condition mentioned earlier, erythroleukemia or red-white-blood condition, the immature, nucleated red blood cells in the bone marrow multiply at a tremendous rate and pour into the blood stream; at the same time the production of mature red blood cells is reduced; and since the immature red blood cells cannot perform the functions of mature red blood cells satisfactorily, one of the inevitable results is anemia, which becomes steadily more severe.

Similarly, each type of white blood cell has its own characteristic malignancies. Leukemia of the granular white blood cells, known as myelocytic (marrow cell) leukemia, is marked among other things by enormous proliferation of the immature and mature forms in the bone marrow where these cells are formed, as well as excessive numbers of granular white cells in the circulating blood. Leukemia of the lymphocytes, known as lymphocytic leukemia, is marked by an uncontrolled proliferation of lymphocytes, enlargement of the lymphoid tissues of the spleen, lymph nodes and other sites where lymphocytes are formed, and the appearance of great numbers of these cells in the circulating blood as well as in various organs and tissues. The property of ameboid movement is a factor which has an unfortunate significance in leukemia, for by this means the cancerous white blood cells are able to leave the blood and lymph vessels and colonize surrounding tissues. This is particularly serious because the leukemic cells often tend to concentrate in the brain where they cannot be reached by most of the drugs used in chemotherapy, since these drugs are stopped by the blood-brain barrier.[2] Furthermore, because in many forms of the disease a large proportion of the proliferating white blood cells are immature types they cannot overcome infections or repair tissue damage; and the inevitable results of the total leukemic process are an increase of secondary infections and persistent hemorrhages.

Leukemia, in all its forms, is still largely—overwhelmingly— a mystery. We know that it can be induced in mice by treatment with different chemicals and by radiation, specifically X-rays, which will also cause leukemia in man (radiologists have five times as much leukemia as the rest of the population). We also know that it can be induced in mice, in fowl, and possibly in other animals such as cattle, guinea pigs, cats and rats, by viruses; but we have no definite information that viruses can cause the disease in man. In an earlier chapter it was pointed out that leukemia of the granular white blood cells in human beings (chronic myelocytic leukemia, one of the more common forms) seems to be associated with an abnormality of one of the chromosomes, known as the Philadelphia, or Ph^1, chromosome: the non-committal qualification, *seems to be associated*, is indicative of scientific caution regarding this finding, for it has not been established whether chromosomal disorders play any part in inducing human leukemia, whether

---

[2] The blood-brain barrier is a complex monitoring and filtering system, imperfectly understood by scientists, which prevents the entry of most harmful substances into the brain.

they are signs that a malignant condition is present, or whether they result from the disease itself.

Innumerable theories have been developed to account for the occurrence of human leukemia: none, so far, has proven satisfactory even as a working hypothesis. The idea that leukemia is caused by viruses has been heavily favored by many scientists all over the world, and in the United States the National Advisory Cancer Council stated in its annual report for 1966, "The possibility that the disease in man may be caused by a virus is so strong that a large portion of the research conducted and supported by the National Cancer Institute is devoted to this particular problem in the hope of eradicating leukemia, as poliomyelitis has been virtually eradicated, by a vaccine. In the past two years Congress has appropriated $27,-000,000 specifically for virus-leukemia research sponsored by the National Cancer Institute. This is a fully organized program for the study of (1) the cause and prevention of human leukemia, (2) the treatment of human leukemia, (3) the nature of animal leukemias and their possible relationships to man, and (4) hazards involved in virus research and methods of controlling them."

The hope of finally establishing that viruses cause leukemia affects the minds of cancer scientists, and those who write about cancer, like strong wine. Even more intoxicating is the possibility of developing a leukemia vaccine, putting an end to the threat of this most deadly of diseases as the Salk and Sabin vaccines put an end to the intolerable threat of polio, and by an extension that is not really too extreme we can then hope for incontrovertible facts that identify viruses as the cause of all or most forms of cancer and fulfillment of the *ultimate* hope: a universal cancer vaccine. The National Cancer Institute has listed a number of points emerging from recent research which implicate viruses as a cause of leukemia, none as yet conclusive but all significant and adding up to an impressive body of evidence. In brief, here are some of them:[3]

---

[3] Condensed from *Progress Against Cancer*, A Report by the National Advisory Cancer Council, 1966.

1) Virus-like particles of two different types can be detected by electron microscopy and, in some cases, isolated from patients of different countries who are afflicted with leukemia or lymphoma. The first, called the "C"-type particle, is identical in structure with viruses known to cause leukemia in laboratory animals. Particles of the second type are similar in size and shape but not identical to herpes viruses, known to cause fever sores or shingles in man, and to viruses found in lymphomas and carcinomas in toads and frogs (but not proved to be the causative agents of the tumor). . . . Work is in progress on determining the biological activity of these herpes virus-type particles in order to elucidate whether they play a role in causing malignancy or are merely passenger viruses trapped by the cancer cells.

2) It is now firmly established that Burkitt lymphoma occurs in African children at a rate higher than that of all other forms of childhood leukemia and lymphoma in Africa combined. . . . The distribution of this type of lymphoma in a specific region of equatorial Africa suggests that an insect may play a role in its transmission. A spontaneous lymphoma in a species of African frog yields virus particles that resemble structurally the particles associated with Burkitt lymphoma cells. Because mosquitoes feed on frogs, there is a possibility that frogs may be a link between the animal tumor virus and the candidate human virus.

3) As part of the over-all plan of study, materials from leukemic patients have been inoculated into more than 600 newborn monkeys and baboons. One type of virus, known to cause cancer in chickens and other fowl, crosses species lines and has been found to induce malignant sarcomas in marmosets, a species of small monkey. . . . Hamsters inoculated with material from Burkitt lymphoma cultures developed proliferative brain lesions after six months (suggesting that human virus has passed to the hamsters).

4) Vaccines like those used to prevent human influenza, polio and measles, are being produced to prevent animal leukemia.

5) It appears from studies of leukemia in cattle, cats and dogs, that at least some leukemias and lymphomas occurring in animals that have prolonged and close association with man are virus-induced. If this can be established unequivocally,

means can be found for prevention or control of such animal leukemias. It will be possible to isolate, treat, or sacrifice animals known to be carriers of their own leukemia viruses.

6) Leukemia induced in a monkey has yielded large quantities of herpes-like virus particles, identical in size, shape, and other characteristics to those found in tissue cultures of human leukemia and Burkitt lymphoma.

By the time this book is printed the great virus program may have reached a triumphant conclusion; but writing before the event it is only fair to point out that the difficulties facing the program are formidable. In the past two or three decades, fully aware that human leukemia bears many signs that it might be induced by a virus, a great many scientists all over the world have devoted themselves to searching for the causative organism, without success; and it appears inconceivable to some observers that any virus could continue to be so elusive, could remain in hiding, in view of such a massive search carried out with the most sophisticated equipment and the most elegant methods. A parallel with poliomyelitis is apt to be discouraging, for Dr. Karl Landsteiner, one of the geniuses of medicine, showed as long ago as 1909 that the cause of polio was a filterable virus; and although the exceedingly difficult techniques for preparing polio vaccines then had to be developed, the first public trials of vaccines took place in 1934 and 1935. These were not altogether successful, but the way had been opened, and large-scale success was achieved in 1952 and 1953 by Salk. The historians of pathology will recall, finally, that the earliest report of a virus-induced leukemia of fowl came from two Danes, Wilhelm Ellermann and Olaf Bang in 1908, almost at the same time that Landsteiner discovered the filterable polio virus in Vienna; and one cannot help speculating why the intervening 60 years should have brought total victory to the polio virus researchers and done so little for those who are investigating human leukemia viruses.

A recent paper by F. C. Chesterman, a distinguished British pathologist, opens with the magisterial statement, "No tumor of man has been shown to be induced or maintained by a virus."[4] Helena Curtis, in her admirable book *The Viruses* (New York, 1965) makes a statement that is no less adamant: "No virus has ever been isolated from a human cancer that has regularly and unequivocally caused a tumor in a laboratory test." The *possibility* that human cancer and in particular human leukemia are the outcome of action by viruses is not denied; all that is lacking is proof. Once proof is established and the virus identified, a leukemia vaccine might conceivably be developed; but certain very significant questions arise to bedevil the investigators.

Perhaps the first question is, *Can we really assume that a specific leukemia virus exists?* The common cold is a viral disorder which might long ago have been made obsolete by a cold vaccine except for the unhappy fact that colds can be caused by dozens of different viruses, and to manufacture vaccine potent against all of them would be virtually impossible. The case against an influenza vaccine is even stronger, for here we have different viruses which have the ability to combine and form new types, so that a vaccine effective against influenza viruses in an epidemic a year ago, or even a week ago, might be useless against a form which came into existence only twenty-four hours ago. It would not be unfair to argue, therefore, that *if* leukemia is virus-induced there might well be a number of different viruses which are responsible for the numerous forms of the disease, and to guard against all of them would require an enormously elaborate vaccine that is probably beyond our present capabilities.

Another element of the argument has to do with the nature of viruses and the nature of leukemia. In any of the common viral infections what seems to occur is this: the invading viruses seek out specific kinds of cells which presumably offer them the materials and facilities they require for reproduction. The polio virus in its dangerous form, for example, seeks out cells in the gray matter of the spinal cord and in certain areas of the brain; the influenza viruses seek out cells in

---

[4] *The Prevention of Cancer.* Edited by Ronald W. Raven and Francis J. C. Roe. Chapter 9, "Viruses," by F. C. Chesterman. Butterworths, London, 1967.

the respiratory organs; the virus of mumps seeks out cells in the salivary glands and in the ovaries or the testes. Once the virus invades the cell it may proceed to take over the cell's chemical stores and machinery, and then replicates itself, sometimes in enormous numbers. One cell may house fifty million or more virus particles of a particular kind; and these at a certain point may rupture the cell wall and burst out into the blood stream. Or there may be a lesser number of viruses which leak out of the cell relatively slowly. The process was described by Dr. R. J. C. Harris: "In mammalian cells the takeover may be partial, just sufficient to maintain adequate production of viruses, leaving the cell more or less intact. These are the cells that leak virus. Occasionally the viruses act catastrophically and blow up the cell, and the virus is poured out. From the evolutionary point of view the successful viruses are those that have been temperate in their habits and have not been so catastrophic. The 'flu virus, for instance, has been temperate: it hasn't killed off all its human hosts—it can't have done so, because we're still here."[5]

Often a virus chooses to lodge peaceably in a cell without causing any untoward disturbance: the polio virus can again serve as an example, for it normally inhabits the intestinal tract and rarely draws attention to its presence. Or the virus may disappear within the cell it has invaded and pass through numerous cell divisions before once again resuming its reproductive cycle—a way of life practiced extensively by the herpes virus, which may remain hidden and inactive for thirty years.[6]

---

[5] The viruses that attack bacteria, the familiar bacteriophages (bacteria-eaters) do so in the catastrophic manner. The virus attaches itself to the outer membrane of the bacterial cell, squirts its core of nucleic acid into the cell; this *nucleic acid* takes over the bacterium's nucleic acid and twenty minutes later the cell membrane bursts open and two hundred new viruses emerge, ready to go off and colonize other bacterial cells in the same manner.

[6] The rubella virus, responsible for German measles, behaves in a manner that seems to be unique. In tissue culture, cells infected with rubella virus seem to be structurally identical to cells that are free of the virus. However, according to a report from the National Cancer Institute, "the infected cells grow at half the speed of healthy cells. This 'reverse cancer'

These conditions, whether the viruses are multiplying furiously or are lying dormant, have one important similarity: the viruses to all intents and purposes retain their identity. They may modify their form; nevertheless they start an infection as viruses and end it as viruses. And, as active viruses, to the best of our knowledge, they have not yet been shown to cause malignancies in human beings, whatever else they may cause. As long as they retain their identity as viruses they are candidates for extinction by one means or another—as a result of action taken by the body's immunological defenses, or of any of various stratagems which man's ingenuity has devised and will continue to devise in the future.

However, for certain viruses there is another destiny. Once they are within a cell they may—temporarily, perhaps—abandon their viral way of life and, for reasons that are still totally beyond our understanding, become incorporated in the cell's own chromosomal material. The cell is thus changed, or transformed; and it is in this condition (among others) that the cell may become malignant. The various immune processes now cannot act specifically against the virus because it no longer exists as a virus: it is simply a particle of nucleic acid which has hidden itself within a complex chain of nucleic acid and which couldn't be recognized, as the saying goes, by its own grandmother. It reproduces not as a separate organism but along with the chromosomal material in which it hides.

If the transformed cell happens to be a white blood cell or a cell in the tissues in which white blood cells are produced, the first step may have been taken toward leukemia. The body's immunological defenses *may* have the ability to take action to suppress this transformed cell: if they fail to do so, the cancerous process will proceed yet another step. Again, in the next division the transformed cells are vulnerable to immunological suppression, but soon a point is reached where the immune defenses are outstripped. They are unable to halt the cancer.

---

effect has been suggested as an explanation for rubella-induced congenital birth defects, for the slow growth of the rubella virus-infected cells results in malformed organs with fewer than the normal numbers of cells."

This, then, is one of the fundamental problems facing the researchers. If leukemia is proven to be caused by a virus, a leukemia vaccine utilizing these viruses might well be developed; but to be effective it would have to destroy not merely a large part of any invading viruses but *all* of them, down to the last one, *before* any virus enters a cell and transforms it. For in acute childhood leukemia the malignant cells may double every four days; and, theoretically, at this rate a single malignant cell will multiply to a trillion in 164 days, which means a child will die.

There is every possibility that the deadly human cancer viruses, if and when they are tracked down, will turn out to be not strange and exotic organisms, never before seen by the eye of man, but familiar viruses which normally play a fairly unsensational part in our daily lives, causing little mouth sores, sniffles or sneezes or various kinds of polka dots, and which only become malevolent in certain very special circumstances. It is even being argued today that cancer may be a chance occurrence, an accidental happening, that sometimes follows a viral infection. This is merely speculation. It exists only on the lofty plateau of cancer metaphysics. A booklet issued in 1966 by the U. S. Department of Health, Education, and Welfare, entitled *Cancer Programs of the U.S. Public Health Service*, states briefly and bluntly where we now stand: "In the present state of knowledge no target date can be set for achievement of the special virus-leukemia research objectives." We can translate this into an even simpler statement: No virus has so far been identified as causing human cancer and consequently a vaccine is nowhere in sight. Yet leukemia is with us here and now, and people—conspicuously children—are dying of the disease in numbers that increase every year.

What we know about the epidemiology of leukemia is of no great help. *Item:* Children afflicted with mongolism are thirty times more likely to develop leukemia than other children. *Item:* Radiation may induce leukemia. *Item:* The risk of developing leukemia seems to be slightly higher for a child whose mother was over the age of forty when he was born than for the child whose mother was under forty. But a survey made in

New Zealand in 1961 showed that all these factors could, at the most, account for only 7 per cent of all cases of leukemia; and we must admit candidly that at the present time we have no idea what causes more than 90 per cent of the leukemias of children and adults, nor do we have any explanation for the many different forms that leukemia takes.

Lacking this knowledge means that there is little we can do to prevent the occurrence of human leukemia; and for the present the chief concern of cancer scientists must be directed toward improvement in the treatment of this disease, which is almost invariably fatal.

The qualification *almost* here is of some importance. It has a history. In 1963 the National Cancer Institute organized an Acute Leukemia Task Force which, among its other activities, began to collect information about patients suffering from acute leukemia, in the United States and other countries, who had survived more than five years after their disease was diagnosed instead of succumbing in a year or less. This Registry of Long Term Survivors, as it was called, was to a large extent the responsibility of Dr. Joseph H. Burchenal, and at last report it numbered 157. Some had survived five years or more and had then died, but there seems to be a strong likelihood that about half will survive for fifteen years and perhaps remain permanently free of the disease. Why 157 sufferers from leukemia should break the pattern is well worth investigating, and the data is being studied carefully. We cannot guess, however, what proportion these 157 represent of the total number of cases of acute leukemia which occurred during the past five or ten years in all the countries participating in the program: it must be an exceedingly small part of one percentage point. No wonder, then, that many scientists have been looking with the greatest interest at progress in the treatment of Burkitt's lymphoma, for here nearly 20 per cent of patients caught in the early stages of their malignancy have experienced complete remissions. To all intents and purposes these patients appear to be fully cured, and (with the exception of choriocarcinoma) there is no other human tumor which responds to chemotherapy in such a striking manner.

Dr. Joseph H. Burchenal's paper, *Burkitt's Tumor as a Stalking Horse for Leukemia*, discusses all aspects of the disease and its treatment in a solid scientific way, with charts, tables, microphotographs, and no fewer than eighty-eight cross-references, many of which go back forty years or more and seem to anticipate some of our latest ideas. Once the scientific data has been presented, Dr. Burchenal proceeds to ask a number of highly pertinent questions:

> These various avenues of research suggest that Burkitt's tumor has broad implications for acute leukemia. Even with the relatively few drugs available in Africa, 15–20 per cent of Burkitt's tumors may be made to disappear for long periods of time. There is a good possibility that, with the addition of certain of the new agents presently available and intensive combination therapy, this rate of successful therapy might approach 50 per cent. Why is treatment more effective and lasting with Burkitt's tumor in Africa than with acute leukemia in Europe and the United States? Does Burkitt's tumor in the United States respond differently than in Africa? What can be learned from Burkitt's tumor that will help in the control of leukemia? These questions call for wide-ranging speculation.

Some of the questions and some of the speculations were discussed in the course of an interview with Dr. Burchenal at Memorial Hospital in New York.

At the outset, some of the essential facts about Burkitt's tumor were briefly reviewed. "In the first place," Dr. Burchenal said, "it's very common in equatorial Africa, where it makes up 50 per cent of childhood tumors. Originally it was thought to occur only around the equator in areas that were below 5,000 feet, in Rhodesia below 3,000 feet, and further south below 1,000 feet. It appeared to require a moist, warm climate, and studies seemed to show a close correlation with certain types of mosquitoes (which, incidentally, cause malaria, although there is not necessarily a connection—it may just be coincidence). The distribution of Burkitt's lymphoma has now been studied outside of Africa, and we find that it occurs in New

Guinea; it occurs in England; it occurs in the United States, in Brazil, and in Colombia.

"In these countries it occurs less commonly than it does in Africa, but it still may be more common than was thought. I would say that this is a new recognition—that the tumor may have been here all along and people are just beginning to recognize it. We may, in fact, have seen a great deal of it here; in other words, most of our lymphosarcomas in childhood may well turn out to be Burkitt's tumor. Where the disease is common in Africa it occurs in younger children, and 70 per cent of the presentation signs will be jaw tumors; whereas in places in Africa where it's less common it occurs in teenage children and young adults; and the presentation signs are predominantly abdominal tumors. The chances are that if it turns up here in the United States, and in Britain and Canada, it will show mostly abdominal tumors rather than jaw tumors. The distribution may be quite different in the United States from what it is in Africa because, obviously, the areas where it occurs here do not have any malaria.

"Now, while Burkitt's tumor makes up half of all cancer in childhood in Africa, here the lymphomas of childhood make up only 8 per cent of all children's cancers—leukemia makes up about 40 per cent to 50 per cent. Of these lymphomas, only a portion are going to be Burkitt's, so it's true that it's much less common in the United States than it is in Africa. But it may be much more common than we thought it was. The big problem is getting the pathologists to make the diagnosis. There is still a question among pathologists as to just how to make the diagnosis, and how Burkitt's differs from other tumors. My position is that I don't care what they call it as long as they can tell us that Case A here is just like the cases that Denis Burkitt and Dennis Wright have reported from Africa, because if they *are* the same then the important thing is to try the same treatment. Try the treatment which cures down there: then if our cases respond as well as the cases in Africa and in 20 per cent of our patients the tumor goes away and never comes back, that will be wonderful. If, on the other hand, it goes away and in all cases it comes back again, we will know there is something different about the African environment, or about the patients in Africa and the patients here, which influences chemotherapy; and this, too, will give us something to work on. Perhaps the heavy infections with malaria, or something like that, make the African patient better able to react to his disease.

"So, this concept of treating the same tumor by the same techniques in two countries with quite different environments, and finding out whether there are differences or similarities, can be extremely valuable and have important implications for all cancer research, and particularly for leukemia.

"For instance, suppose we find the disease is curable in a high percentage of cases in Africa, and it is not curable here.

"Then, suppose we say, Well, maybe it's due to the malaria in Africa; and we take patients here with Burkitt's tumor, once we get them into remission, and give them induced malaria—inject them with malaria. After ten or fifteen febrile (fever) episodes with malaria we give them chloroquine, or something similar, to bring their temperature down; and we find the Burkitt's tumor doesn't come back. The next step might be to try the same treatment with children who have acute leukemia. You can bring them back to complete good health for a period of time, but they always bounce back. However, when they're in remission you can try inducing malaria, and see if it works in leukemia patients as it does in Burkitt patients."

The suggestion that induced malaria might be used to treat patients with leukemia is actually not new, nor is it claimed to be: the technique, known as malariotherapy, or malarialization, has been used in the past for the treatment of syphilis and its grim aftermath, locomotor ataxia. Under yet another name, pyretotherapy (meaning fever therapy) the technique included raising the patient's temperature by inoculation with malarial organisms, by injection of T.A.B. vaccine, or by diathermy; and it is interesting to note that some recent reports describe experiments similar to pyretotherapy for the treatment of cancer, carried out in the United States and Europe with only limited success. References to the beneficial, but temporary, effects of malaria on leukemia and allied diseases, Dr. Burchenal points out in his *Stalking Horse* paper, go back to 1905. Some twenty-four hundred years ago Hippocrates alluded to the way in which many diseases—epilepsy, convulsions, and "maniacal attacks"—were greatly modified by concurrent malarial fever.

"Many people," Dr. Burchenal said, "including Lloyd J. Old and others, have done experiments which show that if you inoculate mice with BCG,[7] the mice will develop large spleens and an increase in the reticulo-endothelial system. In other words, the BCG acts as a chronic infection, and the mice fight it off. In doing so, the reticulo-endothelial system—which is the immune system—gets all set; it's all mobilized and ready to go. When you inject a tumor into these mice its growth is greatly inhibited; whereas in a normal animal, unprepared for this emergency, the tumor grows rapidly and overwhelms the defense. Thus, if you take two sets of mice, one immunized with BCG, the other normal, the tumor grows very rapidly in the normals but more slowly in those that are immunized. The BCG immunization is not against the tumor however.[8] We can compare it to the situation that existed in World War II, when we mobilized to give Britain the tools of war she needed. As a result, we were in a much better shape to fight off the Japanese when that problem came up than if we had been on a purely peacetime basis."

"Could you conceivably extend this kind of non-specific immunization from mice to human beings?"

"Several people are trying BCG at the present time," Dr.

[7] BCG stands for Bacillus Calmette-Guérin, an attenuated bacterium used as a vaccine against pulmonary tuberculosis. The reticulo-endothelial system is an extensive network of cells in the lymphatic tissues, the lining of the blood vessels, the spleen and the liver; these cells act as phagocytes (eating cells) engulfing and destroying invading microorganisms and other harmful particles; they also manufacture antibodies and other substances which participate in providing immunity against disease.

[8] This is referred to as non-specific immunization.

Burchenal said. "Peter Clifford and the group in Nairobi are trying it on patients with Burkitt's tumor, and George Mathé in France is doing the same thing with leukemia.[9] When the patients get into remission, they are then vaccinated with BCG in the hope of stimulating their immune mechanisms nonspecifically. The reasoning is that this may be similar to what happens in the Burkitt tumor patient. As you know, probably half the children in Nigeria and Uganda die in the first five years of life from malaria, dysentery, and other infectious diseases; so those who survive presumably have an immune mechanism which is more effective than the immune mechanism of those who fail to survive. The theory is, the high incidence of malaria (they all have big spleens and a lot of malarial pigment) may somehow enable them to fight off the leukemic stimulus—whatever that happens to be—better than individuals who have not had malaria."

Dr. Burchenal then discussed recent progress in the treatment of leukemia, and hopes for the future.

"New drugs have come up, and the survival time of patients with acute leukemia, particularly children, has been climbing. Quite a few researchers have done important studies using very large doses of drugs. For instance, a group at the National Cancer Institute treated eleven children in a program known as VAMP (derived from the names of the drugs which were used: vincristine, amethopterin,[10] 6-mercaptopurine, and prednisone). The children were treated very intensively for about four courses; then the treatment was stopped. Of those eleven patients, nine relapsed within two hundred days of stopping treatment. But the other two have gone a thousand days without relapsing: they have had no more treatment and are completely free of the disease. One of them has gone more

---

[9] At the laboratories of the Chester Beatty Research Institute in Sutton, Surrey, I was told by Prof. Peter Alexander: "We are doing this here now. All our leukemic children in remission are treated with inactivated bacterial antigens. . . . It is a modification of observations by George Mathé, which are extremely interesting and have a very good scientific rationale."

[10] Also known as methotrexate.

than three years now with no evidence of the disease; the second did relapse after about three years but only with a localized tumor of the ovary which was read (diagnosed) as a Burkitt's tumor. It was not acute leukemia.

"The important thing is that with this intensive treatment 80 per cent relapsed, as you might expect; but 20 per cent went on for a very long period of time. If 100 patients received the same treatment and 18 survived for a long period of time, it would be very exciting. When you get a patient in remission for three years or so, without any further treatment, I think that this patient may be in orbit. In other words, he may not be going to relapse. Our big problem with leukemics is that you can put a patient into a beautiful remission, but then he goes down again with the disease. But there are occasional cases—and we have collected 157 from all over the world[11]— who have come up into a remission and remained in orbit; and have not relapsed for at least five years. These are the long-term remissions. All of them haven't remained in complete remission indefinitely, but about ninety have stayed in remission from five to sixteen years.

"This is a new idea—that leukemia is curable, that if you blast the cells with large doses of drugs you might be able to cure the disease.

"In the past, you treated the patient as gently as you could. You tried to get him into remission and keep him there as long as possible. But it was a somewhat defeatist attitude. You figured that he was going to relapse eventually.

"A lot of people now believe that if you hit hard enough, a certain number of patients will go on for a long time—and, maybe, for ever.

"You can't use surgery for leukemia, and you can't use radiation except on localized lesions. This leaves chemotherapy, treatment by means of drugs. But, in addition, there is another big hope—utilizing the body's own chemotherapy, or immunotherapy.

"I think we are probably not going to be able to cure leuke-

[11] As of April, 1967.

mia with chemotherapy alone. I think we require a defense on the part of the host (the patient). It may be, as in Burkitt's tumor, *a natural defense possessed by the host*. Or it may be as in acute leukemia *a defense we have to stimulate* by giving the patient injections of BCG or injections of irradiated leukemic cells; or, as some people are doing, injecting the mother with the patient's irradiated leukemic cells, developing an antibody, or an antiserum, to the patient's own leukemic cells in the mother, then injecting the mother's serum or the mother's white cells back into the patient."

"Where is that technique being tried?"

"It's being done by a number of groups," Dr. Burchenal said. "We are doing it here, it's being done at Oak Ridge and at various other places; and I think it's a very important way of working. I don't believe that immunotherapy alone can ever be completely effective in leukemia if your patient is full of leukemic cells. On the other hand, if you destroy 999 out of every 1000 cells in the patient, then with immunotherapy you may be able to destroy that last cell, and your patient will remain in remission. This is much the same as the treatment of pneumococcus pneumonia with the sulfonamides. The sulfonamides never sterilized the lungs completely of all the bacteria, but they killed off most of them, and then the body defenses cleaned up the rest. That's what we would like to see in cancer chemotherapy.

"I think this is a great possibility. I think this is what is going to control a lot of tumors. And I think that leukemia and Burkitt's tumor are going to be the first tumors to be controlled in this way."

The prognosis is hopeful, therefore. The implications of Burkitt's tumor, the lessons learned from those African children, may be of vital importance to children in other parts of the world, to the little boy or the little girl in the house next door. We have a stalking horse for acute leukemia, for the lymphomas which are closely allied to leukemia; but we are still in the process of working out precisely how this fabulous animal should be put to work.

The story continues across the Atlantic Ocean. We go to Villejuif.

5

Today and Tomorrow

NINE

Villejuif—London—Boston

Villejuif

It is reached, by Citroën from the center of Paris, in about forty minutes: an assemblage of large somber old buildings, set off by walls and railings and iron gates from a narrow and rather grimy street. One enters the gate of the Hôpital Paul Brousse and begins to walk through endless galleries, like cloisters, bordering wide lawns, inquiring for the *Institut de Cancérologie et d'Immunogénétique*. But most of the people one encounters are patients, or the perturbed relatives of patients: they have never heard of this *Institut*, apparently, and they can only suggest that you proceed directly ahead and turn to the right or possibly to the left. Eventually you pass through a simple door set in a high wall; a sign points to the *Institut* which does not look at all institutional; and in due course you enter, first, the office of the Director's secretary, which is small and crowded, and then the Director's office, which is also small and crowded. Scientists throughout Europe speak of him with considerable respect, almost with awe, because he is doing some extraordinary work; and one expected him, perhaps, to occupy a larger, more imposing office. France, alas, can spare little money for what (in political circles) must be considered superficial trappings. "George Mathé's cancer center clings to survival on a scanty governmental allowance," a French editor wrote to me: "In 1967, the INSERM (*Institut National de la Santé et de la Recherche Médicale*) spent 12,086,000 francs (a little less than $2,500,000) on cancer research. This money was to maintain eight research teams, meet the wages of eighty-five scientists and technicians, and subsidize several independent laboratories. That is why Villejuif, as well as the Hôpital Broussais, has to appeal for private donations to continue with its cancer research program."

Professor Mathé is slender, dark, vigorous: a young man—only forty-five—in terms of what he has accomplished. To a large extent English is now accepted as the international language of medical science,[1] and Professor Mathé speaks it fluently, sometimes explosively.

Villejuif, which he described as "a cancer town in France"—that is, a town specializing in cancer as some other town might specialize in tuberculosis—is notable for three institutes. "One," Professor Mathé explained, at the start of our conversation, "is for basic research, mainly but not completely related to cancer; and this institute belongs to the *Centre National de la Recherche Scientifique* of the Ministry of Education. Then there is a clinical center for diagnosis and treatment of cancer patients, the *Institut Gustave Roussy*. Between the institutes for basic research and treatment is this institute, of which I am the Director, which is concerned with applied research—research *applied* to cancer. This institute is called (in translation) the Institute of Cancerology and Immunogenetics."

Professor Mathé showed me a schedule of the work being done in his institute. It was impressive, ranging from statistical studies, biochemistry, radiobiology, endocrinology, virology,

[1] It is commonly quipped among scientists that the international language of medical science is Broken English, rather as the international language of diplomacy is Fractured French.

genetics, immunology, immunogenetics, molecular biology, studies in carcinogenesis, and—under a separate heading—*Pratique Cancérologique*—the application of these cancerological studies in practice. In some respects the schedule was not dissimilar to those of other great national institutes; it became unique only when Professor Mathé enlarged on his personal concept of cancer research.

"I am Professor of Experimental Oncology,"[2] he said. "And for me experimental oncology is not only oncology on animals but oncology on animals *and* human beings who cannot be cured by conventional methods. I think when one discovers, or one establishes, some new method in animals one must go on to try it in man; and only the research worker who is thoroughly familiar with the method in animals can apply it to man. If the method doesn't work well in man you must return to animals to find out why you failed, so that you can correct what went wrong. You know, we are now able to cure forty per cent of cancer in man, if we include skin cancer and various other kinds of cancer; and all this progress has come from clinicians or applied research workers. None of this progress has come from basic research workers."

A similar remark had been made to me by an eminent epidemiologist in New York, and I quoted it to Professor Mathé: *"Millions and millions of dollars have been spent on basic research into the nucleic acids, and not a single cancer patient has been helped by any of this expenditure."*

Professor Mathé said, "I agree! I quite agree!"

"I'm not sure that I really agree," I said. "I only raise it because it's your point. But whether it is true or not, certainly there now seems to be a trend away from what is called exotic cancer research; more researchers seem to be turning directly to the problems of human cancer, and I have the impression that the work you are doing here is an example of that trend."

"Yes," Professor Mathé said: "Our aim is human cancer; but our approach is variable. We use animals, or we use humans.

[2] Oncology is defined as the study of, or the science dealing with, the physical and biological properties and features of malignant tumors. Here the term also includes the treatment of malignant tumors.

We have here about twenty thousand mice; we have ten thousand rats; we have guinea pigs, we have hamsters, we have rabbits, we have cats, we have sheep, we have pigs, we have monkeys; but we also have five patients."

"*Human* patients?"

"Yes. In aseptic rooms. They are there for investigation."

Aseptic rooms are carefully designed to guard against the entry of any kind of disease-causing organism. The patient, as far as possible, lives in a totally sterile environment. I asked, "Are these patients volunteers?"

"Yes," Professor Mathé replied. "We ask their permission. But in France, patients are very courageous and they readily give permission. It is, after all, for their benefit."

Professor Mathé went on to discuss some of the current thinking in immunology, and particularly the idea that after the leukemic patient has been brought into remission[3] his immune defenses might be stimulated in a number of different ways—by malaria, which can then be controlled by drugs, or by injections of the pulmonary tuberculosis vaccine BCG, or by injections of irradiated leukemic cells.

"We have done that here in cases of acute leukemia," Professor Mathé said.

"So I was told by Dr. Burchenal."

Professor Mathé reached for a pencil and a sheet of paper, and at great speed jotted down some essential figures. "We know that when a patient has a visible leukemia (the disease has reached the point where it is detectable in a clinical examination) he has 10^{12} leukemic cells.[4] First, therefore, we induce

[3] Remission is defined as a temporary abatement of the symptoms of a disease.

[4] This is mathematical shorthand for 1,000,000,000,000. Even for non-mathematical readers it is simple and foolproof. The index gives the number of zeros following 1. Thus, $10^1 = 10$; $10^2 = 100$; $10^3 = 1,000$, and so on. According to the numerical systems used by the United States and France, a billion is a thousand million (10^9) and a trillion is a million million (10^{12}). However, in the numerical systems used by Britain and Germany a billion is a million million (10^{12}) and a trillion is a million billion (10^{18}).

a remission with prednisone (a drug similar to cortisone), and we go from 10^{12} leukemic cells down to 10^8 (100,000,000). Then, when the patient is in remission, we try to reduce the number of leukemic cells still further, from 10^8 to 10^4 (10,000) by giving the patient a series of drugs in sequence. In our trial we had eight patients with this very low number of leukemic cells, and we 'randomized'[5] them in three groups. One group of three patients served as 'controls' and received nothing more. One group of three patients received BCG. The other two patients received vaccines of irradiated (killed) leukemic cells.

"The results clearly demonstrated the value of this form of therapy. The three patients who served as controls relapsed after fourteen weeks, ten weeks, and eleven weeks respectively.

"The patients treated with BCG have not relapsed yet, after twenty-six months, twenty months, and twelve months respectively.

"The patients vaccinated with irradiated leukemic cells have gone eighteen months in one case, and more than twelve months in the other case."

The experimental use of non-specific stimulation goes back more than forty years. It has been suggested that the cells of a cancer are able to proliferate because the immunological defenses against them are weak. Moreover, as the tumor mass expands, the efficacy of this defense becomes less and less. In other words, a rapidly growing tumor *overwhelms* the immunological defense mechanisms.

In 1924 a scientist named J. B. Murphy found that in tumors of laboratory rats and mice, the animals' immune systems could be stimulated by oleic acid (a colorless oily acid prepared from animal and vegetable fats and oils). When the tumors were then surgically removed there was *no recurrence* in 62

---

[5] This means arranging the individuals in a deliberately random manner, as a means of reducing errors in an experiment. The principle of randomization is considered to be fundamental in any experiments or trials involving a number of individuals, and it is vital that there should be an adequate number of "controls."

per cent of the animals tested. Zymosan, a carbohydrate obtained from the walls of yeast cells, was later found to give good results. Repeated injections of live cells of BCG, in the words of Professor Peter Alexander, are a most effective method of stimulating the immune response; and, besides BCG, Professor Mathé has reported that the bacillus that causes whooping cough and another, similar to the diphtheria bacillus, have been shown to be useful as "non-specific active immunotherapy agents in man."

"BCG," Professor Mathé explained, "acts as an adjuvant of the immune system: it *aids,* or *enhances,* the action of the immune system." As a vaccine against tuberculosis it is *specific,* just as a smallpox vaccine is specific against smallpox; but administered to patients suffering from acute leukemia it acts as a *non-specific* adjuvant, fortifying the immune defenses of the body generally and so, in a sense, encouraging them to move against the leukemic cells. The action is not at all powerful or dramatic. Professor Mathé has demonstrated that even when the immune defenses are stimulated by BCG the number of leukemic cells killed is no more than 10^3 (1,000) or 10^4 (10,000); but this may determine whether treatment is successful or not if the leukemic cell count has been brought down to a low level by other means. Permanent remission from the disease means that *every* leukemic cell be eradicated. One leukemic cell, by the simple process of doubling 41 times, will in 164 days arrive at the deadly total of 1,000,000,000,000. BCG could provide the means of killing this one cell.

Specific immunotherapy, in which the treatment is directed to stimulating the body's defenses *specifically* against the disease, consisted of injections of leukemic cells obtained from a pool of donors, all of whom were suffering from acute leukemia. Two of the patients received these injections. The pool of cells did not contain any leukemic cells taken from these two patients. Little discernible difference between specific and non-specific immunotherapy is shown in the final results: both forms worked as expected.

What happened in Professor Mathé's trials, therefore, was that the patients were put into remission with prednisone, which reduced the number of their leukemic cells from 10^{12} to 10^8. The central nervous system was treated by radiotherapy over a period of seven days, concurrently with prednisone therapy, since it is here that relapses frequently begin. The patients then received a series of drugs in sequence, and when this therapy was completed the leukemic cells had been reduced from 10^8 to about 10^4. Chemotherapy was then stopped; and immunotherapy reduced the number of leukemic cells still further. Five patients who completed this program have remained in remission for as long as 26 months.

"*Without any further chemotherapy,*" Professor Mathé said emphatically. "Many people working in this field have patients who have been in remission for several months, but those patients continue to receive maintenance chemotherapy. But our five patients are the first who have received no further chemotherapy, and whose treatment was continued by immunotherapy."

"The point is that intensive chemotherapy is toxic—poisonous—to the patient?"

"Yes," Professor Mathé said. "And it suppresses the immune defenses. To avoid this, we stop chemotherapy as soon as possible."

I said, "I have the impression that in this field for every plus there is only too often a minus. Is there a minus in your treatment?"

"Our problem is that we are not able to take all our patients from 10^{12} to 10^4 cells," Professor Mathé said. "In the trial we have just been discussing, we started with thirty-three patients and we arrived at 10^4 cells with only eight. The others had relapsed in the course of the chemotherapy, before they reached the point where they could receive immunotherapy." Professor Mathé then proceeded to explain why this occurred: "You may give a particular drug for two months. But the patient may become resistant to that drug, and he relapses. Now, the doubling time of this cancer is four days. If the patient has reached the point in his treatment where he is down to 10^8 leukemic cells, and then the drug does not work efficiently because he is resistant to it, in four days he will have twice that number of cells: 2×10^8." From 10^8 (100,000,000) to 10^{12} (1,000,000,000,000) takes only sixty days.

The treatment carried out by Professor Mathé can be termed "heroic": that is, it consists of extreme measures, taken in grave circumstances, to save life. The extreme measures are justifiable because of the nature of the disease. Acute leukemia is considered, to all intents and purposes, incurable. It is a generalized condition: it does not manifest itself, like so many cancers, as a tumor at a particular place or in a particular organ. The tissues in which the cancer occurs are distributed throughout the entire body, and in the present state of our knowledge we cannot catch it early and thereby eliminate it—like other cancers—before it becomes invasive: it is already widely invasive at the time it is first seen in the patient.

Some idea of the severity of the measures taken by Professor Mathé can be gained from his schedule of chemotherapy.[6] Remission is initiated by treatment with prednisone and X-radiation of the central nervous system. The drugs are then given in the following order:

2-month course of methotrexate;
   a course of prednisone for 1 month;
2-month course of 6-mercaptopurine;
   a course of prednisone for 1 month;
2-month course of vincristine;
   a course of prednisone for 1 month;
2-month course of cyclophosphamide;
   a course of prednisone for 1 month;
2-month course of vinleurosine;
   a course of prednisone for 1 month;

[6] This schedule is taken from: The Preliminary Results of the Treatment of Acute Lymphoblastic Leukemia During Remission by Sequential Chemotherapy and Radiation of the Central Nervous System Followed by Active Immunotherapy. [1] Results of Sequential Chemotherapy and Irradiation of the Central Nervous System. By G. Mathé, J. L. Amiel, L. Schwarzenberg, M. Schneider, A. Cattan, J. R. Schlumberger. Institut de Cancérologie et d'Immunogénétique, Hôpital Paul Brousse, Villejuif; Service d'Hématologie de l'Institut Gustav Roussy, Villejuif; and Groupe européen de Chimiothérapie anticancereuse. 1968.

2-month course of methyl-glyoxal-bis (gyanylhydrazone);
  a course of prednisone for 1 month;
2-month course of vinblastine;
  a course of prednisone for 1 month;
2-month course of E39.

This sequence[7] included all the chemotherapeutic drugs that were known *at the time the trial began* (1963) to be active against proliferating lymphoblastic cells (the malignant cells in acute lymphocytic leukemia).

One recalls Dr. Burchenal's remark: *If a hundred acute leukemia patients received the same intensive treatment and eighteen survived for a long period of time, it would be very exciting.* The program at Villejuif resulted in lengthy survival for five out of thirty-three who entered the program at the outset, and this can be projected to read fifteen out of a hundred, which is impressive indeed. Intensive chemotherapy alone was shown to be inadequate, for the three patients who served as controls and who received no immunotherapy, relapsed within ten to fourteen weeks after chemotherapy was stopped—precisely the expected period required for the leukemic cells to double enough times to re-establish the disease fully. It was only by the additional destruction of leukemic cells by immunotherapy, small as this was, that the other five patients were brought into the safety zone. Of these patients who were treated by non-specific or specific immunotherapy, Professor Mathé reported, "They have a completely different pattern of evolution of their disease. They are still in remission twelve to twenty-six months after stopping chemotherapy and their total survival time is at present between twenty and sixty-four months."

Since cancerous cells in the later stages of any given form of the disease usually divide rapidly, they are obvious targets for antimitotic, antigrowth drugs. Unfortunately, antimitotic drugs on the whole are not particularly selective and they will attack rapidly dividing healthy cells, such as cells of the

---

[7] Virtually all of these drugs are highly toxic. The schedule is given here to illustrate the exceedingly severe nature of Professor Mathé's method of treatment.

lining of the intestine and the mouth, hair follicles, the cells of the testes in men and the ovaries in women. Most damaging is their effect upon the rapidly dividing cells of the bone marrow, which results in a depression of the body's defense mechanisms and thus reduces the ability of the body to act against infectious agents and probably, to some extent, against cancer cells. It is part of the curious plus and minus pattern that runs through everything relating to cancer that, at the present time, the more potent a drug is against tumor cells the more toxic it is likely to be to the patient. The results of intensive chemotherapy, carried on relentlessly for many months, must therefore include gastrointestinal disturbances, loss of hair, skin lesions, the constant risk of infections and hemorrhages; and one can readily understand why patients who have undergone this treatment, and who have survived, need to be maintained in aseptic rooms, secure from any possibility of bacterial infection.

Other techniques have been exploited by Professor Mathé to improve the leukemic patient's immunological response. One is the transplantation of bone marrow which (when it is successful) has a long term effect, compared to the relatively short term effect of white cell transfusions. The bone marrow is obtained from healthy donors by means of bone punctures made (under a general anesthetic) in sixty to a hundred sites in each donor. Then, in the form of an emulsion, it is given intravenously to the patient and travels spontaneously to the bones, repopulating the blood and bone marrow with healthy white cells which can participate in the task of controlling the leukemia. The antileukemic effect has proven to be remarkable; but once again a minus intervenes to counterbalance the plus, and the clearance of leukemic cells is accompanied by a severe and highly dangerous complication.

"You know that when we graft a kidney," Professor Mathé explained, "there is a reaction on the part of the host—the patient—*against* the kidney. (The body recognizes the graft as foreign, and attempts to reject it.) The same reaction occurs when we graft a heart: the host reacts against the foreign heart. In these cases there is no reaction by the heart or the kidney against the host. What occurs in a bone marrow transplant is that there is not only the expected reaction of the host against the bone marrow graft but also *a reaction of the graft against the host.* This results in what we call secondary disease, or secondary syndrome. It is extremely serious, and we are not yet able to control it completely."

Yet another aspect of Professor Mathé's leukemia research is concerned with leukemia viruses.

Certain viruses have long been known to cause leukemia in animals. Here the classic postulates of Robert Koch can easily be fulfilled: (1) The microorganism is shown to be present in every case of the disease; (2) the microorganism can be isolated and grown in pure culture; (3) inoculated into susceptible animals it causes the same disease; (4) the microorganism can be isolated from the infected animal, and grown again in pure culture. In the textbook phrase, *The agent under study is thus proved to be the cause of the disease which is being studied.*

In the laboratory, the process consists of injecting mice with a filtrate[8] containing the appropriate virus. Within a few days there will be an enlargement of the spleen; then, in two or three weeks, leukemia will appear.

The spleens of the leukemic mice are removed, cut up and prepared as a cell-free filtrate, and inoculated into another group of mice. In the same period of time these mice will develop identical symptoms—enlargement of the spleen followed by leukemia.

Since no leukemic cells were transplanted from the first group of mice to the second group, the leukemia is demonstrably induced in the second group of mice by virus in the cell-free filtrate.

If we assume, though, that certain forms of leukemia in human beings are caused by viruses, we are faced with a peculiar

---

[8] The filtrate is termed "cell-free." It has been passed through exceedingly fine filters which hold back any mammalian cells (or other cells of this size.)

problem: how can we *prove* that viruses cause the disease, and how can the infective process be studied? For, clearly, Koch's postulates cannot here be met. Leukemia is essentially a fatal disease; and we cannot inject viruses suspected of causing leukemia into disease-free human beings in order to see what happens (although at least one scientist is alleged to have tried the experiment on himself, with negative results). Nor can human leukemia be cultivated in laboratory animals.

The answer found by Professor Mathé is blunt and simple: the species must be transformed.

To establish the method and to show that it is viable, a first step is taken: rats are transformed into mice.

This is accomplished by bone marrow transplants. The rats receive grafts of bone marrow from mice. Those rats which survive will then themselves begin to produce mouse bone marrow. Proof that this occurs is revealed by examination of the chromosomes: the bone marrow cells manufactured by the rat following the transplant will have mouse chromosomes, which are different in number and aspect from rat chromosomes. These animals are referred to as rat-mouse heterochimeras.[9]

The next step is to inject mouse leukemia virus, which is species specific—causing leukemia only in mice. A number of the transformed *rats* will then proceed to develop *mouse* leukemia.

"Now," Professor Mathé told me, "we are trying to transform monkeys into human beings—at least, as far as their bone marrow is concerned."

"How do you do that?"

"In the same way: by bone marrow grafts."

"Will monkeys accept human bone marrow?"

"We do everything we can to make it take. But so far we have only been able to keep the monkeys alive for 40 days, and that is not enough. We need two years."

He gave the impression that the necessary technique would

[9] In ancient mythology the chimera was a female monster represented as having a lion's head, a goat's body, a dragon's tail, and a goat's head rising from its back. Biologically, a chimera is defined as an organism having tissue characteristics of two or more types, especially a hybrid produced by grafting. Heterochimeras are hybrids made up of different species—as in this case, rats and mice.

inevitably be found, and he would then have an experimental tool of enormous potential value. "There are some leukemic patients who are very, very rich in virus particles," he said, "and one must work on these patients and learn more about these particles." Are the particles actually viruses that play a part in causing leukemia? Are they merely passengers, which thrive in the leukemic environment? We cannot experiment on human patients, but it is permissible to experiment on transformed monkeys, monkeys with human chromosomes—a concept that takes us back to H. G. Wells at the beginning of the century, and *The Island of Dr. Moreau.*

George Mathé is one of the geniuses of present-day cancer research. He is restless, impatient with delay, anxious to see results. I said to him during our talk, "What strikes me is that you move faster from the laboratory animal to the human being than, say, your American counterpart." He replied, "Yes. That is our aim. We want to move fast. And we want the same doctor who treats mice to treat human beings, because if you have different people working on mice and human beings you lose a lot of time, *a lot of time.* Our people work on mice, on monkeys, on human beings. They must be able to work on *any* animal, studying the same problem."

What emerges, among other things, is the terrible recalcitrance of acute leukemia: its resistance to the most extreme, the most heroic measures. The observer cannot help recalling almost with envy the comparative ease with which Burkitt's lymphoma responds to a handful of pills or a single injection. George Mathé, assaulting a more heavily fortified position, may yet have the same good fortune.

London

We have seen that one (and only one) of the problems of treating acute leukemia is that the patient will frequently respond in a most encouraging manner to a particular drug, and will then—possibly within a few weeks, or less—fail to sustain this response. It has been suggested that what occurs is a form of natural selection. Some of the leukemic cells are unaffected by the drug being used, and these quickly take over the leadership of the entire leukemic process, multiplying with the fearful rapidity characteristic of acute leukemia. In a short period of time a leukemic cell population comes into being which is almost totally resistant to that drug and can flourish without any restraint, and the patient relapses. The physician then proceeds to employ another drug, aware that the same sequence of remission and relapse will almost inevitably be repeated and, indeed, in the present state of leukemia therapy *must* be repeated. But although the ultimate outcome is nearly always tragic, the patient's life can be significantly extended, as Mathé and a host of other scientists have shown, by treatment with a variety of antileukemic drugs, drugs which have different properties and act in different ways and thus circumvent the deadly phenomenon of cellular resistance. What the physician requires is an arsenal of drugs, providing him with the widest possible range of choice.[10]

In 1963, a limited number of drugs were available to Professor Mathé (and other scientists treating acute leukemia). It comes as something of a shock to learn that in 1968 the situation was substantially the same. Although some promising new drugs have appeared, it is probably true to say that only

[10] The subject being considered here is chemotherapy, but there are other factors of great importance in the treatment of leukemia. Dr. C. Gordon Zubrod, of the National Cancer Institute, has listed three obstacles which must be overcome if we are to achieve complete control of the disease: the first obstacle is the lack of a method to detect the presence of the last few thousand leukemic cells following therapy; the second is the serious danger of infection, often leading to death; the third is the fact that modern therapy can today be carried out in only a few special centers. "The modern management of leukemia is complex, difficult and potentially dangerous," Dr. Zubrod said in a speech given in September, 1967: "Even when money is abundant, and physical and other resources adequate, and even when full knowledge, and enthusiasm and autonomy are present, it takes from five to ten years to build the total medical team and give them what they need to treat leukemia optimally."

one of them is of outstanding significance—L-asparaginase, which is still undergoing tests and is exceedingly scarce.

Criticism of established programs is healthy, necessary, and (in this era of dissent) unavoidable. Science, more than any other human activity, is dependent upon ceaseless self-questioning, and we are dealing with a branch of scientific inquiry that directly affects many lives. In the years between 1963 and 1968, some seventy thousand men, women and children died of leukemia *in the United States alone.* For the world at large that figure can be multiplied by ten. It is not surprising, therefore, that many scientists have expressed concern about the present position of cancer chemotherapy. Foremost, they say, is the need for new drugs and new concepts of what drugs should do. One of the leading authorities on choriocarcinoma, Dr. K. D. Bagshawe, told me in London, "I don't think we can carry our success rate very much higher with the agents we have at present. I think we really must have new chemotherapeutic agents or we must have some very different approach. . . . All generalizations are likely to come unstuck, but I think the pointers at the moment are that chemotherapy is useful but that it is likely to prove of limited use in its present form. It has had some success in prolonging life; and in a couple of tumors (Burkitt's lymphoma and choriocarcinoma) it is producing what are certainly cures, with a substantial number of patients who have gone on now for ten years, free of disease. Unless there is some major alteration in the type of chemotherapeutic agents available, I don't think we can expect very much more from them. . . . Perhaps as we learn more about immunological methods and start to apply these, we may find that we have to bring both immunological and chemotherapeutic agents into use together in order to achieve more success than can be achieved by either of them alone; but this will not be easy, because they oppose each other's action to some extent—at least, the chemotherapeutic action is likely to oppose the immunological action by depressing the immune response."

Dr. J. A. Stock, of the Chester Beatty Research Institute, in a lengthy survey entitled "The Chemotherapy of Cancer,"[11] eloquently describes some of the factors inherent in the problem: ". . . The fault may lie largely in our concept of drug design. We were early encouraged by the huge success of chemotherapy in bacterial disease, but we have not properly shaken ourselves free of the ideas which engendered it. This is partly because experimental cancer chemotherapy has in some ways been too easy; we have been able to make, by the score, compounds which (aided to an unknown extent by host defense mechanisms) inhibit various experimental tumors, and this pursuit has tended to become an end in itself. The performance of the agents in the clinic has, however, often disappointed us. Why the disappointment? Why should we expect these compounds to be specific in human cancer? . . . We must not expect the cancer cell to cooperate in quite the open-handed way the microorganisms have done, giving us gross metabolic differences to exploit. We shall have to find, as it were, an extra dimension of specificity."

Other scientists, notably T. A. Connors and F. J. C. Roe, have argued with great force that our current approach to cancer chemotherapy may be based on obsolete and false concepts of what should be expected of anticancer drugs, and furthermore, that the screening program and the drug development program of the Cancer Chemotherapy National Service Center of the U. S. Public Health Service are inadequate and based upon the wrong criteria. The concluding chapter of *The Biology of Cancer,* contributed by the editors, F. J. C. Roe and E. J. Ambrose, states: ". . . Very large programs of work (in cancer chemotherapy) have been undertaken in the absence of a sound biological basis, and even on a complete misconception of the probable biological nature of the disease. In the first place, cancer has been regarded as though it were a type of micro-biological infection—the cancer cells acting as parasites in the host. This approach entails the tacit assumption that the cancer cells are different from the host cells in a *constant and potentially exploitable way.* In the second place,

[11] *The Biology of Cancer,* D. Van Nostrand Company Ltd., London, 1966.

it has been assumed that the special attribute of cancer cells is their rapid rate of multiplication. . . . All the biological screening tests for cancer chemotherapeutic activity are, in effect, screens for antigrowth or antimitotic activity. It is not surprising, therefore, that most of the drugs so far available tend to be most effective against rapidly growing tumors and to have the drawback that they damage those tissues in the body which are normally the most mitotically active. In fact, the cell generation times in many cancers are longer than those in the gut mucosa or bone marrow. In such cases, cytotoxic drugs may damage those tissues more than the cancer."

It is only fair to point out that critics of any aspect of cancer research inevitably enjoy the benefits of hindsight. Cancer has proven to be a problem of such unexpected proportions that nobody could possibly have anticipated a fraction of the roadblocks that still impede our progress; and nobody, twenty-five years ago, could have laid down a research program that would be viable, fully productive, and totally critic-proof today.

Changes were, in fact, made in the chemotherapy screening program procedures in 1965; but here we encounter another difficulty—anticancer drugs are not produced overnight. According to the National Cancer Institute,[12] "A review of drug testing in the national program disclosed that an average four-year gap intervened between the time a test material was acquired for screening until (if found active) it entered clinical trial. The time required for determining its clinical effectiveness (or lack of it) was at least several years. Thus a seven- to ten-year interval was estimated as the average time between a material's acceptance for screening and knowledge of its clinical effectiveness."

In terms of the lives at stake an interval of seven to ten years seems inordinately long, and this statement seems to supply ammunition for the critics. However, steps have been taken "to advise the National Cancer Institute on criteria

[12] *Special Report: Cancer Chemotherapy Program.* February, 1966. Public Health Service, U. S. Department of Health, Education, and Welfare.

for advancing the most promising (anticancer) materials more rapidly from the screen into the clinics and to undertake definitive clinical trials."

An eminent cancer scientist (his name is omitted here for obvious reasons, but it is to be found in nearly every modern history of medicine) said to me in a London office, fully aware that his words were being recorded on a tape recorder, "There is too much money in cancer research and not enough brains. Consequently, with all this money available, you have the administrators floating up to the top, and they administer cancer research in such a way that it is good for administration but not really good for research into cancer. Empires are built; and this is the curse of cancer research today . . . There's an idea that if you pump millions of dollars into research, you will get millions of dollars' worth of results; but it doesn't work like that. It's rather like going to the Director of a college of music and saying, Here are twenty-five million dollars (or pounds) a year for the next fifteen years: find us another Beethoven. You can't do it. . . . Several scientists have even gone so far as to propose that we abandon cancer research as a thing in itself. Abandon the big cancer institutes. They were a mistake. The work should be done in the universities, where the material pressures aren't so intense."

On the subject of chemotherapy, this scientist expressed himself even more forcibly: "Chemotherapy? I'm afraid I'm a little heretical on this matter, and I share the heresy with innumerable other cancer research workers. Chemotherapy is an absolute farce. At one time the Americans were testing (or screening, as they called it) thirty thousand compounds a year. How on earth can you really *test* thirty thousand compounds a year against a disease that's as complex and variable as cancer? Many cancer people call the screening program nothing more than a lucky dip. It's a shameful waste of money and time, and quite the wrong attitude to cancer research."

Since the days of the Pharaohs, administrators have been bitterly assailed by non-administrators, not merely as empire builders but as quenchers of man's dreams, his creative spirit, and his immortal soul. But no matter how much one has suffered at their hands one cannot really condemn them *en masse;* one has to concede, grudgingly perhaps, that there may be good administrators as well as bad administrators; wise and capable administrators as well as brutal, insensitive administrators. And a case can be made for the view that in any kind of medical research it serves the administrator's interests to encourage his research people in every possible way, for it has been shown time and time again that an institution doing indifferent work is likely to be treated with indifference by the public (which, after all, supplies the funds to support administrators and researchers alike), while an institution that is lively and productive will attract public support as honeysuckle attracts bees.

The vehement condemnation of the chemotherapy program by this anonymous scientist was one of the themes in a conversation with Dr. Francis J. C. Roe[13] at the Chester Beatty Research Institute. The question was put to him in very broad terms—more accurately, within the framework of a series of questions: Any person reading a book (such as this one) dealing in general with cancer, may ask, *Suppose I develop this disease, what can be done for me? What can I expect from surgery, from radiotherapy, from chemotherapy? And what are the prospects for the immediate future? Can I look for new developments in, say, surgery and radiotherapy, or have the surgeons and the radiologists reached the apex of their skills?*

[13] Francis J. C. Roe is coeditor with E. J. Ambrose of *The Biology of Cancer* (D. Van Nostrand Company, Ltd., London, 1966), and with Ronald W. Raven of *The Prevention of Cancer* (Butterworth & Co., London, 1967). Dr. Roe is the Head of the Department of Experimental Pathology at the Chester Beatty Research Institute (which itself is a part of the Institute of Cancer Research of the University of London), and an Associate Pathologist of the Royal Marsden Hospital. He told me that he is greatly worried by the present organization of cancer research, and spends much energy in trying to influence the present organization of the subject. He feels he is able to do this to some extent through his membership of a number of committees and through his editorial work for various journals.

"I think," Dr. Roe said, "it is certainly true that we have advanced very close to the ultimate in radiotherapy. The limitation here is destruction of normal tissue. What the radiotherapist is trying to do, of course, is destroy 100 per cent of cancer cells, with the least possible destruction of normal cells. One can reach the point of 99 per cent kill of cancer cells, and still fail to achieve a complete cure. To achieve 99.9 per cent kill of cancer cells the radiation dose might have to be increased tenfold, and yet still fall short of being completely curative while causing greatly increased destruction of cells.

"Even if you increase the radiation dose *again* tenfold, which will mean very considerable destruction of healthy tissue, you still may not bridge that tiny but all-important gap between 99.9 per cent destruction of cancer cells and 100 per cent—the destruction of all the cancer cells—no matter what fancy way is dreamed up of delivering the rays to the affected area. So there seems to be an absolute limitation here, and I very much hope we will in our lifetime see the day when radiotherapy is no longer used, when other methods take its place, because one just doesn't like to destroy normal cells in this way.

"In surgery I think the horizons are perhaps a little brighter than they were five or ten years ago. At that time it seemed that we were close to the ultimate, but we have new techniques in anesthesia and in hypothermia (the technique of lowering the body temperature below 98.6°F) which have made possible more radical surgery. Transplantation surgery hasn't yet come into its own in the treatment of cancer; whether it ever will is difficult to say, but the people who are engaged in it seem very hopeful. Substitution surgery, involving the replacement of cancerous organs by artificially-made parts, has perhaps a greater future than transplantation surgery. This remains to be seen. In any event, I believe surgery will continue to edge forward."

"Isn't there a tendency to say, We must try to avoid surgery at all costs, and if possible eliminate it?"

Dr. Roe said, "I believe it would be much healthier to eliminate radiotherapy."

"What about radiotherapy in conjunction with chemotherapy?"

"That seems to me just gimmicky. There is no real evidence that it provides any great advantage. And chemotherapy is at present, I think, the most blunt tool we have for treating cancer, though it certainly offers the brightest hopes for the future."

"In what sense is chemotherapy a blunt tool?"

"The surgeon can *focus* on the tumor, so to speak, with his knife. The radiotherapist uses special mechanical means to focus on the tumor. The difficulty with chemotherapy is that it cannot be focused in this way. You can only focus it if you have a chemical agent which will home in (or zero in) on the cancer cells, and it yet remains to be demonstrated that this is feasible. In certain experimental situations, where there is a definite, distinct, constant difference between tumor cells (particularly in transplanted tumors where nearly all the tumor cells have a known defect, or some characteristic that distinguishes them from normal cells) it is possible to dream up a chemical substance which will home in—focus—on tumor cells."

"Doesn't something of that kind happen in choriocarcinoma and Burkitt's lymphoma?"

"Those are special forms of cancer. At the present time I think there is no reason to hope it can occur with the common types of cancer, say of the stomach or of the lung. The problem there," Dr. Roe said, "is that these tumors seem to be very like the host who bears them. There is very little difference between the normal host cells and the tumor cells; and very little margin in relation to the design of chemical agents which will *selectively* attack the tumor cells and avoid the normal host cells.

"Not only that: if you look under the microscope at these tumors, different parts of the same tumor look different; they behave differently; and many of the cells may have different numbers of chromosomes. So there is every reason to think that they would respond in a different manner to a given chemical agent. Furthermore, these tumors are changing all the time, throwing off new types; they are very unstable; and we are a long, long way from finding chemical agents which at any one time can kill off all the cancerous cells in a mixed population of cells."

"Isn't there always a possibility of finding such chemical agents by screening a very wide range of materials?"

"I would have thought this process had a very poor hope of success," Dr. Roe replied. "It has produced very little, and the cost has been tremendously high."

We had been discussing earlier the good fortune that seems to pursue certain scientists, a phenomenon that Dr. Michael B. Shimkin describes as serendipitous. Dr. Roe suggested that this might bear upon the cancer chemotherapy screening program in a somewhat *negative* way. He said, "Much of the work that has been done up to now has been farmed out in the United States to contract research organizations. Now, these are geared to avoid serendipity, which essentially depends on having a highly competent observer present who is able to make an observation, who can evaluate what he has observed, and who has the judgment to choose to follow up that observation. It is the exercise of choice that is so important. . . . If research is routinized, as has been done in the screening program, and conducted at the level of the average technician, the technician is not likely to do anything more than the minimum, and certainly not more than he can fit into a working day. The result is that anything which departs from the normal pattern of negative or positive is a nuisance to him, and he tries to lose it in the system—and usually succeeds in doing so. This is perhaps the biggest tragedy of the screening program: we have no way of knowing, of being certain, that the enormous number of substances which have gone through routine screening are really of no use in cancer therapy. We cannot be sure that, used properly, some of them might not be of the greatest value. And what makes it doubly unfortunate is that there is little chance funds will ever again be made available to examine all these materials in a more scientific manner."

"You believe, in other words, it is impossible to test half a million different materials by routine laboratory methods?"

"Such a large number couldn't be tested adequately," Dr. Roe said. "The cancer chemotherapy screening program may or may not have been justified at the time of its inception (1955). But it is my belief that the fact that so little has come out of the program after so many years should lead one to suspect that the question being asked was incorrectly phrased."

"You think, statistically, more should have been found by now, thirteen years later?"

"Yes. If the problem, as it was originally conceived, had been rightly stated, then more should have come out of the program because of the amount of work that has been done. And *if* so little has come out of the program, then we must have started with an incorrect idea of what that problem was —and we are persisting with that incorrect idea. I thought the problem was wrongly phrased in the first place; and that, I now think, is quite certain."

The conversation then turned to so-called natural remedies and the substances synthesized in the laboratories. "Throughout the world," states the report issued by the World Health Organization, *The Chemotherapy of Cancer,* "there are folk remedies in use against cancers, ulcers, and slow-healing sores. Many of these are extracts prepared from identifiable plants, and many have now been tested under controlled experimental conditions to discover whether they possess any general or specific antitumor activity." Considerable success has been obtained with drugs called vincaleukoblastine (vinblastine) and leurocristine, derived from the humble little periwinkle (and other drugs derived from this plant have now come into use). Colchicine, derived from meadow saffron (autumn crocus) and a synthetic derivative called demecolcine or colchamine have been found effective: colchamine ointment (the report states) can bring about a cure of skin cancer in the early stages. Yet another drug considered to be useful is podophyllotoxin, obtained from the May apple, which is also known as vegetable calomel, American mandrake, umbrella plant, or duck's foot.

Periwinkle, it appears, has been in use for centuries in India as a cancer cure. Western scientists learned of it, proceeded to test it and found it to be effective in the treatment of lymphomas, including Hodgkin's disease, and leukemia (periwinkle derivatives are among the drugs used by Professor Mathé, for example). "But this is not, strictly speaking, *screening*," Dr. Roe pointed out, "because the scientists started out with a lead, suggesting that the substance had some sort of curative effect." In other words, if the scientists had not heard of Indians using preparations of this insignificant trailing herb with its blue and white flowers, there is little likelihood that they would have discovered it for themselves. A similar lead from India gave us rauwolfia, a genus of dogbane (literally, *dog poison*), from which our first tranquilizers were fashioned. And it was a lead from an old, old woman (who might have come out of *Hansel and Gretel*, except that she lived in a Shropshire cottage) that led William Withering, M.D., of Birmingham, England, to make use of a brew of the leaves of the foxglove for the treatment of dropsy, resulting in a drug which has been of immeasurable benefit all over the world in the treatment of heart disease: digitalis. (For the record, the common foxglove, *Digitalis purpurea*, is considered to be one of the poisonous plants, and it is known variously as fox-and-leaves, fox docken, fairy finger, fingerflower, and fairy bell.)

A curious state of affairs. Why, for some of our most effective drugs, must we go back to the Dark Ages, to old herb women, to tribal medicine men, to gibbering witch doctors? Dr. Roe, on the spur of the moment, proposed that these people, having no other resources, can only make use of natural products —substances, for the most part, obtained from plants. And it is from plants that we still derive some of the most active materials used in our pharmacology.[14] It can be argued, there-

[14] Such substances are present in plants *because* they are pharmacologically active, having evolved (Dr. Roe suggested) as cogs in the

fore, that the medicine man or the witch doctor has available to him a great range of materials of considerable pharmacological potency; some of these *might* be of interest in cancer (and, of course, have actually proven to be valuable) and a great many would certainly be of general medical interest.

"By comparison," Dr. Roe said, "our present source of drugs is the synthetic chemical laboratory where chemists and technicians go through all the possibilities in the book of fitting together carbon, hydrogen and oxygen atoms. Perhaps in the first instance they produce a variety of compounds; these are then fed into a number of biological test systems; and if things go well, something positive may come up. Everything else is then dropped, and the chemists produce a series of closely related chemical compounds, or analogues. The further they move away from the broader forms of research, the more they concentrate on following one line of chemical products, the less likely they are to find something which has high pharmacological value. Over billions of years, nature has screened the limitless possibilities of organic chemical structures and selected a relatively small number because of their pharmacological activity. Thus the witch doctor who goes out into the jungle collecting a great variety of plants and roots is more likely to come up with substances of pharmacological interest than the synthetic chemist." Dr. Roe paused, and added, "This is a little jocular. But underneath it there's something really very serious."

Serious enough, indeed, to demand consideration from another viewpoint.

---

ecology of nature. One way or another they are of survival value to the plant species—killing or driving off natural enemies or providing an unusual source of energy.

Boston

Not long after these interviews in London I visited Boston (Mass.) to talk to Dr. Sidney Farber. Dr. Farber is one of the most eminent cancer scientists in the United States and, for that matter, in the world. He belongs to a legendary group of American cancer workers who inaugurated a marvelous age of research and discovery—Peyton Rous, Richard E. Shope, Charles B. Huggins, Cornelius P. Rhoads. He is Professor of Pathology at Harvard Medical School, Chief of the staff of the Children's Hospital in Boston, and was recently named President-Elect of the American Cancer Society.

As long ago as 1948 he had published a paper entitled *Temporary Remissions in Acute Leukemia in Children Produced by Folic Acid Antagonist, 4-aminopteroylglutamic acid (Aminopterin)*,[15] a classic of cancer literature, for it provided some of our earliest evidence that chemotherapy could be beneficial in the treatment of human leukemia.

Dr. Farber and his group at Children's Hospital had for some time been investigating dietary factors in cancer, and they had observed that folic acid—one of the Vitamin B_2 complex—improved the health of children suffering from acute lymphatic leukemia, but the improvement was of short duration for the folic acid appeared to increase the rate at which the leukemia developed. Dr. Farber then decided to make use of substances which very closely resembled folic acid but which were, in effect, counterfeit, with the result that rapidly-dividing leukemic cells taking up the counterfeit folic acid (or, in scientific terminology, folic acid antagonists) were unable to carry out certain vital metabolic functions and were

---

[15] The paper appeared in the *New England Journal of Medicine*, No. 238. Dr. Farber's co-authors were L. K. Diamond, R. D. Mercer, R. F. Sylvester, Jr., and J. A. Wolff.

thus killed. First results with antifolic drugs were so spectacular that many people were convinced that the ultimate cure for acute leukemia was imminent. Unfortunately, as the title of Dr. Farber's paper indicated, the remissions were temporary, and patients developed resistance to the drug only too quickly. Nevertheless, aminopterin has been of profound importance not only for the practical benefits it brought, but for the observation, the reasoning, the philosophy that originally led to its introduction. It subsequently underwent minor chemical changes; the later form is called amethopterin (better known as methotrexate), considered by many authorities to be the best antifolic drug available at present, and one of the most widely used drugs in cancer chemotherapy. In recent years Dr. Farber has made extensive use of actinomycin D, an antibiotic of natural origin, in combination with X-ray therapy for the treatment of several forms of cancer, particularly Wilms' tumor, a kidney tumor of children.

We spoke first about new directions in cancer research. Was a change of direction, in fact, necessary? Should there be greater emphasis on the more common tumors of man, rather than on what are referred to as the more exotic forms? Different scientists had given me different answers: some were enthusiastically in favor of a total pragmatic approach, others felt that any attempt to impose direction on cancer scientists might prove to be disastrous. Dr. Farber said, "This question of the choice of direction in cancer is something that can be talked about endlessly, with different answers coming up at every discussion by the same group of people. The answer is that to begin with one follows ideas where they lead; or one takes a problem that is forced into one's hands, as in the case of Burkitt's lymphoma. Once Burkitt made his observation, the problem just had to be worked on. And, despite the fact that it is a so-called exotic tumor, it attracted the interest of many scientists.

"Or, you may have a new anticancer agent such as actinomycin D, and find (at the time, in 1954) that it is the most powerful anticancer agent by weight, when used against mouse cancer systems. You then must go to man; and you cannot say, *I will choose an exotic tumor,* or, *I will choose a common tumor.* You take this new material to man, when you know you can do it safely, and try to give assistance to people who will die because you have nothing else to offer. In the course of such a trial—before you have any idea of the agent's mechanism of action, or the kind of tumor in man that it might affect, since we have no good predicting system now —you might find that cancer of the breast will not respond, nor will other common cancers, of the lung, of the intestinal tract, the prostate, the uterus, and so on. And then, after a series of failures, you find that a tumor which is not common, the Wilms' tumor of the kidney in children, will respond almost selectively.

"No predicting system could have led us to that; and it occurred—not on a hit or miss, or trial and error basis—but as a product of the total care of the patient suffering from cancer.

"First, you do everything that can be done with methods of treatment of proven value. Then, finally, when you have nothing more of proven value that can help that patient, you must try something that has not yet been proven, if the new treatment is not worse than the untreated disease. And, in doing so, you uncover leads. It requires the study of each individual patient in depth, in accordance with an experimental design you work out with great care that (first, I repeat) will not harm the patient, and (second) might give you the greatest amount of information about what that chemical will do to a patient.

"That is how we discovered the action of actinomycin D on pulmonary metastases[16] in a Wilms' tumor, although the mechanism of action was not known for seven years afterward. But if we had not been alert to the changes (which could have been missed in a cursory going-over) in a child who was dying of multiple metastases of Wilms' tumor, to whom we had given actinomycin D less than three weeks before, we might have missed it. *One child gave us the whole clue.* One child, *carefully* studied."

[16] Secondary tumors in the lungs. Multiple metastases means widespread secondary tumors.

I asked Dr. Farber, "What led you to give actinomycin D to that child?"

"There were two reasons," Dr. Farber answered.

The first was the outcome of a policy decision he had made very much earlier, in 1946. It was then known from experience that certain tumors, whose life history and biological behavior had been established, would respond in a statistically predictable manner to treatment.

Thus, in the case of Wilms' tumor it was known that surgery and local irradiation of the kidney bed—as performed in the best of clinics—would save 40 per cent of children suffering from the disease, while 60 per cent would die. "You could not tell on Day 1, when you operated," Dr. Farber said, "whether the child would be one of the 40 per cent, or one of the 60 per cent. But if the child were given a chemical (which had been carefully studied in animal tumor systems and for toxicity), and we continued the use of that chemical even in the absence of proof of cancer elsewhere in the body, we could tell within two years whether we were making any headway by using that particular chemical against that particular tumor, *because we could compare the results against that 40 per cent base line, which we had never exceeded.*

"Beginning January 1, 1947, as a policy decision, every child with Wilms' tumor received not only surgery and radiotherapy locally but, in addition, the best chemical we had available at the time which could destroy cancer of any kind. The drug might have been nitrogen mustard, it might have been methotrexate, and so on. From 1947 until 1954, every single child who came to us with Wilms' tumor received this treatment; but we still did not change the 40 per cent survival figure. Until, in 1954, we used actinomycin D."

The second reason, Dr. Farber explained, was this: The percentage of cures that can be expected statistically, following surgery and X-ray treatment, is known for many kinds of cancer. Some of the percentages are fairly high—as in the case of skin cancer—so that the statistical chances of recovery for a patient are good. Some of the percentages, though, are small

—5 per cent for lung or stomach cancer, an over-all rate of 30 per cent for cancer of the breast.

"Now, what are you going to do for those patients who have failed to respond to surgery and X-ray?" Dr. Farber asked. "Well: you can hold the patient's hand and give sympathy and nothing else—and that has been all too common as a result of the pessimism prevailing in the medical world that if the surgeon can't cure it right away then the patient will not be cured.

"But, as an alternative to that, you can make vigorous attempts to use anticancer agents in addition to surgery. You take away nothing that has saved life before—in 30 per cent, or 10 per cent, or 5 per cent of the cases, according to the kind of cancer the patient has; but you *add* something. In other words, you take as your problem in an institution such as this the patients who are *failures* to surgery and to radiotherapy. You continue to use surgery or radiotherapy to alleviate symptoms; but by practicing this aggressive approach to cancer treatment, by adding anticancer agents, you may find that eventually you get regression of one kind of tumor—let us say, cancer of the breast by the use of hormones, or cancers of the liver and gastrointestinal tract by the use of 5-fluorouracil. The use of chemical agents in this way, in a scientific environment, as part of the total care of the patient, gives you an opportunity to do much more for each individual patient; *and the patient knows that something is being done for him, he has not been abandoned.* This, alone, has proven to be one of the great contributions of cancer chemotherapy.

"But in addition, this kind of approach gives skilled research workers the opportunity to look for leads. You may take a patient who has many metastases, as was the case with this child I just talked about with Wilms' tumor. It may not be possible to save that child. Even if you had an agent that could destroy every tumor cell in the body within one hour, you would still lose that child because so much tissue has already been destroyed and his death is inevitable. But the fact that you were able to get certain results using actinomycin D gives you a lead, a solid basis on which to plan a new experimental attack on all patients with Wilms' tumor.

"So these are the two roads we have followed. In the first instance we began with an attempt to prevent metastases—the spread of the cancer throughout the body—by using chemical anticancer agents after surgery and irradiation. In the second instance we sought out leads by taking the patient who has 'incurable cancer'[17] in the late stages; if we could produce some effect, if we were able to destroy some of that cancer, it gave us the courage to start much earlier, and on a broad scale, the treatment of all patients with that particular form of cancer. We take every child, because that is what we were organized for; we select the adults on the basis of those we can help most."

We spoke for a few moments of work being done elsewhere, and about the very intensive programs of chemotherapy now being followed by some scientists. Dr. Farber said, "we have very strict rules which we follow in our clinical investigation. They are very simple. I teach them to my younger men. The first is that when trying, or studying, a new form of treatment the patient must not be deprived of anything *of proved value* that might save his life. Even though I might hate like fury to see a leg removed for osteogenic sarcoma (a form of bone cancer) if that might give the patient even a 20 per cent chance of survival, I have no right to say the leg will stay on if I have nothing of proved value to offer instead.

"The second rule is, anything that is done or given to a patient in clinical investigation must be primarily for the good of the patient. That is restating the first rule, but it explains it a little further, and we are very strict about it.

"The third rule is, never give anything to a patient when studying new methods of treatment that in itself is worse for the patient than the untreated disease—except for short peri-

---

[17] Dr. Farber's actual words were: *"by taking the patient who has, quote, incurable cancer, unquote."* He was, in fact, expressing disapproval of the term "incurable cancer."

ods of time when you give something that may be temporarily toxic to try to save the patient's life.

"And, finally, to make it very simple for young investigators, when they ask, How do you make a decision in a given case, I reply, Never do anything to a patient that you would not like to have done to your mother, father, wife, sister, brother, or children; and that makes it very simple. I think these are rules of clinical investigation which, in the field of cancer particularly, must be lived up to if we are to make progress against the disease and also if we are to make progress as human beings. The M.D. is not a hunting license."

I asked, "Isn't it true that most of the anticancer drugs available today are antimitotic drugs—that is, they attack cells that are in the process of dividing?"

"Yes," Dr. Farber replied. "But it is not the antimitotic effect that I am afraid of, because there is a differential effect which we know exists although no one has yet explained it fully: we are still unable to say why an anticancer drug—any one of the antileukemic drugs, for example—will kill the leukemic cell and not the patient. It may kill normal cells; it may cut down on mitotic activity of normal tissue; but the most delicate indicator we have of good health is growth of a child, and we have given an antimitotic drug *daily for eight years* to a child with no effect on the growth rate—the growth has increased in the expected pattern. This is the best proof we have that there is a differential: that you can kill the tumor and not the normal tissue. But there are chemicals that kill the normal tissues so fast that you have no chance to see if they can kill the tumor. Mitomycin C, for example; a Japanese antibiotic. They use a great deal of it in Japan against cancer of the stomach and some other forms of cancer, but it is a material you must give with the utmost care—you must make sure it doesn't leak into the tissues or there will be great necrosis[18] and scarring, and so on."

---

[18] Necrosis is defined (*Stedman's Medical Dictionary*, 21st ed.) as the pathologic death of one or more cells, or of a portion of tissue or organ, resulting from irreversible damage to the nucleus.

Dr. Farber, according to a short biography prepared by the American Cancer Society, is recognized internationally as the founder of modern pediatric pathology; his research helped spark the great developments in the chemotherapy of cancer, notably in the treatment of leukemia; he has been Chairman of the Subcommittee on Cancer of the President's Commission on Heart Disease, Cancer and Stroke since 1964. As perhaps the leading authority on chemotherapy in the United States, I asked him to discuss the issue raised earlier: that chemotherapy is the most blunt tool we have for treating cancer.

"It is a blunt tool," Dr. Farber said, very gently and patiently, "only if the wielder has a heavy hand. Chemotherapy *can* be a blunt tool. It can be a very cruel thing if one uses it that way. But chemotherapy as I define it is all-inclusive: it ranges from the use of the chemicals and hormones we have now, to the ultimate—that is, when we have pinpointed the chemical abnormality that we call cancer, identified it very clearly within the nucleus of the cell, and can fashion a chemical that will selectively correct that biochemical abnormality. Now, this is not a blunt tool. This is the most delicate of delicate approaches to cancer chemotherapy."

"Are we in sight of accomplishing that?"

"Oh, yes. We are doing it today. There are now a number of chemicals whose mechanism of action is fairly well—although not completely—understood. Take as an example actinomycin D. It acts by interrupting the DNA-related RNA.[19] We know the structure of DNA. We are now, in our

[19] Some readers may wish to have a somewhat fuller explanation. DNA and RNA are, of course, nucleic acids found in living cells. DNA is the substance making up the chromosomes, carrying all genetic information. RNA, apparently under the direction of DNA, is responsible among other things for the synthesis of proteins within the cell, and thus governs growth. Actinomycin D appears to combine with DNA in such a manner that the formation of RNA is inhibited (held back); and so the growth of the cell is inhibited, preventing the cell from functioning properly and also interfering with cell division. When actinomycin D combines with the DNA of malignant cells, therefore, tumor growth is inhibited.

molecular biology division, working on the structure of a model of RNA to go with the Watson-Crick model of DNA. On another floor we have a famous organic chemist, whom I brought here to synthesize actinomycin D. With the structure of RNA and its relationship to DNA understood, as well as the mechanism of action of actinomycin D, we are now going to fashion a series of analogues of actinomycin D, until we get just the structure that will interfere with each particular tumor at the molecular level.

"This," Dr. Farber said, "is chemotherapy with intelligence. This is chemotherapy on a rational basis. This is not the kind of chemotherapy that entails going to a factory and saying, *You have ten thousand drugs and chemicals on your shelves; give me the ten thousand and I will try them against every mouse tumor.* There was a time when we had to do that because we had no rational basis for research. But what we learned through systematic studies of that kind has enabled us to utilize information now coming to us from molecular biology, and from biochemistry, and from organic chemistry. This is the chemotherapy of today, and of tomorrow."

"In a sense, this program you have been describing is unique?"

Dr. Farber replied, "No. Nothing is unique once you have talked about it and lectured about it for a number of years, and written papers about it. Then you find that other men have been thinking along similar lines, and you find a group here and a group there working with the same aim. One of the finest minds of this kind is Professor Franz Bergel, who recently retired from Chester Beatty; he has been here for six weeks as a consultant, and he has written about the fashioning of compounds in this way. We have a whole program, now, with Dr. E. J. Modest, who is making compounds on a purely rational basis.

"That is why I react to the statement that chemotherapy is a blunt tool. There can be no more delicate tool if it is the proper kind, if it is honed properly. What we have to find out is why actinomycin D did *this* to the Wilms' tumor cell, and did not do it to the breast cancer cell or the lung cancer cell. What are the molecular differences between those tumors and the Wilms' tumor? It should not be impossible to find out. We're going along with it very rapidly now. Then we can go ahead and fashion our chemicals on the basis of these differences.

"So, in the most simple terms," Dr. Farber said, "my dream of the solution of the cancer problem is this: First, we must have a universal diagnostic test, a test that can be carried out inexpensively, simply, rapidly, and with complete accuracy on the population as a whole. A drop of blood. Or a drop of saliva —which would be the easiest of all, since you wouldn't even have to prick a finger. The purpose of the test would be to tell us only one thing—that somewhere in the body normal cells are being transformed into malignant cells.

"I don't even want to know if it's in the liver, or in the lung, or the brain. I don't have to know that, with this program of mass screening. I want to find the presence of the cancer *before there is a tumor*, before there is a swelling, before an organ has been destroyed, or the body interfered with in its normal functioning. And when I have evidence that somewhere cells are being transformed because an abnormal biochemical principle is at work, because an abnormal biochemical substance is present in the cells, I want to introduce this tailor-made biochemical material into the body to correct that transformation and *retransform it back to the normal state* in the case of each cell.

"That is the ideal way to handle cancer. To take care of it by chemotherapy before there is a destructive tumor. I think that day is going to come. We won't have unphysiological treatments such as surgical removal of a leg, or of an organ. No surgeon is happy about this method of treating cancer. It's unphysiological; it's taking something away. We don't even want lifesaving radiotherapy, because at best it's a killer of tissue—normal tissue as well as cancer. We don't want some of the chemicals we have now, like nitrogen mustard, which *are* blunt instruments, which *are* crude and heavy, although they may be lifesaving today; and we do want simple chemicals— maybe an enzyme like L-asparaginase, or something of very much smaller molecular size—that we can introduce into the body in the form of a tablet or a pill, which will go through the body to the abnormal cell and correct that biological abnormality.

"This is an oversimplified picture of our hope for the control of cancer," Dr. Farber said. "Can it be achieved? Yes. This is the underlying thought of all cancer men."

The differences of opinion reported here may not be as profound as, on the surface, they appear to be. One scientist expresses concern about the present status of chemotherapy and about a program of research that has brought us a preponderance of antimitotic drugs which exert their effect on both healthy and malignant dividing cells. The other scientist expresses confidence in the future of chemotherapy, in the fashioning of drugs which will exert their effect in a highly specific manner only on malignant cells.

It is indisputable that chemotherapy today plays a valuable part in the treatment of cancer, that the cancer patient has available many drugs which will relieve the effects of his disease even though they will not provide a permanent cure. The difficulty is that these drugs may affect normal tissue. Nitrogen mustard, for example, which is used in the treatment of Hodgkin's disease, lymphosarcoma, and chronic leukemia, is exceedingly dangerous, as might be expected of a war gas. Vincristine, derived from the gentle periwinkle, is a potent nerve poison and may cause paralysis of the bowel wall (paralytic ileus), various forms of palsy, and an extremely painful condition called peripheral neuritis.

At the present time, then, in the words of Dr. J. A. Stock, "there is universal agreement that improvement is sorely needed." On the other hand, when the molecular biologist and the biochemist have completed their work we may indeed enter a golden era of cancer chemotherapy, with a wide range of drugs that are exquisitely selective, attacking only cancer cells, bypassing healthy cells. In the near future? The distant future? Ten years, fifty years, a hundred years? Nobody can say.

6

Defense

TEN

But Immunologists Speak Only to Immunologists

Immunology is the branch of medical science that deals with immunity to disease. Immunity is the condition of being resistant to a specific disease. Immunotherapy is the treatment of disease by immunological methods.

These are simplified, and therefore incomplete definitions. They serve in this context only to introduce what appears to be (to many people) by far the most complex and incomprehensible of all the disciplines concerned with disease, particularly cancer.

Immunotherapy is the fourth of the various methods by which cancer can be treated. The other methods are surgery, in which malignant tissue is physically removed: radiotherapy, in which malignant tissue is subjected to radiation that will either kill the tumor cells or sterilize them so that they are unable to divide; and chemotherapy, the treatment of cancer by chemical compounds. Compared to these three, immunotherapy is wrapped in mystery; and even the vocabulary of the science is bewildering. "Immunologists speak only to immunologists," a scientist once told me: "And even then it is open to question whether one immunologist knows what another immunologist is talking about." A slanderous statement, no doubt; but it expresses a view that is widely held.

At the same time, the current role of immunologists perhaps permits them certain intellectual luxuries: although their direct intervention in cancer therapy has not so far been outstandingly effective, they are playing a vital role in relation to tissue and organ transplantation—procedures that will undoubtedly become more and more important to cancer patients in the future. The surgeon, with his elegant techniques, may install a new heart, a new kidney, or a new lung in a dying patient; it is the immunologist who bears the responsibility of keeping the new organ—and the patient—alive. But a long and wearisome apprenticeship has been spent by the immunologists to bring them to their present eminence. "Hardly any other branch of science," says Charles Oberling, referring specifically to the early study of cancer transplants, "has demanded such infinite patience of its disciples, or subjected them to such a bitter ordeal." And it was in relation to cancer transplants that Paul Ehrlich said to a young colleague, "You wish to work at experimental cancer? Do not think of it. I have wasted fifteen years of my life in that way."

Just as the *beau idéal* of the epidemiologists is John Snow, who proved his worth in the Broad Street pump episode of 1854, the *beau idéal* of the immunologists (or, at least, the first to emerge as a *beau idéal*) is Edward Jenner (1749–1823), described by Fielding H. Garrison as "the typical English country gentleman, blond, blue-eyed, of handsome figure." "He wore his hair in a sort of wind-swept bob, tied in a club at the back," says Greer Williams in *Virus Hunters:* "He was neat in dress. Commonly, when he called on patients, he wore a broad-brimmed hat, blue coat with yellow buttons, buckskin pants, well-polished jockey boots, and silver spurs. In lieu of the gold-headed cane that was the mark of the city doctor, he carried a good whip with a silver handle." The whip was necessary because he traveled from patient to patient on horseback, like the early American country doctors (and presumably early country doctors everywhere).

In 1780, Edward Jenner was already thinking seriously about a common legend that milkmaids who contracted a relatively mild disease, cowpox, were mysteriously protected against an extremely dangerous disease, smallpox. In 1789 he made his first attempt to test the legend: he transferred some material taken from a pig suffering from a disease called swinepox into the arm of his ten-month-old son. Within eight days the child became sick and pustules appeared.

Jenner then proceeded to carry out a rash and hazardous experiment: he inoculated his baby son five or six times with smallpox material. As luck would have it, the smallpox did not take, and no other illness occurred. But the same procedure, attempted more than a year later, resulted in the child developing fairly severe inflammation in his arm, possibly a bacterial infection. Happily (for the child, the father, and mankind) little Edward recovered. Whether this experiment affected his health nobody can say: he was sickly, mentally retarded, and he died—apparently of consumption—at the age of twenty-one. No doctor, no researcher, in his right mind would dare to try anything so perilous today.

In 1796 Jenner performed his most famous experiment. It was equally rash, but no alternative was open to him: he could only experiment on human beings. The leading characters were a young milkmaid, Sarah Nelmes, suffering from cowpox, and an eight-year-old boy, James Phipps. The scene was a small thatched garden house. Jenner extracted some matter on a lancet from a cowpox pustule on Sarah's wrist, and made two scratches with the lancet on James' arm. Several days later James complained of uneasiness in his armpit, and two days still later he had a headache and chills; but during this time a single pustule appeared on his arm—the first vaccination, officially recorded, to take. A scab then formed and in due course fell off, leaving a small indented crater. After six weeks Jenner made the critical test: he inoculated James Phipps with smallpox matter. Nothing happened, except slight inflammation; and in similar tests over the next twenty-five years James Phipps continued to demonstrate that inoculation with cowpox provided immunity against smallpox. Jenner then went on to demonstrate that cowpox matter could be taken from a person who had been inoculated with it and passed directly to another person; it could then be passed from the second recipient to a third, and so on—apparently—in a more or less endless progression. This technique is now known as serial passage, and it has been of great importance in the development of vaccines and in the investigation of disease-causing organisms, particularly viruses.

Because *vaccinia* is the medical name for cowpox (from the Latin, *vacca*, a cow) the process of transferring the cowpox material into a patient became known as vaccination, and the material itself was called a vaccine. Inoculations of widely different kinds are still referred to as vaccinations; materials used for inoculations are still called vaccines although they may have come, not from a cow, but from a horse, a rabbit, or from the embryos of ducks or fowl. With improvements in technique, Jenner's method of inducing infection has led to the control of a number of diseases previously catastrophic to man, and also to the control of diseases just as catastrophic to his domesticated animals. Smallpox heads the list of human afflictions (and the vaccine is still obtained from vesicles of cowpox); among the others we can count cholera, diphtheria, influenza (only partially controlled by vaccines), measles (only partially controlled), mumps, whooping cough, plague, polio, rabies, tetanus, tuberculosis, typhoid and paratyphoid, epidemic typhus and yellow fever. Jenner needs no other memorial. He is one of the great men of medicine.[1]

---

[1] Garrison (*History of Medicine*) points out that "the mere idea of innoculation is apparently as old as the hills." Human inoculation is mentioned (of course) in ancient Indian writings, and was known to many Oriental peoples. Lady Mary Wortley Montagu had her three-year-old son inoculated in Turkey in 1718; her five-year-old daughter was inoculated in England in 1721. The merit of Jenner's work (again in Garrison's words) was that "he transformed a local country tradition into a viable prophylactic principle." A comment by Benjamin Waterhouse (1754–1846), a Harvard professor of medicine, throws a strange light on conditions in America before Jenner's discovery became known; he says that prior to the introduction of vaccination, the fear of smallpox compelled the New Englanders—"the most democratic people on the face of the earth"—to endure "restrictions of liberty such as no absolute monarch could have enforced." Castiglioni (in *A History of Medicine*) comments, "One cannot imagine the emotions aroused throughout the civilized world" by the publication of Jenner's account of vaccination in 1798. Nor can one imagine the emotions aroused throughout the civilized world by the announcement of some similar procedure to control cancer.

All the diseases that can be controlled by vaccination have one factor in common: they do not arise in man, so to speak, spontaneously, as the result of a peculiar change within any of the thirty trillion cells that combine to make up the human system. On the contrary, they are always, without exception, the result of invasion by foreign organisms, and each disease is due to invasion by a very specific foreign organism—specific viruses, or specific microorganisms of a number of different kinds. The virus of smallpox causes only smallpox, never whooping cough; the tubercle bacillus causes only tuberculosis, and not influenza or typhoid. We are literally surrounded by these miniature forms of life; all of them are compelled (as we ourselves are) to strive to survive and multiply; and there is no way we can totally isolate ourselves from them. Their prevalence is stupendous: it has been calculated that *by weight* they exceed all animal life on earth twenty times. Their *numbers* are incalculable and beyond comprehension.

Despite these odds, we have managed to survive, and for several reasons. Not all the microorganisms in our environment are hostile; many are indifferent to us and greatly prefer other living things; a few have joined forces with us and have become indispensable to our well-being. Then, the hostile microorganisms are not waging ceaseless war against us: many, like the influenza viruses, attack only occasionally. Some of these microorganisms in a few densely-populated areas of the world have to a large extent been exterminated, so that they pose a minimal threat. But by far the most important reason for our survival is that each human being, by the time he or she is a few months old, has acquired an armamentarium of highly efficient defenses, capable of dealing effectively with a considerable number of the more common invaders; and this armamentarium can be reinforced, when necessary, to subdue many of those microorganisms against which our natural defenses are inadequate.

Our first line of defense, of course, is the skin; it is to all intents and purposes impregnable except when it is broken by a wound. Chemical substances on its surface increase its defensive capabilities. There are, however, some microorganisms which can in certain circumstances damage the skin, invade the deeper tissues and enter the blood stream, causing very serious infections.

A parallel line of defense takes the form of a variety of enzymes and other chemical secretions in the mucous membranes of the various bodily orifices, together with the cilia—myriads of tiny hair-like processes that trap encroaching microorganisms and other foreign particles, and sweep them away from sensitive areas. One of the tragedies of the habit of cigarette smoking is that it tends to paralyze the cilia lining the upper respiratory tract; consequently they are unable to combat those microorganisms that have a liking for the warm, moist respiratory passages, thus leading to bronchial ailments; at the same time the cilia are powerless to expel the cigarette tars carried down to the lungs in the smoke, thus promoting the possibility of lung cancer.

A second line of defense is also chemical. Injuries to body cells trigger the release of histamines and other substances which act against bacterial invaders. Histamine is a vasodilator —that is, it causes the distention of blood vessels, an effect of great importance in the defensive procedure. Another chemical participating in defense is interferon, a protein discovered by the British virologist Alick Isaacs in 1957. This appears to be manufactured by all normal body cells, and it "interferes" with the reproduction of many viruses (though not all) within the cell. More interesting is its second mode of action: it alerts neighboring cells to the danger of infection, so that they can begin to manufacture a protective protein. Interferon has received a considerable amount of attention in recent years, but it is difficult to resist the thought that—from the prevalence of viral diseases—its efficacy in reducing susceptibility to infection is not particularly high. Presumably without it, however, we would be even more vulnerable to viral diseases than we already are. Dr. Isaacs' death in 1967, at the early age of 46, was a great loss: he might have helped to find means to increase the activity of interferon, so that it would tackle those viruses to which it now seems rather indifferent.

But all the defense systems so far described are relatively weak compared to the extraordinary array of internal defenses made up of white blood cells circulating throughout the body, plus an extensive network of fixed cells lining strategic positions, plus ten thousand (or so) different forms of antibodies.

The white blood cells, or leucocytes, have the responsibility of attacking and destroying all kinds of invading microorganisms and particles. They are thus non-specific. They regard all foreign invaders (or nearly all) as enemies.

Some, the granulocytes (containing relatively large granules in the nucleus) are described as cells of the myeloid series, which means they originate in the bone marrow; and the type most commonly seen are called polymorphonuclear leucocytes, an alarming term which only means that the nucleus appears to have several lobes, usually from three to five. (Nobody should allow himself, or herself, to be intimidated by medical terminology. It is usually absurdly simple, even naive, when it is broken down into its components. Here, for example, *poly* = many; *morpho* = form or shape; *nuclear* = of the nucleus; *leuco* = white; *cytes* = cells.)

Lymphoid cells are manufactured in lymphatic tissue of the thymus (particularly during childhood), the spleen and the lymph glands (or nodes). The latter are structures composed almost entirely of lymphatic cells, found throughout the body. They include aggregates of lymphocytes in the tonsils[2] and the appendix.[3]

[2] The tonsils are generally taken to be the faucial, or palatine tonsils at the back of the throat, but there are numerous structures of the same kind that are also, technically, termed tonsils: the lingual tonsils on the upper side of the tongue; cerebellar tonsils, on the under surface of each cerebral hemisphere of the brain; tubal tonsils, in the Eustachian tubes from the middle ear to the nasopharynx; the pharyngeal, or so-called third tonsil, in the nasopharynx, which sometimes becomes enlarged and causes the condition known as adenoids; the *tonsilla intestinalis*, an extensive collection of lymphoid nodes in the mucous membranes of the small intestine. Similar nodes are found throughout the gastrointestinal tract, and are very conspicuous in the caecum (a blind pouch formed where the small intestine terminates and the large intestine begins).

[3] In the course of an interview in London with Professor Peter Alex-

The white blood cells are mobile: they are carried through the blood stream and in the lymph, and they perform their task by engulfing the foreign particles they encounter; for this reason they were named by Elie Metchnikoff, in 1884, *phagocytes*, or eating cells. The dilation of blood vessels—one of the results of histamines being released by injured tissue cells—enables the phagocytes to seep through interstices in the walls of the capillaries, and reach foci of infection in surrounding tissues; and where the infection is substantial, battalions of white cells will hasten to the area, literally like shock troops. What stimulus alerts them, why they respond to the stimulus, how they find their way to the scene of the conflict, are biological mysteries.

In addition, vast numbers of fixed phagocytes participate in defense. These comprise the reticuloendothelial system. (*Reticulo* means in the form of a network; *epithelium* is a layer of cells lining blood vessels, lymphatic tubes—through which the lymph flows—and the internal cavities of the body.) The liver, spleen and lymph nodes are profusely supplied with these immobile, ever-alert, cellular watchdogs.

And, finally, we have the system of antibodies: molecules of protein manufactured in lymphatic tissue by specialized lymphocytes called plasma cells. While the white blood cells are on the whole *non-specific,* attacking wherever possible any kind of foreign invader they encounter, antibodies are highly specific, precisely matching specific foreign particles. This is so much so that if a particular antibody is found to be present in the blood it is virtually certain (with a few exceptions) that the matching foreign particle is present too, or was present in the past and has been eliminated.

It is at this point that the non-scientific reader is apt to find himself floundering in a sea of confusion, for immunology is encumbered by a wretched and baffling vocabulary un-

---

ander I asked if the appendix plays a part of any importance in the immunological system. His answer deserves to be quoted. "It depends on whether you are a rabbit or a man. In the rabbit, unquestionably it does. In man, the proportion of lymphoid tissue to the whole is so small that it's neither here nor there. . . . I do not feel that I myself have been placed in hazard by losing my appendix."

matched by any other science. Antibody does not mean what at first glance it seems to mean: a substance that acts against the body. On the contrary, it means (to compound the confusion) a substance that acts against *foreign bodies* that act against the body.

Furthermore, a given antibody has a precise reason for its existence: it was produced to oppose a specific adversary (which might be a certain virus, a certain bacterium, a certain molecule of a particular pollen). A specific antibody, then, is created when an antibody-manufacturing plasma cell encounters some new foreign substance; and immunologists call such a substance (or the microscopic parts of the substance that induce the manufacture of antibodies) *antigens.* Again we have an inept noun: antigen means "against producer," which is senseless in this context. It acquires meaning only if we insert *body* between the two halves of the word: *antibodygen*, or stimulator of antibody production. This is, indeed, the simple definition of antigen—*any of numerous substances such as toxins, enzymes, or foreign proteins that cause the development of antibodies.* Yet another immunological ineptitude is the term antiserum; and this, when one untangles it, reveals itself not as a substance that acts against blood serum, but as serum containing antibodies.

The unborn child may acquire antibodies from its mother; but after the first few months of life the general rule is that antibodies are made by plasma cells in response to invading antigens.[4] The antibody molecule is so constructed that it fits

[4] Antibodies obtained by the child from its mother during pregnancy are said to be passively acquired—"passive" indicates that the unborn child did not participate in manufacturing them. Antibodies against a specific infection can be manufactured externally (as a rule, by utilizing animals such as horses or rabbits under carefully controlled conditions) and then administered to a patient suffering from that particular infection. They provide short-term immunity lasting only a few weeks, because they are rejected by the individual's immune system. Those antibodies manufactured by the individual himself, or herself, following an infection, are termed active specific antibodies.

Readers of this book may be interested to learn that there is, in process of formation, a group of desperadoes who plan to seize scientific power and then to send all immunologists to special kindergartens where they will be taught to write and read the English language.

the antigen molecule as a key fits a lock; the union of the two immobilizes the antigen (and any foreign body to which the antigen belongs, or is attached), permitting its ultimate destruction by any of the fixed or circulating phagocytes. The pattern of key and lock seems to be tucked away in the files of the immunological system, for the next time the same antigen appears there is an immediate and vastly more vigorous antibody response; and it is this that accounts for the success of most types of vaccination. The vaccination is relatively mild, and serves to establish the antibody pattern; any subsequent infection is then met by overwhelming antibody resistance.

Viruses, bacteria, the skin or the kidney or the heart of another individual, are all foreign. The immunological defenses are mounted to reject them and to drive them out of the body. Sometimes the foreign organisms grow too rapidly to be controlled; or the immune mechanisms may be depressed or inactivated by drugs or radiation, permitting the foreign invader to establish itself. Otherwise, the immunological process is rigid and intolerant.

This lengthy preamble serves to lead to a very simple question: Why do the complex, sophisticated, sensitive, wide-ranging defensive mechanisms of the body tolerate a cancerous growth which, in due course, will lead to the body's destruction?

This question is really of vital importance to our understanding of cancer and to the treatment of the disease; but although a number of different answers have been suggested they are all hypothetical, and none appears to be completely satisfactory.

One hypothesis—currently out of favor—is that in normal circumstances the immunological defenses do indeed respond to the appearance of cancerous cells in the body, do indeed regard them as foreign, and attempt to eradicate them. Only when, for some reason, the defenses fail in this attempt does cancer become manifest. Cancer may thus be viewed as an outcome—possibly rare, possibly common—of immunological failure.

Professor Peter Alexander commented about this:[5] "It's quite clear that people with advanced cancer generally have impairment of immune responses. Do they have advanced cancer because they have impaired immune responses, or vice versa? I think the feeling now is that the impaired immune responses are a *consequence* and not a *cause* of cancer. There is no indication at all that the early cancer patient has an impaired immune response, nor is there any evidence that those who have a poorer immune response do worse, or have worse prognoses (that is, forecasts regarding the course of the disease) than those who have a good immune response. The theory (that cancer may be related to impaired immune responses) is still occasionally stated because it would be so nice if it were true, but there is no evidence to support it at all. . . . In the case of leukemia, lymphomas and other malignancies involving the immune system itself the situation is very complex, and it is just conceivable that when the tumor actually involves the immune system an impairment of the immune response might precede the disease. But even that isn't clear."

Another hypothesis starts with the assumption that a cancerous growth consists of an individual's own cells. Consequently, these cells are privileged, like all the other cells in that individual's body, and the immune system will not, or cannot, discriminate against them. Furthermore, since they are "self" and not foreign, they contain no constituents capable of acting as antigens; they cannot induce antibody production, and they do not provoke attack by lymphocytes. They are thus secure from immunological intervention and can proliferate freely.

This theory has the virtue of being simple and logical; but evidence exists that seems to contradict it. For example, almost twenty years ago a young woman in a Baltimore hospital underwent surgery for the removal of a small tumor, an operation from which she is said to have made a satisfactory recovery. Laboratory tests then revealed that in tissue culture this tumor grew at an astounding rate; the total weight of the cultured tumor must now be many times the weight of the *patient*

[5] In an interview at the laboratories of the Chester Beatty Research Institute in Sutton, Surrey.

when she had her operation, and the material is used as a standard by cancer researchers all over the world. The fact that this tumor was quite small when it was removed seems to suggest that the patient's immunological defenses played a part in slowing down the growth of the tumor cells.[6] When the immunological (and other) restraints were no longer in effect the growth could proceed at full speed, producing a tumor mass of bizarre proportions.

Again, the idea has been put forward that in the tremendous population of cells comprising the human body—thirty trillion, or more—some, purely on the basis of statistical probability, may undergo changes that eventually lead to malignancy. It has been suggested that these cancerous, or precancerous, cells come into existence with great frequency, perhaps many times every minute of a person's life. Cancers rarely result from cellular accidents of this kind, it is assumed, because the abnormal cells are swiftly suppressed by the immunological defenses. To test this hypothesis, animals have been treated so that their immune systems were completely unreactive; tumors should then have sprung up at a very high rate. But, as one immunologist expressed it, "This crucial experiment turned out to be completely negative, and the very nice hypothesis has consequently lost some of its appeal."

Another immunological dilemma is whether cancer antigens do, or do not, exist in human beings. It is similar to the puzzle that has baffled virologists since the beginning of the century: *Where are the human cancer viruses?* We know that certain viruses cause certain specific forms of cancer in certain animals; we believe therefore that some viruses almost certainly cause some forms of cancer in human beings. Yet, in spite of a tremendous concentration of effort all over the world, human cancer viruses still have not been identified (although a few are under suspicion). If they *were* found, we *might* be able to make a vaccine that would be effective against them; at the very least, new prospects of research and treatment might be opened up.

[6] It is also possible that other agents affecting growth, such as hormones, were involved.

The discovery of human cancer antigens could be even more fruitful, because methods might then be devised to enable the body itself—through its immune mechanisms—to deal with tumor cells carrying any specific antigen. The prospects are not altogether encouraging: the situation is summed up in a couple of sentences by two of the world's leading immunologists, Dr. Lloyd J. Old and Dr. Edward A. Boyse: "One of the most important problems of the present time is to demonstrate that human tumors, like tumors in experimental animals, possess specific antigens. Although numerous attempts have been made, there is no certain evidence for the antigenicity of any tumor in man."[7] Professor Alexander has stated the case in much the same terms: "On general grounds there is little doubt that some human cancers contain (tumor specific) antigens, but we do not know whether this is a common or a rare occurrence. As yet, the presence of tumor-specific antigens has not been unambiguously established in any case of human malignant disease."[8]

The potentialities of immunology in cancer therapy have received a great deal of publicity in the past few years; and as George Mathé has shown (and other scientists) the method is valid. It works. It extends the life of dying people. But Mathé himself has said, "If immunotherapy develops as an effective therapeutic method it will, probably, remain a method which will be difficult to manage. . . . It is still too early to foresee the future development of leukemia immunotherapy and its eventual indications. Certain of the techniques which are the most active are not free of risk: however, the same could probably be said of certain other procedures at their outset."

The issue was put even more strongly by Professor Peter Alexander during our conversation in one of the laboratories of the Chester Beatty Research Institute in Sutton, Surrey. At

[7] "Specific Antigens of Tumors and Leukemias of Experimental Animals," *Medical Clinics of North America*, Vol. 50, No. 3, 1966.
[8] "The Role of Tumor-Specific Antigens in the Genesis, Development and Control of Malignant Disease," *The Biology of Cancer*, London, 1966.

the outset, Professor Alexander explained that his primary interest had been radiobiology—the effect of radiation on cells. A study of radiation and animal tumors led him, around 1959, to an investigation of immunological methods of treating these tumors. "When we started this," he said, "the field was more or less empty, but recently it has become popular, perhaps excessively popular. What seems to be happening is that many people are abandoning their own line of work, thinking that the field of immunology is more promising; but I'm afraid we may have a great disillusionment. These things tend to go in cycles. People are excessively optimistic and then excessively pessimistic. . . .

"I think the first consideration about any form of immunotherapy in cancer is that even if everything goes in one's favor there is no reason whatever to believe that immunotherapeutic procedures will constitute anything akin to a magic bullet. They will at the very best be an adjunct to existing forms of therapy. I think it is inconceivable that they will be a form of therapy on their own, but they may be an adjunct to be used after surgery, after radiotherapy, possibly after chemotherapy, to take care of some residual cells. I think immunotherapy has no place at all in treating the very advanced case who is near the end of the road—one will not be able to snatch anyone back to life as one can with penicillin, two days from death. So, even at the most optimistic estimate, it could only be an additional tool in the hands of the doctor treating the cancer patient."

It is ethically impermissible to inoculate a healthy human being with leukemic cells taken from a human leukemic patient. Nevertheless it has been tried. Leukemia is almost invariably fatal; its course cannot be predicted or controlled; and if the transplanted cells somehow established themselves the recipient would literally be condemned to death. The transplantation of solid tumor cells from a cancer patient to a healthy human being has been tried frequently; a notable series of experiments was carried out by Dr. Chester M. Southam of the Sloan-Kettering Institute on convicts in the Ohio State Penitentiary: more than 100 convicts (a progress report, dated June 1958, described them lyrically as "men who bore some of society's ugliest labels: murderer, rapist, swindler, thug,") responded to a call for volunteers in the prison newspaper. Of the hundred volunteers, fourteen were selected for initial tests. In all cases the cancerous implants were rejected.

Again, it would be ethically impermissible to implant cells taken from a human cancer patient in a healthy human being *if there were any possibility of the implantation becoming invasive and forming secondary tumors (metastases)*, for here again a healthy human being is placed in peril. The legal consequences of such an experiment, if the implantation proved fatal, might be substantial. One or two unfortunate incidents in the past have aroused public anxiety and controversy, even when the transplants were made in patients who had entered the terminal stage of their illness; and, generally, scientists today are reluctant to engage in experimental procedures involving cancer transplants between human patients and healthy human recipients.

There is one form of cancer, however, which might be described as a natural experiment in cancer transplantation: choriocarcinoma. The most notable fact about this disease is that it is essentially a condition in which cancerous tissue of one individual grows inside another individual—hence the similarity to a transplant. Equally notable is the fact that, like Burkitt's lymphoma, it can be cured by chemotherapy alone; and the cure rate so far achieved is considerably higher than in the lymphoma. One difference in the treatment of the two diseases is that in Burkitt's lymphoma successful results have been obtained with what Denis Burkitt calls "minimal" doses, whereas in choriocarcinoma the drugs must be given in substantial amounts, and drug resistance may develop if the dosage is inadequate with the tragic result that the tumor then may fail to respond to all chemotherapy.

Choriocarcinoma is broadly described as a malignancy related to pregnancy. When it occurs it usually follows pregnancy or miscarriage, and the interval between the end of the pregnancy and the appearance of the tumor may be as much as four months, although in some cases (when the tumor grows slowly) the interval is considerably longer. The disease seems to be fairly rare in Western Europe and America: in the United Kingdom, for example, in a population of 54 million, there are between thirty and forty cases a year, and the incidence seems to be about one in thirty thousand pregnancies. The frequency is very much higher—perhaps a hundred times—in Asian countries such as Malaya, Indonesia, Taiwan, the Philippines, Japan, parts of China, India, and even in some parts of Africa and the Middle East. In these areas it is now regarded as one of the more common cancers of women of menstrual age. No epidemiological explanation has yet been found for the difference in geographical distribution: this aspect of the disease remains a mystery. But scientists have been digging into the many peculiarities of choriocarcinoma, and recently they have come up with some remarkable findings. Here, once more, we have a narrative that reads like a detective story.

In the issue of April 1, 1967, under the heading *Hypothesis*, the British medical weekly, *The Lancet*, published a communication with the title (forbidding, as usual, but in this case curiously metrical) "The Masking of Antigens on Trophoblast and Cancer Cells." The authors were G. A. Currie, M.B. Lond., M.R.C.P., and K. D. Bagshawe, M.D. Lond., M.R.C.P.

As a general rule, communications of this kind are written, or assembled, in a dry, objective, noncommittal style, as befits a scientific document; but this particular communication was, in places, unusually assertive. For example, the first paragraph ended, "These observations call for a re-evaluation of some fundamental biological concepts"—a claim that must have caused the raising of many a Harley Street eyebrow. Later, even more boldly, the authors wrote, "If our hypothesis is substantiated, it is inevitable that the mechanism outlined will have important effects not only on the control of cancer but also on the prevention of tissue-transplant rejection and the treatment of autoimmune disease. It will also contribute to our understanding of fundamental biological processes."

A short time after the appearance of this communication I visited Dr. Bagshawe at Fulham Hospital, London, and he described some of the work that preceded publication of *The Lancet* article, and also some of the implications of the hypothesis.[9]

"It all began with choriocarcinoma," said Dr. Bagshawe. "I first became involved with this tumor about ten years ago —accidentally, because I wasn't pursuing a line of interest in cancer at all. My first contact with choriocarcinoma was in a young girl of 19 who was brought into St. Mary's Hospital, Paddington (London), as an emergency. She was breathing so heavily that the doctor who saw her in the emergency room was told she was in some sort of hysterical state of 'overbreathing.' Obviously this wasn't the explanation; but at the time we were unable to find out what was wrong with her. We knew she had a strain on the right side of the heart due to something in the lungs, although there was no evidence of tumor of the lungs in the ordinary sense.

"The disease progressed, unfortunately, and she died within four or five days. At autopsy we found a very unusual form of choriocarcinoma which was confined entirely to the blood vessels in the pelvis and to the pulmonary arteries; and I became interested in the tumor as a result of this one case. By an extraordinary coincidence another case was admitted only six months later and we were able to diagnose what was wrong with this patient. Meanwhile I had seen a preliminary report from the National Institutes of Health by Dr. Roy Hertz and his colleague Dr. Min Chiu Li that methotrexate was effective in some cases of choriocarcinoma. We didn't know *how* effective at that time; only that it produced some sort of remission. Our second patient was given methotrexate, and another drug,

---

[9] The conversation lasted nearly two hours. Transcribed from the tape recording it occupies about thirty pages of typescript. Like other interviews in this book (which is intended for the general reader) it has been condensed somewhat, omitting some of the more technical material discussed by Dr. Bagshawe.

6-mercaptopurine, and she recovered. In fact, she is still alive and well today, ten years later, having been *in extremis* when she was diagnosed.

"There were several things about this tumor which seemed particularly interesting to me at that time. One was the fact that the tumor itself produces a hormone that we can measure relatively easily now, although ten years ago methods were relatively crude. Because the hormone is related to the amount of tumor in the patient we were able to follow the course of the tumor very much more accurately than we could follow the course of any other tumor.

"The second thing about it was that it responded to treatment rather better than almost any other tumor. A significant number of the patients who had this tumor could be cured.

"Thirdly, this is an exceptional tumor by any standards, in that it's a tumor of one individual which is growing in another individual—that is, it's a tumor of *fetal tissue* growing in the mother."

Several questions, Dr. Bagshawe explained, arose from these special characteristics of choriocarcinoma. Why was this tumor curable by drugs, and why did no other tumor (at that time) respond anything like as well? Why, indeed, was this tumor able to grow at all, since we know that if tissue is transplanted from one individual to another individual it is rejected by the graft rejection process? But this, in a way, is only half of a question because it immediately raises the problem of why the fetus is not rejected by the mother in mammalian pregnancy. The fetus is a foreign individual in the womb of the mother, and we still cannot say for certain why its presence is tolerated.[10]

Linked to these questions was the evidence accumulating (in the late 1950s) that experimentally-induced tumors and naturally occurring tumors in animals, and possibly human

[10] The fetus (in immunological terms) must be "foreign" to the mother since it develops from the fusion of two germ cells, one contributed by the mother, the other contributed by the father. Thus—as an example of "foreignness"—the child and the mother may belong to different blood groups.

tumors were antigenic to the host. That is, the host recognized them as foreign in certain ways. But again this posed a question: why is the tumor *not* generally rejected, whereas a skin graft from one individual to another—or a kidney transplant, or a heart transplant—*will* be rejected?

"So this seemed to be a tumor that provoked several interesting questions," Dr. Bagshawe said, "and the problem was how to go about studying it. First we had to arrange some way in which we could make systematic studies; and over the course of several years we developed here a special unit into which we receive most of the cases of choriocarcinoma occurring in the United Kingdom. Altogether, there are probably 30 to 40 cases a year, and we treat about 25 of them."

"Other people, of course, have been interested in this fetal-maternal relationship," Dr. Bagshawe continued, "and numerous explanations have been given for it. Perhaps the uterus is a sort of privileged site which accepts foreign tissue and permits it to grow. Perhaps in pregnancy the mother's immune state is depressed. All kinds of possibilities have been suggested, but one by one these have been eliminated, and it all appears to come down to a particular tissue—the so-called trophoblast. It is this tissue that gives rise to choriocarcinoma: it consists of a layer of cells on the surface of the placenta, it is fetal in origin, and it abuts onto maternal tissue. So what is apparently a sort of fetal-maternal relationship is, in effect, the trophoblast-maternal relationship."[11]

[11] A slightly fuller explanation may help to clarify the relationship of trophoblast and maternal tissue.
Trophoblast first appears as a layer of cells covering the blastocyst (an early stage of the embryo, when it is merely a small cluster of cells).
The function of the trophoblast is of the greatest importance at this point, and without it mammalian life as we know it could not exist, for the trophoblast penetrates and erodes the surface tissue of the uterine wall with the result that the cluster of cells becomes attached to the uterus.
Moreover, the eroding action of the trophoblast damages and thus opens up some of the uterine blood vessels, providing a source of food materials, and it is through the trophoblast that the embryo at first

Trophoblast, therefore, is a foreign tissue in contact with maternal tissue which is not rejected by the mother in the same way that foreign tissue is normally rejected. Obviously, it has some peculiar property; and the suggestion was made that trophoblast differed from all other cells by *not* expressing its foreignness. It was neutral: a sort of neutral thing which just did not have individual antigens in the ordinary sense.

"In that case, what would be its purpose?"

Dr. Bagshawe answered, "*This* could be its purpose: *to be neutral*. Quite a lot of evidence has been produced to indicate that this is so. You can isolate mouse trophoblast fairly easily and make it grow in other animals; you can take it from one strain of mouse and transplant it to another strain of mouse, and it will grow quite happily in the kidney or in various other sites. It grows for the normal period of gestation, and then dies out. It isn't rejected in the same way that a graft of any other tissue is rejected."

---

receives nutriment. (*Tropho* means nutritive, *blast* means the precursive, non-mature stage of a cell.)

Later, the trophoblast becomes two-layered. The outer layer, consisting of a mass of cells without separate cell membranes, is called the syncytial layer (or by some scientists, the syncytiotrophoblast, or syntrophoblast). This manufactures a wide range of hormones.

The inner layer is called the cytotrophoblast. These cells have membranes.

The two layers form finger-like processes extending into the placenta—the organ through which the interchange of nutritive substances and wastes takes place during pregnancy; and these processes are known as the chorionic villi. The chorion is the outermost of the membranes enclosing the embryo, and the villi are said to abut on, or to be in close association with, the part of the placenta formed by the maternal tissue, called the decidua basalis.

There is, of course, no direct blood or nerve connection between mother and embryo. All exchanges occur in the placenta by diffusion—nutritive substances, including oxygen, diffuse *into* the chorionic villi and are carried to the fetus; fetal wastes diffuse *out* of the chorionic villi into the maternal blood and are then carried away in the maternal blood stream.

Another point about trophoblast is that it acquired its name before its functions were fully understood. It does play an important part in the nutritive process (*tropho*) but it is by no means a precursive or non-mature cell (*blast*). On the contrary, because among other things it can manufacture a number of highly complex hormones, scientists refer to it as a very sophisticated cell.

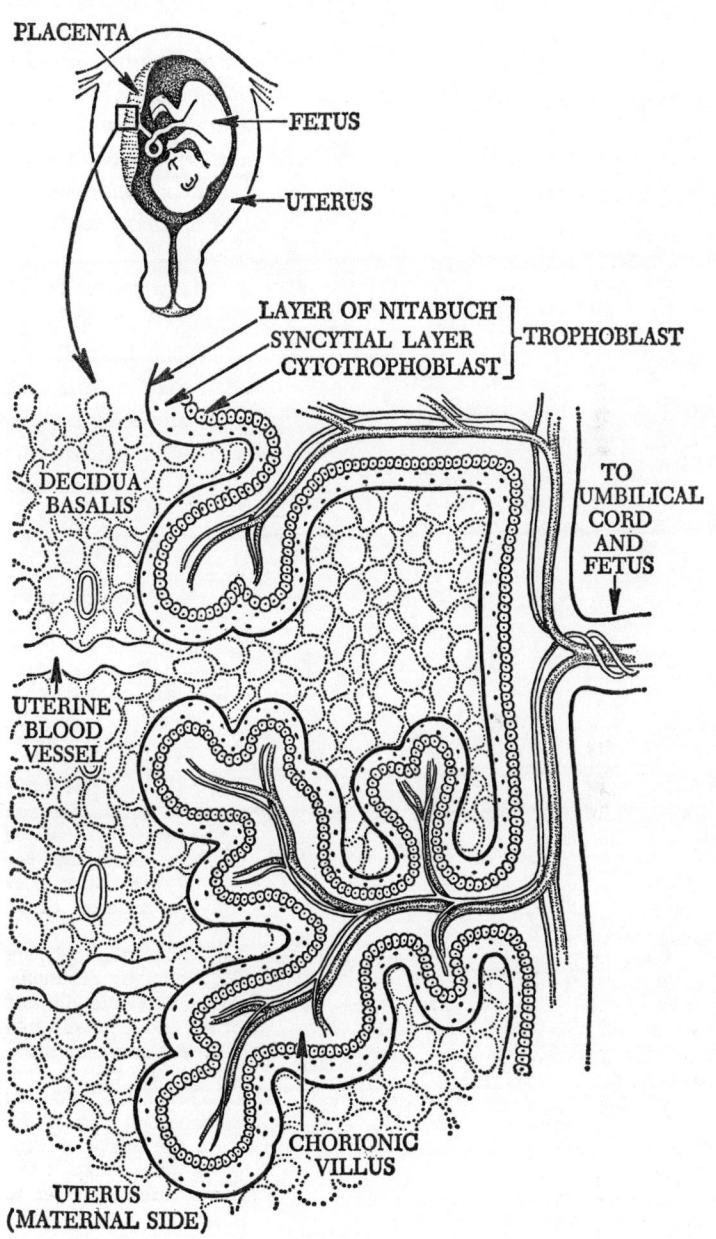

The particular fascination of what one can call the Bagshawe-Currie hypothesis is that as it is expounded one finds oneself —somewhat like Alice in Wonderland—traveling through a landscape in which the details become finer and finer and curiouser and curiouser. There is, for example, the matter of the trophoblast and the antigens it *might* or *might not* possess: an academic point, one could say, yet it is of critical importance to the entire argument.

Some scientists (the anti-antigen group, so to speak) had expressed the view that trophoblast is deficient in antigens. Since it is the antigens that provoke the immune response, *a deficiency of antigens* would explain why the immune response ignored the trophoblast, tolerated it in the uterus, took no action to expel it. A highly plausible explanation, apparently, which neatly disposes of an awkward problem.

But Dr. D. R. S. Kirby and a group of scientists at Oxford, who had been working on fetal-maternal relationships, put forward a contrary view; and here we get down to some rather fine embryological detail. They drew attention to a substance called fibrinoid, which has been known for at least a hundred years: a non-cellular, pinkish-staining material found in the placenta. At the end of the last century a German physician named Raissa Nitabuch had observed that there was a thin layer, or coating, of this material over the surface of the placenta, between the trophoblast and the maternal tissues; and it was, in fact, named for him—the layer of Nitabuch, or Nitabuch's stria. It had never attracted very much attention, which is understandable when one considers the enormous complexity of the placenta; but it is a standard feature described in textbooks of anatomy.

Seen by light microscopy (that is, by means of a microscope utilizing ordinary light) the layer of Nitabuch appears to be broken up, or discontinuous, not applied evenly over the surface of the trophoblast. However, examined by the electron microscope, and using special staining techniques, Dr. Kirby and his colleagues claimed that it was present around all trophoblastic cells, and that each trophoblastic cell appeared to have a coat of this material—the old neglected layer of Nitabuch. The Kirby group now made the startling suggestion that this coating served as a barrier to prevent the escape of antigens from the embryonic tissues. The layer of Nitabuch, or fibrinoid, holds back any trophoblastic antigens; and for this reason the mother's immune response cannot be stimulated into taking action against the foreign tissue growing so rapidly in the mother's uterus.

Without the layer of Nitabuch, consequently, the trophoblast would be attacked and destroyed by the immune forces, the blastocyst would never have an opportunity to attach itself to the uterine wall; and there would be no mammalian life on earth.

All this, of course, is theoretical. The decisive factor, for or against, was whether the trophoblast did or did not carry antigens. Kirby and his group said, Yes: the antigens were there, but they were masked by the coating around the trophoblastic cells. Other scientists (the anti-antigenists) said, No: this layer had no special significance because the trophoblast is intrinsically non-antigenic and *itself* serves as a barrier between the embryo and the mother. "The situation was obviously one where you had to find out whether the trophoblast had antigens or whether it didn't," Dr. Bagshawe said to me; and it is well to remember that he is a physician who treats women suffering from a grim form of cancer. He is not a theoretician; he is not purely a laboratory researcher. To the non-scientist this question of antigens or non-antigens might appear to be something of a quibble, purely intellectual and far out, like disputing how many angels can stand on the head of a pin. But the answer might play an important part in determining whether it shall be life or death for a great many young, frightened human beings.

"In April, 1966," Dr. Bagshawe said, "Dr. Currie came to join me and we went to work on this problem." The detail now becomes just a little finer; and we brush the margins of other scientific disciplines—physics, organic chemistry, electrodynamics.

"It had been observed by Professor E. J. Ambrose and his colleagues at the Chester Beatty Research Institute that cells of the Ehrlich ascites tumor[12] had, on their surface, a very high negative electrostatic charge. The electrical charge is measured in a small tube with electrodes at each end, called a micro-electrophoresis chamber. The cells are suspended in a suitable liquid medium; they are within an electrical field of known strength; and their electrical charge can be estimated from the rate at which they travel toward—usually—the positive electrode. Most cells have a net negative charge (which is why the positive electrode attracts them), but some (as in Orwell's *Animal Farm*) are more negative than others, and this applies to the Ehrlich ascites tumor—its net negative charge appears to be very high."

Dr. Bagshawe made a brief foray into organic chemistry.[13] "But the Ehrlich ascites tumor cells also appear to have on their surface a substance which has staining reactions similar to the material—fibrinoid, or the layer of Nitabuch—present in the placenta and around the trophoblastic cells.

"The substance around the Ehrlich ascites cells is known variously as acid-mucopolysaccharide, or mucopolysaccharide; and a component of many mucopolysaccharides is a compound called sialic acid. In its turn, the sialic acid carries what is known as a carboxyl group; this carboxyl group ionizes; and it is the ionization of the carboxyl group that confers a negative charge. If the cell surface carries numerous chemical groups which ionize, the result is that the cell has a high negative surface charge.

---

[12] This is a standard experimental tumor found in cancer laboratories all over the world. It was started by Paul Ehrlich more than sixty years ago. The cells are generally freely suspended in the peritoneal fluid (in the abdomen) of the experimental animal.

[13] Readers whose knowledge of organic chemistry and physics is scanty, or even non-existent, are urged to grit their teeth and bravely carry on through the next few pages. The effort will be well worthwhile for what is unfolding here is a marvelous mystery. The key phrase is *a high negative surface charge.*

"Unfortunately, you can only measure the surface charge of cells readily if they are blood cells, or similar to ascites cells (because they must be able to float freely in the liquid in which they are suspended), and it is difficult to measure the electrical charge on trophoblast because the cell is relatively fixed in the tissues, and if you try to break up the cells in order to separate them you are likely to damage the surface.

"It is known, though, that leukemic white cells tend to have a higher negative charge than the corresponding normal white cells, and if we reduce the negative charge they will clump together. Probably the negative charge is *of necessity* high on circulating cells—it's one of the means whereby they remain separate, and if the net negative charge is reduced the cells tend to stick together. This aspect has been fairly intensively studied by L. Weiss at Roswell Park and by E. J. Ambrose and his co-workers here, and it is known that there are several forces which tend to draw small particles *together*, whether they are blood cells, tumor cells, or any other type of cell: van der Waals' forces of interaction, hydrogen bonds, dipole interactions, and various others—"

I said, perhaps a little unhappily, "Here you get into physics."

"This involves the physics of the contacts of small particles," Dr. Bagshawe said, an apologetic note in his voice. "I'm not a physicist. One just has to pick up a few fragments about it. . . . But according to Professor Ambrose, the only force known to *repel* cells is the electrostatic negative charge. As everybody knows, similar charges repel. If the negative charge on the surface of two opposed cells is comparatively high, the two cells when they come to rest will be relatively far apart because of the force of repulsion. If the negative charge is smaller, the two cells will tend to come closer together."

Dr. Bagshawe now branched off into immunology and described a simple procedure which serves to explain what happens in the first stage of a graft rejection.

"We can construct a small chamber with walls that are pierced by microscopic pores that allow non-cellular substances to enter but are too small to permit the entry of cells.

If we put a piece of foreign tissue into this chamber and transplant it into an experimental animal, the foreign tissue will grow quite happily inside the chamber—graft rejection doesn't take place. However, if we make the pores big enough to allow cells to enter the chamber, the foreign tissue will be destroyed by graft rejection. There is a lot of evidence of a similar kind to suggest that in the rejection process some sort of *direct cell to cell contact* must occur; and the evidence also suggests that the host cell which makes the direct contact with the foreign tissue is a white blood cell—the lymphocyte.

"What the lymphocyte does when it establishes contact is not clear. Some message goes back to the lymph gland in the area, with the result that there is a proliferation of lymphocytes in the lymph gland. These are specialized lymphocytes, which can then move in to attack the graft; and there may also be a secondary process in which antibodies are produced.

"The first step in recognizing the foreign tissue, then," said Dr. Bagshawe, "is the cell to cell contact. Once this occurs, the whole process of immune responses goes into action. But if the lymphocyte (which itself has a fairly high negative surface charge) opposed a cell with a high negative surface charge, then it might not be possible for the lymphocyte to make the appropriate contact."

And if the appropriate contact were not made, no message would go back to the nearest lymph gland, no specialized lymphocytes would be produced to attack the foreign tissue (whatever it happened to be) and it would have freedom to flourish without intervention by the host.

"Various bits of evidence," in Dr. Bagshawe's words, seemed to support the idea that the substance found on the surface of trophoblast (now known by a variety of names: the layer of Nitabuch, fibrinoid, mucopolysaccharide) played a key role in this phenomenon whereby lymphocytes were unable to make direct contact with foreign tissue cells. It has long been known, for example, that foreign tissues—even human tumors —can be grown in the cheek pouch of hamsters, which has a dense layer of mucopolysaccharide. Cartilage can be transplanted readily from one person to another, and cartilage has a very high content of mucopolysaccharide.

It was also established in various ways that antigens were present on trophoblast, and that the antigens were *masked* by the surface layer of mucopolysaccharide. As long as this layer was intact, the trophoblast would not be attacked by the mother's lymphocytes. When this layer was removed (by treatment with an enzyme called neuraminidase) lymphocytes from the mother attacked and destroyed her own trophoblast. Controlled experiments seemed to provide conclusive evidence that the masking of antigens by the layer of Nitabuch, or fibrinoid, or mucopolysaccharide—whatever you called the substance—effectively prevented the direct cell to cell contact between lymphocytes and foreign tissue.

One vital result of this masking process, of course, is that the mother's lymphocytes do not attack the embryo in her womb; and because of this physiological mechanism—consisting merely of a microscopic layer of pinkish staining material—mammalian life can come into existence.

"And this would also seem to be related to choriocarcinoma," Dr. Bagshawe said. "The choriocarcinoma cells, also, have a surface layer of mucopolysaccharides, similar to normal trophoblast, and this might account for the failure of the host to reject the tumor.

"Perhaps of even greater interest is the possibility that the same type of mechanism may exist in other types of cancer cells."

What, precisely, is this mechanism?

It is simply the high electronegative charge produced by (or resulting from) the coating of mucopolysaccharides around the cell. The lymphocytes, which have the duty of destroying foreign cells (and perhaps all cells which jeopardize the life of the individual) also have a high electronegative charge. *But negative charge repels negative charge,* and thus the lymphocyte cannot make the direct contact necessary to identify the foreign tissue. "You know how it is when you have two magnets suspended by pieces of string," Dr. Bagshawe said: "They'll wobble close to each other, but they're unable to touch, to make contact."

The ultimate and deadly biological consequence is that in these circumstances the foreign tissue can grow freely, secure from intervention by the host's immune defenses.

I said to Dr. Bagshawe, "When I read your communication in *The Lancet* it seemed to me that you and Dr. Currie had established a sort of hopeless situation—a natural phenomenon which cannot be overcome. This is one of the most elementary laws of Nature—similar electrical charges repel each other; thus tumor cells with high negative surface charges will repel lymphocytes with high negative surface charges. Is there any possibility of changing the polarity of the charges so that the lymphocytes could reach the tumor?"

Dr. Bagshawe replied, "I want to stress that this is still only a hypothesis. It seems fairly certain that there is something which interferes with the recognition of foreignness of some tumor cells and probably also of the trophoblast, something on the surface of these cells. . . . Certainly, one can alter the surface charge by means of enzymes, by the use of *electropositively* charged substances, but there are difficulties about doing this in practice. For instance, there is no question at all of injecting these substances into patients with tumors because the first effect they'd have would be to reduce the surface charge on the circulating (blood) cells and on the substances lining the blood vessels, and this would produce clumping of cells and thrombosis.

"But there are other possibilities, such as removing pieces of tumor, perhaps producing suspensions of the cells from these tumors, then reducing the surface charge and injecting them back into the patient so that they can then be recognized as foreign cells. In this way one might be able to initiate a strong immune response.

"It's still uncertain whether the immune response would be adequate to control or to produce regression of an established tumor. From some of the work we've done in experimental situations it looks as if this might be the case (the tumor can be controlled); but I think it would be quite wrong to say that this would necessarily occur in the human situation. . . .

"There are three aspects to the immune response. The first is recognizing the enemy; the second is building up forces on a big enough scale to attack; the third is carrying out the attack effectively. But it appears that certainly in the fetal-maternal situation, possibly in some tumors or in all tumors, recognition—the first prerequisite—can't occur because the enemy is behind a smokescreen. If we can get rid of the smokescreen, recognition can occur and the subsequent stages of the immune response can take place."

The hypothesis remains to be proven. But it is backed by a formidable amount of evidence; it is simple; and (a factor which is not scientifically valid but has its own particular validity) it is intellectually satisfying. It is, furthermore, a superb example of the process of cancer research in action. It may not help the cancer patient today; it may do a great deal for him tomorrow.

7

The Hidden Toxins

ELEVEN

"... A New Kingdom of Medicine"

The Hotel New Otani is one of the most impressive hotels in Japan and thus, by extension, in the world. It was built for the Olympic Games of 1964, and structurally it consists of three tall, slab-like wings, each pointing in a different direction. Superimposed on the three wings is an immense circular restaurant which revolves slowly, providing its patrons with a superb panoramic view of Tokyo—unfortunately, from the air, a rather drab city. The grounds are charming, bubbling with tiny streams and waterfalls, shaded by graceful trees, ornamented with mysterious rocks and stones. The Japanese order these things very well. In a cramped, airless little room of this luxurious hotel (reserved, presumably, for scientists, writers, and other third-class citizens) I sat one Saturday morning conversing with Dr. John Higginson, and heard him talk about the nitrosamines and the aflatoxins—obscure substances that may influence the destinies of a great many human beings.

John Higginson is tall, dark, highly strung. In some ways his career resembles that of another Irishman, Denis Burkitt. He was born in Belfast, received his medical degree in Dublin, then studied pathology in Glasgow and South Africa. At the age of thirty-six he became Associate Professor of Pathology at the University of Kansas Medical School; and three years later he was appointed American Cancer Society Professor of Geographical Pathology at the University of Kansas. When I met him in Tokyo he had been, for about three months, Director of a newly-formed organization, the International Agency for Research on Cancer—so new, indeed, that although its headquarters were in Lyons, France, any building to house the headquarters was still nonexistent. We were talking about his plans for the agency when the nitrosamines[1] and aflatoxins entered the conversation.

This chapter, by its nature, must be full of digressions, and it is worth digressing briefly at this point to tell the story of how Dr. Higginson's agency came into existence because, apart from everything else, it is an excellent example of the emotionalism that has harassed cancer scientists for more than a quarter of a century.

At the end of World War II many intelligent, well-meaning people were apt to declare that if the huge sums of money spent by the United States to develop the atom bomb had been spent on a crash program of cancer research, the cure for cancer would quickly have been found and, instead of producing a hideous weapon which might lead to the total extinction of all life on this planet, mankind would at last possess the means to overcome its most fearsome enemy. Television addicts may occasionally see an old motion picture with Gary Cooper in the role of a scientific genius, stating this case in a bitter and accusing voice. "We could have the cure for cancer in a year," he announces grimly.

The belief in a crash program to solve each and all of our ills dies hard. The truth is, a cancer research program in 1945 on the gigantic scale of the Manhattan Project would have been largely a waste of money and effort. Medical science was not ready for a program of this kind. The roadways had not

---

[1] For those who have not encountered it before, this is a somewhat tricky word. It is pronounced *nitros-a-meens*. Aflatoxin is fairly straightforward.

been laid out, the road signs were not up. Years of unspectacular spadework remained to be done.[2]

One of these periodic outbursts of emotion came to a head on November 8, 1963, when "thirteen distinguished French intellectuals" (the information comes from *The International Journal of Cancer*, which does not name the thirteen; one of them, of course, was Jean-Paul Sartre) "signed an appeal to General de Gaulle, President of the French Republic, requesting that a minute fraction—one half of one per cent—of the military budgets of the United States of America, the USSR, Great Britain and France, be made available to finance cancer research (and research on other chronic diseases)."

One cannot avoid an uneasy feeling that General de Gaulle must have been delighted at being presented with such a splendid scheme for embarrassing his former friends and allies. For, technically, it was unworkable. It represented the kind of mushy idealism that one thought had gone out of fashion with Esperanto. Nonetheless, since other nations were certain to reject the scheme General de Gaulle could well afford to support it, thereby gaining acclaim as the champion of suffering humanity.

Accordingly, on November 9 (*one day after the thirteen intellectuals presented their appeal*) "General de Gaulle endorsed the proposal and asked his Minister of Health to take all necessary steps in the matter. In December, 1963, and again in February, 1964, delegates of the Federal Republic of Germany, Italy, the United Kingdom and the United States of America met in Paris at the invitation of the French government."

[2] R. J. C. Harris, in his excellent handbook, *Cancer* (Pelican Books, 1964), has stated the case admirably: "It has frequently been suggested that cancer research would proceed much faster if very large sums of money were made available for it. The argument is often taken from applied science rather than pure. If you know how to separate U_{235} from U_{238} and it will cost, for example, $100,000,000 to build a plant on a sufficient scale to separate enough to explode over Hiroshima and Nagasaki, then you must have your dollars if you want your bomb. On the other hand, if you are not sure how to achieve your result, too much money is just an embarrassment." Dr. Harris is himself the head of a large and highly respected cancer research institute.

The result could have been anticipated. *At the conclusion of the first meeting* "it was clear that the French concept of a massive assault on cancer could not be supported."

The language of diplomacy does not conceal the impression that at least some of the delegates must have found the brainwave of the thirteen intellectuals fairly close to lunacy. We can assume that a couple of years (at least) would be spent in preparations for launching the scheme—signing agreements, obtaining suitable quarters, assembling a staff, acquiring equipment. The United States of America would then be obliged to contribute half of one per cent of a military budget of approximately sixty billion dollars—that is, three hundred million dollars; the USSR would be obliged to contribute an amount not substantially smaller and perhaps substantially larger; the United Kingdom would add some thirty million, France would add about the same. Approximately seven hundred million dollars *per year* (more than six times the total budget of the United Nations) would be available to be spent —by whom? On precisely what? Under whose control? Under what guarantees?

The proposal was not rejected completely. After a certain amount of infighting and after several somewhat acrimonious discussions, the International Agency for Research on Cancer came into existence in May, 1965, supported by eight governments and occupying a niche of its own in the World Health Organization. The annual contribution of each member country is not one half of one per cent of its military budget, but the modest sum—perhaps rather too modest—of $150,000.[3]

[3] Opinions about this curious episode remain divided even today. In Washington, a scientist who had been a representative of the American government throughout the negotiations told me, "We were opposed to the original French proposal because we already had an extensive foreign grant program, and we preferred to determine ourselves where, and to whom, our foreign grants should be made, rather than leave the decisions to the international agency. . . . But some countries in Western Europe, which receive insufficient research funds from their own governments, hoped that if the United States and Russia put up hundreds of millions of dollars, their chances of getting funded would be improved. The amount of money would really have been staggering."

On the other hand, the counterpart of this scientist in London told

At 2:30 in the afternoon of this particular Sunday an event of considerable importance was due to take place in Tokyo: the opening of the Ninth International Cancer Congress by Dr. Tomizo Yoshida, in the presence of Their Imperial Highnesses Crown Prince Akihito and Crown Princess Michiko. The elaborate ceremonies (which included the staging of a Nō play) were to take place in yet another giant building put up specially for the 1964 Olympics, the Nippon Budôkan. About forty-five hundred cancer scientists from sixty-three countries[4] would be in the audience; on the platform with the Crown Prince and the Crown Princess there would be a select group of renowned cancer scientists, including Dr. Higginson who was to make a brief speech.

One of the Tokyo newspapers had appeared that morning with the headline: *Eyes of World Are On Cancer Congress;* and sitting in the small room in the Hotel New Otani I could not resist quoting it to Dr. Higginson. The implication of the headline, of course, was that the world would be awaiting the announcement of spectacular advances—why, otherwise, should so many cancer experts come all this way?—and I wondered if, in fact, anything of a spectacular nature might emerge.

Dr. Higginson deplored the public's hope for spectacular discoveries. He said, "Major breakthroughs were quite possible fifty or sixty years ago, such as—for example—the discovery of the first arsenical preparation that killed the pathogenic agent of syphilis in man. Penicillin was another breakthrough, al-

---

me, "This was a wonderful scheme which was castrated by governments. I hope it will still progress and do well, but it is just a shadow of what it should have been. . . . They didn't have the guts to support it fully, and they didn't have the guts to withdraw from it. . . . It could have been a most dramatic and worthwhile thing on the highest level. I think political considerations came into it very early, and that is what finished it." This authority did not indicate precisely who *they* were.

[4] This figure was later revised to sixty-two. Cancer scientists from Communist China had been expected to attend the Congress, having filed application forms; but I was told that none arrived because they had been denied permission to travel—a tragic example of bureaucratic monomania.

though we shouldn't forget that it took ten or fifteen years for its potential to be recognized. Theoretically, the atomic bomb became possible after the work of Fermi and Nils Bohr in the early 30s, but again its development only came with the outbreak of a world war and the pooling of the scientific resources of several Western nations.

"So, roughly, over a period of about fifty years we had a number of exciting discoveries. We have had a similarly exciting period during the last fifteen years as we have learned more about the cancer cell. But actually all that we are beginning to do is develop the tools which enable us to break into the cell in a way that was not possible earlier. Every advance we make in this process is itself a major accomplishment, because of the difficulties involved; yet the actual gain, when it is presented to the public, doesn't appear spectacular. In practice, we can say that each advance is another brick in an archway and none of us can say how many bricks that archway is going to require.

"I think there are going to be many major discoveries in the next five years. The trouble is, in cancer, each discovery throws open the door to a much vaster world, as it were, rather than to a definite summit. . . . It is now no longer possible for any one individual to cover more than a small field. One of the dangers—and it is becoming a very serious danger—is that our scientists come to know more and more about less and less. Cross-fertilizing between the different disciplines, therefore, is tremendously important; and large cancer congresses such as this one—where scientists can meet each other and there is an opportunity to exchange ideas—make cross-fertilization a possibility."

On a variety of other subjects Dr. Higginson was equally lucid and enlightening. He spoke as a scientist of wide experience; and very clearly, as he stated earlier, he had no use for the dramatic, the sensational, or the spectacular.

It is not surprising, consequently, that nothing of a dramatic, sensational, or spectacular nature emerged until the interview was almost over; and what struck me as a bombshell went off in response to a simple, rather pedestrian question, when I asked Dr. Higginson if he could tell me something about the work he would be doing in his new agency.

His immediate task, he explained, was to obtain a first-class staff—by no means easy. "Then," he went on, "the first function of the agency will be to interest itself in all aspects of the environmental biology of human cancer. In other words, there is a very definite feeling among the governments who have sponsored the agency that it should pay special attention to human cancer, that there is already enough emphasis at the present time on some of the more esoteric aspects of research but all too often practical studies in human cancer are being ignored.

"Secondly, we will be making studies of, for example, cancer of the esophagus, which is suddenly becoming pandemic (that is, affecting a large proportion of the population) in parts of Africa; cancer of the liver in Africa; and other forms of cancer where international collaboration is clearly required.

"We shall also have laboratory studies, where necessary, to determine particular aspects of carcinogenesis (the origin, or production, of cancer) which are still unclear.

"For instance, we have a great deal of doubt about the danger of 'one dose' carcinogens, and we want to know what the theoretical implications are. We know experimentally that certain substances—which may be significant in human cancer— will cause cancer after one dose; and this is, really, a very considerable problem."

"Substances that will cause cancer *after one dose?*"

"Oh, yes," Dr. Higginson said. "It's becoming quite alarming."

"Can you name any of these substances?"

"I can name two," Dr. Higginson replied. "One is a group of substances called the nitrosamines. The world expert on this subject is Professor Druckrey. You can produce cancer[5] with a single dose of a nitrosamine. The alarming thing is that there is a possibility that nitrosamines may form in foodstuffs such as cereals, and the question is now being asked whether

[5] The reference here, of course, is to producing cancer in experimental animals.

these substances may be involved in certain areas where pockets of cancer (that is, an unusually high incidence or concentration of the disease in a particular district) seem to arise."

Dr. Higginson continued, "The second of these substances—quite different from the nitrosamines—is aflatoxin; and aflatoxin is probably one of the hottest subjects in cancer research at the moment."

The leads—as Dr. Sidney Farber remarked on another occasion—had to be followed up. First, the nitrosamines.

One takes the TransEuropean express in Basel, crossing from Switzerland into southwest Germany. The trip lasts about half an hour. Vineyards cover the steep mountainsides, and occasionally one sees charming little farmhouses and churches sparkling in the air as if they had just been dry-cleaned. Freiburg im Breisgau is the chief city of this region. It is the gateway to the Black Forest, it is famous for its twelfth-century cathedral and its university, and it is known to all cancerologists as the location of the department headed by Professor Dr. H. Druckrey, officially designated Forschergruppe Praeventivmedizin am Max Planck Institut für Immunbiologie.

Professor Druckrey is tall, courteous, soft-spoken. At one point he described himself as a pharmacologist and toxicologist—that is (a) a scientist who deals with the sources, chemistry and action of drugs in general, and (b) a scientist who deals with the sources, chemistry and action of poisons, and their antidotes. His scientific qualifications, a little unexpectedly, go hand in hand with creativity, with imagination, with poetic insight. And it is important to make clear at the outset that all the threads of this conversation are significant. Everything has a point, everything leads to an inevitable conclusion which is best described as, not ominous or threatening, but awesome.

He began with the observation that the most striking feature of the carcinogenic process is that like the process of aging it is irreversible. It is the sum of many separate effects, and it occurs only after a latent period (or induction time) of many decades in human beings—or, to be exact, after a certain *percentage* of the individual's life expectancy.

He then went on to point out that with the proper approach it is possible to make comparisons between human beings and experimental animals—for example, rats.

The life span of a human being is of the order of sixty to seventy years. For the rat it is of the order of two years. These periods are comparable: one year in the life of a rat would equal thirty to thirty-five years in the life of a human being. Animal experimentation can be extremely valuable, therefore, because the same things that happen in human beings in thirty, forty or fifty years can be studied in rats over a greatly reduced period of a year or two.

But one of the greatest difficulties in animal experiments has been that researchers could only produce certain forms of skin cancer or liver cancer in rats and mice, *which do not play a role in human cancer.* "The human cancers," Professor Druckrey said, "are entirely different. We have cancer of the esophagus, cancer of the lungs, cancer of the brain, and so on; and these have never (or only very rarely) been produced in experimental animals."

For this reason, one of the first tasks he and his colleagues set themselves was to study whether or not it was possible to produce in experimental animals the same types of cancer that are common in human beings.

"To control a disease we first need an adequate fund of knowledge about it," he said. "This means that we must be able to produce the disease in animals regularly, so that we can explore its laws and mechanisms. We can then try to *cure* the disease in experimental animals, and we can learn how to *prevent* the disease by eliminating the factors that cause it. This approach has been used to control many infectious diseases: for example, we still do not have a drug that is effective against cholera, yet it has been possible to eliminate cholera in many parts of the world by prevention only.

"I am deeply convinced that many diseases of unknown cause are, in fact, caused by toxic substances with irreversible effects (specially on the genetic materials of the cell).

"I am also deeply convinced that when we have learned more about these toxic substances and their mechanism of action, and when we have learned how to eliminate them, we will have opened the way to a new era in preventive medicine which will provide mankind with even greater benefits than the prevention of infectious diseases. *A new kingdom of medicine lies before us.* What we are now doing is the pioneer work, and it has already proven of value in the control of certain toxic food additives and the elimination (in some places) of certain air pollutants. The next generation of scientists will have the task of carrying this work further."

The first step was to learn whether it was possible to produce cancer experimentally in *all* organs, and not merely in a limited number of sites. Other researchers, for the most part, had done their work on mice. In 1937, Professor Druckrey selected the rat as his experimental animal, and after inbreeding for more than a hundred brother-sister generations he developed strains of rats which, in his words, "are like a precision instrument to us. They are like twins. I have known them now for 30 years; I can speak to them, I can put my hand between the teeth of any one of my 8,000 rats and they will only be pleased."

In due course, as he planned, he was able to produce malignant tumors in practically all organs of his rats. *Most important, this could be done in a very specific way.* One substance might produce cancer of the esophagus; and no matter how the animal received it—by subcutaneous injection (that is, under the skin) or by inhalation (in the atmosphere it breathed) or in its food—the result would always be cancer of the esophagus.[6]

[6] I am indebted to Professor Dr. H. Hamperl, who explained the situation more fully to me during a most helpful interview in the Pathological Institute of the medical school of the University of Bonn. Professor Hamperl has been working closely with Professor Druckrey. He said, "It started as a chance finding by an Englishman, P. N. Magee. . . . Then Druckrey continued the research, and his chemist produced a large number of different nitrosamines with different chemical struc-

"This means," Professor Druckrey said, "that cancer of the esophagus is not necessarily caused by something we swallow. It may be caused by something rubbed into the skin—a cosmetic, for example. It means, too, that even air pollution can lead to cancer of the esophagus.

"A similar substance given, let us say, intravenously, will specifically cause cancer of the lung. *Only* of the lung. If we make a small change in the molecule of the substance we will get, not cancer of the lung but cancer of the brain—which, like cancer of the esophagus, has never before been produced experimentally. Furthermore, this cancer of the brain will show clinical signs[7] in the rat strikingly like those in human beings."

"What is the induction time of these tumors in the rat?"

Professor Druckrey replied, "About 300 days—less than half its life span. You may calculate that 120 days in a rat corresponds to ten years in man; 300 days in a rat would mean an induction time in human beings of about twenty-five years."

More than sixty-five different nitrosamine compounds have been investigated by the group at Freiburg. "They are synthesized here," Professor Druckrey explained, "because they are

---

tures—small modifications of the molecule here and there. We found that these substances will seek out a special organ. If you give the animal one modification it will get cancer of the liver. If you give it a different modification it will get a brain tumor. It is like aiming a gun: you can fire a bullet at this organ or at that organ, according to the nitrosamine you use. . . . At least, for research purposes it is very useful to have a substance with which you can produce a tumor in a specific organ. Previously, it was almost impossible to produce experimental tumors of the esophagus, for example. How would you do it? You cannot paint the esophagus. If the carcinogen is in the food it passes through the esophagus too quickly, and nothing happens. But now we can get tumors of the esophagus, if we want them, in about 90 per cent of the rats who are given these special substances. If you need tumors of the brain, you make a slight modification, and this only affects the brain. Another modification will work only on the eyelid, and another modification will work only on the ear."

[7] In a strict medical sense, a *sign* is any abnormality indicative of a disease observed by a physician (or research scientist) in the course of an examination. A *symptom* is any abnormality indicative of disease experienced by the patient. Thus it has been said that symptoms are what the patient complains of, and signs are what the doctor fails to observe.

not available commercially, and we send them (like our rats) to research institutes all over the world."

"Are nitrosamines found in any natural state?"

"Yes. They may occur as a result of simple chemical reactions in growing plants, and in some foodstuffs. About five years ago, Professor Ender of Oslo, Norway, was asked to investigate widespread deaths of minks on mink farms. Sheep were affected in the same way, and so were foxes. The cause was found to be herring meal, which is produced in Norway on a very large scale and is a cheap food material. Professor Ender found nitrosamines in some of the herring meal, and this was the toxic agent in the death of these animals."[8]

But the danger is rather more immediate than the poisoning of minks. In certain areas of the Transkei in South Africa, specially the regions of Umtata, Butterworth and East London, cancer of the esophagus has become very common among the Bantu; and here we have some of those "pockets of cancer" to which Dr. Higginson referred earlier. "Before 1950," Professor Druckrey said, "this malignancy was practically nonexistent in the Bantu. Now about 20 per cent of all hospitalized Bantu have the notorious *black spider*, as they call cancer of the esophagus." The cause has not yet been found, but there is a possibility that a deficiency of molybdenum in the soil of these regions may facilitate the formation of nitrosamines; and some of Professor Druckrey's rats with an established susceptibility to cancer of the esophagus have been sent to South Africa to help in experimental studies of the problem. The raised incidence of nasopharyngeal cancer in the Kikuyu of the hilly

[8] This (as Professor Druckrey pointed out) is similar to the aflatoxin story, which is told in the next chapter. There is no chemical relationship, however, between nitrosamines and aflatoxin.

In 1961, the same situation occurred in Britain. According to a report in the British Journal of Pathology and Bacteriology (Carter, Percival and Roe), minks on a number of fur farms died unexpectedly of severe liver damage, and subsequent investigation showed that the epidemic coincided with the incorporation of a consignment of Norwegian herring meal in the animals' food. In some circumstances, a nitrosamine known as DMNA (dimethylnitrosamine) may be formed when herring are processed to produce meal, and minks seem to be unusually sensitive to this toxin.

regions of Kenya may possibly result from exposure to nitrosamines produced by the burning of cattle excreta in their unventilated huts. We have to recognize, though, that the danger is widespread, and that it exists in more highly developed areas of the world, for the *combination* of various chemicals discharged into the atmosphere by industrial plants may result in the production of nitrosamines and other carcinogens—a dismaying example of how man may induce cancer in man. We see great steel and concrete buildings in our cities blackened and corroded by atmospheric pollutants; is it surprising that the lungs of city dwellers are blackened and damaged by the same pollutants? Most of the fish and most of the plant life in our rivers have been exterminated by industrial wastes: some of these toxins must inevitably reach man. We have been terribly careless, terribly indifferent, about our relationship to the natural world. We have set ourselves above it, as if it were ours, to dispose of as we please. We have given ourselves permission to dump our refuse wherever it suits our convenience; but we have forgotten one of Nature's immutable laws—to each action there is *inevitably* and *always* an equal and opposite reaction.

Recently, Professor Druckrey has been working with other compounds, notably a group of very potent carcinogens called hydrazines; and again, as with the nitrosamines, he found striking organotropic effects (which means that a particular compound will have an affinity for, or seek out, specific organs). One of these compounds regularly and specifically produced colon and rectum cancer in rats—the first time this had been accomplished—identical in every respect to colon and rectum cancer in human beings. With slight changes in the compound's molecular structure different forms of cancer were produced: of the brain, of the mammary glands, of the liver, and even leukemia.

There are substances, then, which will specifically produce cancer only in one organ; and in no others. There are substances which will produce cancer in two, three, or four organs; but invariably in the same organs and no others. A knowledge of the mechanisms involved in this specificity may be of the utmost importance in the development of chemotherapy—as Dr. Sidney Farber termed it, "the chemotherapy of tomorrow, chemotherapy with intelligence."

"In the future—that is, in ten or perhaps twenty years," Professor Druckrey said, "we will learn how to produce a drug which acts specifically to cure cancer of the lung; another drug specifically to cure cancer of the prostate gland; another specifically to cure cancer of the liver; and so on. The very concept of chemotherapy implies specificity. Nobody would think of using the same drug to cure tuberculosis *and* typhoid *and* syphilitic infections. You need different drugs. The same is true in cancer chemotherapy: we must develop *organ specific* drugs.

"But in order to develop this kind of specific cancer chemotherapy, you must have the proper subjects on which to carry out your tests. You require experimental animals with cancer of the esophagus, cancer of the ovaries, cancer of the mammary glands, cancer of the lungs. That is the only way you can study the therapeutic effects of your drugs.

"At the present time[9] the chemotherapy development program of the National Cancer Institute utilizes a screening system of different tumors which occur by chance in mice and rats. But what we require is a systematic approach; and this means we must have lung cancer in the screening program, we must have mammary cancer in the screening program, we must have all types of leukemia in the screening program, we must have cancer of the esophagus, of the liver, of the bladder. It is essential to produce all these types of cancer in experimental animals in order to carry out your chemotherapeutic studies. I don't know when it will come, but it *will* come, because it is indispensable."

Finally, Professor Druckrey went on to discuss some of the problems of carcinogenesis—that is, the induction of can-

[9] This interview was held in Freiburg on January 3, 1968.

cer; and now we arrive at the "one dose" carcinogens, which Dr. John Higginson described so vividly.

For a number of reasons, Professor Druckrey and his colleagues had come to the conclusion that carcinogenesis is more likely to occur when the genetic material in the cells of an individual (a human being or a rat) are highly active. The time when the greatest activity takes place, of course, is during prenatal development—before birth.

"Therefore," Professor Druckrey said, "we administered certain carcinogenic substances to pregnant rats *only once*." He repeated this so that there could be no mistake: "Only one dose. A single dose only."

The result was that *all the offspring* died of cancer at ages corresponding to 10 to 50 years in human beings. Long after they were born, the animals developed cancers of types that had not previously been induced in experimental animals—cancers of the nervous system, of the brain, and of the spinal cord.

I asked, "What were the substances that produced these malignancies?"

"One was methyl-nitroso-urea—a compound every chemist is working with. We could inject these compounds; we could give them by the oral route (in the rats' food), and the result was always the same. The result was the same even if the rats inhaled the compounds, and this means that air pollution may contribute to cancer when any of these substances is present.

"We began with high doses. Then, step by step, we gave smaller and smaller doses. We have now found that a single dose as small as 0.3 of a milligram, given to a pregnant rat, is sufficient to induce cancer in the progeny." Again Professor Druckrey repeated his statement: "A single dose of *0.3 of a milligram*."[10]

He went on, "The cause of cancer, therefore, is not necessarily found in post-natal life—after birth. We are highly susceptible during the period of development *before* birth,

---

[10] An exceedingly minute amount: approximately 1/100,000 of an ounce, considerably less than a grain of sugar.

particularly—as our experiments showed—to the induction of cancer of the nervous system, which is one of the most common of childhood cancers.

"It is terrible to learn that such a small dose can have these effects. The dose is too small to produce symptoms of any change in the mother. The rats are born—apparently—completely normal. Nevertheless, we know they will die of cancer. We know what type of cancer they will have. We know when they will die."

"How long does the process take?"

"As a rule, between 150 and 250 days. But some of our rats now live for only 40 days, and others live as long as 600 days."

Professor Druckrey proceeded to explain some of the implications of these experiments. "In a human being, a very small dose of one of these substances might work so slowly that it would take a thousand years for a cancer to be produced. Since the lifetime of a human being is much less than a thousand years the cancer would have no chance to develop. But there is one exception to this rule, and it relates to the germ cells (the ova, or egg cells in women, and sperm cells in men). If the carcinogen affects the germ cells, then it may be carried over from one generation to the next; and that is what we are now studying. We are giving extremely small doses to pregnant rats, insufficient to cause cancer during their life span; and we are giving the same dose to the next generation, and the next, and so on; and we are waiting to see what will happen.

"But we do know this: to produce cancer of the nervous system in adult rats we require a certain quantity (150 milligrams per kilogram body weight) of this carcinogenic substance, methyl-nitroso-urea. In prenatal life, before the rat is born, the dose required is one-hundredfold smaller. In other words, the susceptibility in prenatal life is one hundred times greater than it is in an adult.

"That is why I warned the Director-General of the World Health Organization that in judging the so-called margin of safety (relating to the hazards of carcinogens) we must bear in mind pregnant women, the children they are carrying, as well as newborn children. For," Professor Druckrey concluded, "the protection of the health of future generations is by far our most important duty."

It is good, and necessary, to know about these problems. Is there anything we can do about them?

The only answer, clearly, is to exclude certain carcinogenic substances from the human environment.

To do so, it is essential first to have a thorough understanding of their effects, and how they occur, and the full extent of the danger they pose; and this is the work that Professor Druckrey, and others, are doing so admirably.

Second, it is essential to regard the human environment—the total environment—with respect, and to cease abusing it. Whether the human race is capable of learning this simple fact remains to be seen. The evidence, at present, is not encouraging.

TWELVE

The Case of the Depraved Turkeys

The aflatoxins enter medical history in a manner that is unique. One has the sense of witnessing a happening, or a series of happenings, satirical and baffling. A considerable number of animals take part in the action, none of them the animals one customarily encounters in the experimental laboratory: turkeys, trout, pheasants, sheep; and when, ultimately, human beings appear they are Zulus and Matabele, followed by distressed Orientals.

Turkeys were the first to come onto the scene, and the historian of this period is W. P. Blount, T.D., Ph.D., F.R.C.V.S., F.R.S.E., Director and Chief Poultry Advisor, British Oil and Cape Mills, Ltd. Early in 1961, Dr. Blount published an article entitled "Turkey 'X' Disease," in *Turkeys*, the magazine of the British Turkey Federation. This has become a classic. It opens with the innocence and skill of a mystery novel by Agatha Christie:

> The first real suspicion we had that anything might be wrong with turkeys last season was in May when there were several comments by well-known farmers that their birds were not

finding their turkey rations as palatable as usual. . . . In June there were reports from the field that young turkeys were dying in large numbers and no typical disease features were in evidence.

Dr. Blount's first direct encounter with the disease was at the beginning of July when he visited a farm in Berkshire, where about eight hundred out of a thousand young turkeys, or poults, had died within two weeks.

> They succumbed literally like flies before your eyes. . . . The birds were nearly all dull and lifeless, many being semi-comatose, and within half an hour more than a dozen others had died. Here indeed was a problem.

The problem continued to grow worse. In the middle of August, the London *Times* reported that several breeders had lost thousands of turkeys, with as many as five thousand deaths in a single flock. "Scotland Yard Forensic Laboratory is helping in the matter," the *Times* announced, "and the Animal Health Society has called a special meeting to discuss the matter." But Scotland Yard and the Animal Health Society were of no immediate help; the mystery of how this epidemic had arisen remained completely unresolved; and it was in fact so baffling to the experts that they simply labeled the sickness Turkey "X" disease and left it at that—the "X" representing an unknown factor.

For the most part, Turkey "X" disease singled out the younger turkeys. Poults under two weeks of age were not affected, as a rule, nor those over eighteen to twenty weeks. The illness was brief. Few poults survived more than a week after the first signs of the sickness became evident.

> During this time [Dr. Blount writes] the bird would lose its appetite completely, but before doing so evidence of depravity was commonplace—the poults pecking at and eating their litter, with subsequent impaction of the gizzard. . . . Lethargy was generally very marked and also a particular weakness of the wings, which could be seen hanging down on either side of the bird's body. The feathers were ruffled and in some cases broken off, or curled upwards. . . . Another of the char-

acteristics of the disease was the attitude adopted by the poults when they died. The neck would be arched and the head drawn back (opisthotonos), and the legs stretched (extended) fully backwards.

Autopsies revealed the kidneys to be congested and enlarged, and the liver sometimes displayed "pale necrotic lesions." Turkey "X" disease also attacked growing pheasants and ducklings; the pheasants developed enteritis and nephritis, while the ducklings had purple or blue discoloration of the feet and legs, a typical symptom of kidney involvement.

There were suspicions from the beginning that the birds' feed might have been poisoned, by error or deliberately, and this may very well have been one of the reasons for the entry of Scotland Yard. Testing for dangerous chemical substances and for certain specific poisons took place at many laboratories, including those at the Tropical Products Institute, in the Department of Scientific and Industrial Research, London; at the Biological Unit of the Chemical Defence Experimental Station in Porton, Wiltshire; and at the Royal Botanic Gardens, Kew. Feeds were examined for the presence of arsenic, antimony, barium, cyanides, lead, mercury, phosphorus, thallium, selenium, tungsten, zinc; for DDT and strontium 90; for digitalis, helibor (or hellebore), oleander, squill; for croton oil (croton tyglium), jatropha curcus (which bears the physic nut, *containing a drastic oil,* says Webster, *poisonous when taken in large quantities*), and other purgative drugs; for Datura stramonium, or Jimson weed, which has narcotic and poisonous properties; for santonin, which is a poison capable of producing disturbances of the vision (not unlike those produced by some so-called psychedelic drugs) derived from the herb wormwood. There were tests for a variety of microorganisms, including Leptospira, which frequently originates as a result of contact with the urine of wild rats.

The results of all these tests were negative. Not one supplied any hint as to the cause of Turkey "X" disease.

For a while, in a manner that has become quite fashionable in recent years, suspicion turned to the United States. Turkeys are susceptible to fowl pest, or Newcastle disease, but this had been ruled out early in the epidemic. However, an American turkey disease called Bluecomb, which up to this time had not occurred in England, bore certain similarities to Turkey "X" disease. Bluecomb is caused by a virus, and it is infectious; but this, too, had to be ruled out because birds suffering from Turkey "X" disease could not be prevailed upon to transmit the disease to healthy birds. "Even," Dr. Blount comments, "if the contents of the inflamed intestines of ailing birds were fed to healthy birds, no disease followed."

There was still another new American viral disease, infectious hepatitis, which some British authorities regarded with suspicion, particularly since lesions of the liver were so often found in Turkey "X" disease post-mortems. Several research workers tried diligently to transmit the virus to turkey poults; but again the results were negative. Willy-nilly, the United States could not be incriminated, nor, at this stage could any other country, or any known infective agent, chemical, viral, or bacterial.

The birds continued to die. Once they had contracted the disease there was no way to save them. Altogether, more than a hundred thousand turkeys died before the end of August, in a period of a little less than three months.

From the beginning, a curious feature of the disease was that it appeared to be contained in an area of the southeastern counties about a hundred miles from London. No cases were reported, according to Dr. Blount, in Northern Ireland, Scotland, Wales, or the West Country; and only a few isolated or scattered cases were reported in any northern counties.

Gradually it was becoming clear that the disease was somehow related to the birds' feed. In one feeding trial there was no reaction: none of the birds died. In a second feeding trial a few birds died of causes that were not typical of Turkey "X" disease. In a third feeding trial, twenty-five out of twenty-five poults died within three weeks of receiving a certain feed; when this trial was repeated with the same feed, twenty-six out of twenty-six day-old poults died, once more, within three weeks. The available evidence showed that all the early outbreaks of Turkey "X" disease were associated with feed that had come from a London mill, but there was no evidence to show what was wrong.

The break came at the end of August. Six turkey poults in Cheshire developed Turkey "X" disease—an apparently trivial event at a time when one hundred thousand had died. But Cheshire is in the West of England, adjoining North Wales. Its county seat, Chester, is 185 miles from London. Suddenly, a completely new and separate area of investigation opened up, and at once some vital information became available.

Poultry feeds for this part of the country—those feeds, at least, that could be linked to the disease—had come from a mill in Selby, Yorkshire. The investigators could now check back and forth, from Selby to London, from London to Selby, and all they had to do was establish a common factor, a common ingredient, in the feeds manufactured by both mills.

It was quickly discovered. The ingredient common to feeds from the London mill and the Selby mill was peanut meal, or, as it is usually called in Britain, groundnut meal. More specifically, it was groundnut meal that had been imported from Brazil. Dr. Blount put it concisely:

> Wherever that ingredient (Brazilian groundnut meal) was used, Turkey "X" disease broke out; whereas when feeds were manufactured containing no Brazilian groundnut meals, or groundnut meals from other sources, no outbreaks occurred. It was as simple as that!

Dr. Blount's company had bought, in 1960, some five thousand tons of Brazilian peanut meal. Chemical analysis at the time this shipment was delivered showed that it conformed to the guarantee and it was distributed among four of the company's mills. Once this meal was implicated, more than twenty feeding trials were carried out, using various samples and percentages; and mortality, among turkey poults and ducklings, averaged 69 per cent. Precisely why Brazilian groundnut meal killed turkey poults and ducklings remained unclear.

To obtain more information Dr. Blount made a trip to Brazil where, he reported later, he found the Brazilian authorities fully cooperative. The Brazilians themselves had been experiencing problems with their livestock and poultry, and these problems were related, in a way that nobody has defined precisely, to the use of "various vegetable proteins including groundnuts." Turkeys were not involved to any great extent for the good reason that Brazil had no large-scale turkey industry.

Those vague "problems" experienced by the Brazilians had arisen "particularly in connection with the wet season's crops." Apart from this—and at the time it appeared of little significance—the Brazilians were unable to provide an explanation for the toxicity of the groundnut meal that had caused the disaster in Britain. A few suggestions were made, without any supporting evidence, that the groundnut meal might have been contaminated by insecticides, caffeine, urea, coffee beans, coffee meal, or cocoa; but none of these, on Dr. Blount's return, could be identified as the causative agent of Turkey "X" disease. An added complication was the discovery that Brazil did not stand alone as the source of toxic groundnut meal. Outbreaks of Turkey "X" disease had been reported from other countries, notably Kenya, where a number of ducklings had died as a result of eating feeds containing groundnuts from neighboring Uganda. Poultry farmers must have had the sense that a totally new pestilence had suddenly appeared on earth, coming from nowhere.

Groundnuts, or peanuts, or monkey nuts, or goobers, grow very conveniently in the ground. The plant, an annual, has two forms: a trailing vine, or a sort of bush or clump about a foot high. In either form the plant bears small yellow flowers which wither after pollination; the flower stalk then elongates and forces its way underground where the pod develops, a process called geocarpy, or earth fruiting.

The benefits which the lowly peanut brings to mankind are largely unknown and unsung. Western man eats it salted, or as peanut butter, or perhaps as peanut candy, but the weight-conscious adult tends to shun it because of its great calorific value—a pound of peanuts is almost the equivalent of a pound of bacon. Peanut oil, extracted from the seeds, or kernels, is used for margarine, cooking oil, soap, and numerous industrial purposes. More than three hundred uses for the peanut were in fact invented by the great American Negro agriculturalist, George Washington Carver, and for decades this has been praised as one of his major contributions toward improving the economy of the South.

For use in animal feeds the peanut kernels are generally ground into a meal and added in proportions that vary from 2.5 per cent to about 20 per cent. This is not merely a matter of making use of a cheap natural product. Nearly half the total substance of the kernel—48 per cent, to be precise—is protein, an unusually high proportion; and the nuts also supply valuable amounts of vitamins, principally the B complex, and minerals.

Because of its high protein content the peanut has become in recent years vitally important as a food supplement. It is invaluable in the treatment of kwashiorkor, a disease of children that is almost endemic in underdeveloped countries where infants are weaned on starchy paps and do not receive an adequate supply of proteins or essential vitamins. The appearance of these children is distressing beyond words. A year old child has the sunken cheeks and the anxious eyes of an old person approaching death.[1] A protein diet based on flour made from peanuts, with the addition of skim or half-cream milk, will quickly bring that child back to life.

[1] This was written before kwashiorkor became all too familiar as a result of the terrible events in Biafra. No animal is as relentlessly cruel and vicious as man.

The next installment of the story of Turkey "X" disease must have come as a considerable shock to a number of people whose training enabled them to grasp its implications. We now begin to move away from the rather confining landscape of turkeys and peanuts. We are a little closer to home, in more familiar country.

On December 16, 1961, two communications appeared in the British weekly magazine *Nature*, possibly the most distinguished of all scientific journals. Both dealt with the same topic and they were printed under a common heading: *Toxicity associated with Certain Samples of Groundnuts*. Some time later, a doctor writing in the *Sunday Times* made the inflammatory statement that pressure had been put on the editor of *Nature* by the British government to withhold publication of these two communications. This was denied by *Nature;* but there is no question that publication was delayed for at least a month, and possibly longer, at the government's request.

There had been some stirring developments in the laboratories in the year since Dr. Blount made his profitless trip to Brazil. One of the communications in *Nature*, from a group of scientists working at the Tropical Products Institute in London (aided by a scientist from the Ministry of Agriculture) reported that the toxic factor—in other words, the actual substance responsible for the poisoning of turkeys, ducklings, and other animals—had been extracted from Brazilian groundnut meal and concentrated 250 times. It was described as crystalline and almost colorless; in ultra-violet light it emitted a bright blue fluorescence. Twenty millionths of a gram of this fluorescent substance given orally to a day-old duckling caused death in twenty-four hours, with the characteristic liver lesions of groundnut poisoning.

There had been up to now considerable confusion about the origin of the toxic factor. Were the groundnuts producing the poison, or was it something that had been added in some way to the groundnuts? The scientists supplied the answer. "It was suspected that the toxic substance might be a fungal metabolite since a highly toxic sample of nuts which had been associated with the deaths of ducklings in Kenya was seen to be heavily contaminated with fungi. . . . After seven days at room temperature, extracts prepared from (the) visibly moldy nuts were shown to contain the blue-fluorescent material and to be lethal to day-old ducklings, producing the typical liver lesions."

This finding, that a fungus and not the peanuts or the groundnut meal produced the toxin, was critical for all future developments. The fungus was easily identified. It proved to be *Aspergillus flavus*, a common mold which is found virtually all over the world, in the air, on the ground, in stored foodstuffs. It grows rapidly in tropical and semi-tropical conditions, and given high humidity and moderately high temperature the toxin is readily produced.

The scientists from Tropical Institute ended their communication on a disturbing note: "Since strains of *Aspergillus flavus* are among the commonest fungal contaminants of cereal grains, it would not be surprising if some grain samples were found to be contaminated with the toxic metabolite described. We intend to study this problem." It was a hint that other foodstuffs contaminated by *Aspergillus flavus* might conceivably carry the potentiality of a large scale epidemic like Turkey "X" disease.

The other communication contained information that was even more disturbing. A group of scientists at the Unilever Research Laboratory in Bedford reported on a series of tests in which rats were fed contaminated groundnut meal under laboratory conditions.

Weanling rats on a diet containing 20 per cent of the Brazilian groundnut meal did not show the same quick response as turkey poults. However, the response was only delayed, and rats killed after nine weeks showed typical signs of liver damage. What followed, apparently, was rather startling. In the words of the scientists: "After six months feeding of

20 per cent Brazilian groundnut meal in a purified diet, 9 out of 11 rats developed multiple liver tumors, and 2 of these had lung metastases. This finding indicates that this diet is carcinogenic." The communication ends on a slightly bemused note: "We think that these unexpected preliminary results are of general interest."

These unexpected preliminary results were indeed of general interest, even of explosive interest. One can understand why the British government requested *Nature* to postpone publication (or, as Dr. Margerison claimed in the *Sunday Times*, to withdraw the communications). The two reports taken together might, in the words of another scientist, open up a hornets' nest. Somebody needed time to think about the implications of the findings. It might be catastrophic to spread the news that groundnuts, a popular and common foodstuff consumed by human beings as well as farm animals could, in certain conditions, cause cancer, if only (so far) in turkeys and laboratory rats. The cultivation of groundnuts is a basic industry in many parts of the world. Several of the emerging African nations are almost wholly dependent upon the production and export of peanuts and peanut oil; they have special ties to Britain, and the British government would undoubtedly be reluctant to see them severely hurt as the result of some uncommonly brilliant research by British scientists.

Meanwhile, a name was devised for the colorless, fluorescent substance. From *Aspergillus flavus* experts abstracted a few letters and coined the word *aflatoxin;* and it was found that aflatoxin was a complex of closely related compounds of which one, labeled B_1, appeared to be the most toxic. Investigators moved out to East Africa to learn how groundnuts became infected by *Aspergillus flavus* and the conditions which led to the production of aflatoxin. Perhaps to the surprise of a few government administrators the bottom did not fall out of the groundnut market after the two communications appeared in *Nature:* people went on buying and eating peanuts, the emerging nations continued to emerge, and the world went on very much as it had gone on before. Except, of course, that aflatoxin was here to stay. Aflatoxin was a carcinogen. It caused cancer in turkeys and rats.

Only in turkeys and rats?

THIRTEEN

The Case of the Tumorous Trout

To all intents and purposes, aflatoxin was a totally new discovery. The toxin produced by *Aspergillus flavus* had never before been isolated, it had certainly never been named, and presumably its existence had never even been suspected. *Aspergillus flavus* must have been manufacturing the substance for two billion years or so, but it had only now come to the attention of mankind. It is extraordinary, therefore, that in the same year there should be at least three outbreaks of aflatoxin poisoning—one in Great Britain, another in East Africa, the third in the United States.

The historians of the American episode are Dr. H. F. Kraybill and Dr. M. B. Shimkin, who, on behalf of the National Cancer Institute in Bethesda, Maryland, compiled a massive report entitled "Carcinogenesis Related to Foods Contaminated By Processing and Fungal Metabolites," which appeared in *Advances in Cancer Research*, Vol. 8, 1964. Just as the Turkey "X" disease story has a noticeably British flavor, the American story has a noticeably American flavor, opening with a scene that might have come from a Wild West movie—"the seizure of a large shipment of diseased Idaho hatchery-raised trout at a California border station."

Many of these fish were found to be suffering from hepatic carcinoma—that is, cancer of the liver.

The species involved was the rainbow trout, which is greatly esteemed both by fishermen and gourmets. Now, it is not generally realized that few wild trout remain in the United States. The point is made clearly by that splendid writer, Brian Curtis, in *The Life Story of the Fish:*

> You can no longer tell, from the fish that you take out of the water, whether you are angling in Vermont or in California; you may get eastern brook, rainbow, or European brown in either, or you may take all three fish out of the same stream. . . . Each season's fishing strips the popular streams bare. Hardly a fish is left at spawning-time to produce another generation. If it were not for the state and Federal hatcheries, there would be few trout and little trout-fishing.

Kraybill and Shimkin make the same point, with a significant addition:

> Essentially all trout populations in the United States have their origin in large federal, state or commercial hatcheries. . . . [Following the seizure in California] an epidemiological survey of state and federal hatcheries revealed the occurrence of the disease in most trout-rearing areas of the country. The prevalence was highest in healthy, fast-growing older fish, the highest rate of hepatomas being in those beyond 3 years of age. The frequency of hepatomas in some hatcheries reached levels of 50 to 75 per cent of the population.

For many years it has been known that rainbow trout appear to have a tendency to develop cancer of the liver, whereas in similar environments their cousins the brook trout and the brown trout seem to be less affected by the disease, or more resistant to it. Various suggestions have been put forward to explain this curious difference: one, that the brook and brown trout do in fact develop hepatomas at the same rate but at a later age than the rainbow trout; another, that rainbow trout raised in hatcheries tend to accumulate in the liver an excessive amount of fat which is not utilized by the fish and may in due course lead to cancerous changes. Infection by viruses has also been suggested, but healthy fish maintained in the same hatchery troughs as diseased fish do not seem to acquire hepatomas, nor have the hepatomas yielded any signs of the presence of viruses.

Since the rainbow trout is of considerable importance, intensive studies were begun after the California incident, and it soon became clear that the exorbitant rate of hepatic cancer among these fish was in some way related to diet. In past years, hatchery-raised rainbow trout had been fed a so-called wet production diet consisting of by-products obtained from packing houses and fisheries—liver, tripe, spleen, lungs and scraps of beef, hog, sheep and horse, with the viscera of carp, halibut, tuna, hake and other fish. But there had been increasing demand for this valuable animal protein to supplement livestock feeds and, as a result, the hatcheries had turned to cheaper rations in the form of dry pellets which were composed of steam or flame-dried fish meal, cottonseed meal, meat scrap meal, wheat shorts, and dried milk.

> In the early months of trout rearing, prior to release into streams [according to Kraybill and Shimkin] there is exposure to commercially prepared rations. Practically no population of trout in the United States is now reared exclusively on a so-called wild or native diet. . . . Diets of unprocessed products [wet diets] were not known to produce hepatomas. . . . The marked increase in hepatomas appeared to coincide with the utilization of dry pelleted rations in place of wet production diets in hatchery operations.

This epidemic was notably different from Turkey "X" disease in one respect: peanuts were not used in making up the dry pellet feed. Something else in the diet of the rainbow trout carried the agent responsible for the widespread liver cancer, and although the findings have not been explicitly stated and remain (perhaps deliberately) ambiguous, it seems certain that the infected component of the pellets was cottonseed meal which had been contaminated by aflatoxin, the metabolic byproduct of the ubiquitous mold *Aspergillus flavus*.

The list of animals tested for response to aflatoxin was now considerable; and a new and puzzling feature was the unpredictable variability of response. In general, younger animals were more susceptible. Among poultry, ducklings showed the greatest sensitivity, turkeys were somewhat less sensitive, followed by pheasants, pigeons and chickens. Among the larger farm animals, pregnant sows and piglets were the most sensitive; calves were fairly sensitive; but sheep showed no obvious signs of damage after being fed contaminated peanut meal for nineteen months. Rats were highly sensitive, mice considerably less sensitive. Rainbow trout, of course, were exquisitely sensitive, while catfish showed inexplicable tolerance. A disturbing observation was that the cow, normally an excellent filter, passed aflatoxin in its milk; but this occurred only under laboratory conditions, and no aflatoxin has been found in commercial milk supplies either in Britain or the United States.

A catalog of this kind cannot remain confined to the farmyard. We are led inevitably to the final, and the most pressing, questions: If man has indeed been receiving doses of aflatoxin, large or small, through one medium or another, how is *he* affected? What is *his* level of sensitivity and response? Are *his* young in general more susceptible?

We do not know the answers because, so far, we have not gathered any reliable data. We cannot feed aflatoxin to human beings and measure the various reactions: such experiments are prohibited. This, therefore, as one scientist put it, is the area of the educated guess. Anything we say in the next few pages about aflatoxin and man can only be speculative, and when we speculate about cancer we must be exceedingly cautious.

There are numerous varieties of *Aspergillus,* and several are identified by their color—among others, *Aspergillus niger,* or black; *A. ruber,* or red; *A. glaucus,* or blue green; *A. carneus,* or flesh-colored; and even *A. versicolor,* variegated or of changeable color. Some species are harmful to plants and animals. At least one, *Aspergillus fumigatus,* is responsible for a lung disease in human beings which may be extremely serious.

Aspergillus flavus is a yellow species of the mold. Given suitable conditions—nothing much more than fairly high humidity and temperature—it will grow on peas, soybean products, flour, fermenting corn, cottonseed, peanuts, rice, on dried foodstuffs and, in the laboratory, on a wide range of artificial media. In the right conditions, according to S. S. Bampton of the Tropical Products Institute, "growth of the mold and production of the toxin is extremely rapid, and groundnuts which are uncontaminated at harvesting can contain detectable toxin within 48 hours."

One has an impression of Nature like some monstrous Lucrezia Borgia preparing her malignant poison and sitting back in the shadows to await the arrival of her victims, in this instance the birds of the air and the beasts of the field. The picture is exaggerated, of course, and untrue. Aflatoxin is not part of an armory of offense or even of defense, like the venom of the cobra. It is in a sense a metabolic accident, manufactured by some strains of *Aspergillus flavus* and not by others. Furthermore, even in the tropical and semi-tropical conditions which are favorable to the growth of *A. flavus* there is no wild abundance of the fungus or its toxin. One does not see whole areas overrun by this tiny mold: it is ubiquitous but it is not a plague. In groundnut territory, for example, it singles out those pods which have been damaged during harvesting or which have been broken into by termites or other peanut-loving predators. The healthy, unbroken nuts are safeguarded by their shells, by the seed coat, and—some scientists think—by a protective factor, posssibly chemical, which repels the fungus. Nuts which have been invaded by *A. flavus* (whether the toxin has been produced or not) become shriveled and discolored, and are identified without difficulty. They are obviously "bad" nuts; and as anybody who has accidentally bitten into a bad nut knows, the taste is extremely unpleasant. One instinctively spits the fragments out, and even the tiniest piece, if it is swallowed, causes a long-lasting feeling of nausea. Most animals are sensitive and fussy, and they do not, on the whole, eat foodstuffs that have been contaminated by fungi—they even seem to have the ability to detect mold when humans cannot. It is unlikely, then, that in tropical or semi-tropical areas where food is relatively abundant, animals will consume sufficient *Aspergillus flavus* and its attendant toxin to cause the death of the animals either from general poisoning or hepatic cancer. In the strict terms of biostatistics we have no data to inform us about the menace of aflatoxin as it affects wild or undomesticated animals in the natural state; but we can reasonably assume that the creatures which exist outside man's magic circle are not in any great danger of being swept by epidemics similar to Turkey "X" disease.

For Turkey "X" disease, and rainbow trout hepatoma, and possibly a host of related but unrecognized diseases (such as an epidemic among cattle in 1883) could not have occurred without man's intervention. They were man-made epidemics, and since they are associated with cancer they assume a special importance in medical history. We can see now—because it was established only after the event—what Dr. Blount was unable to see on his visit to Brazil: those problems the Brazilian farmers experienced with their livestock "particularly in connection with the wet season's crops" were undoubtedly brought about by *A. flavus* enjoying the high humidity which suits it best. Contaminated nuts were milled indiscriminately with healthy nuts; any signs of contamination disappeared in the grinding and mixing process; and when the groundnut meal was received in Britain it passed all the then traditional chemical tests, "conforming to the guarantee," and a hundred thousand turkey poults died in three months.

Something of the same kind happened to one or more of the ingredients of the pelleted rations for rainbow trout, and something of the same kind must have happened countless times in countless different places. Although it is found in soil and will sometimes, like the field fungi, attack growing plants, *A. flavus* is essentially a storage mold, and seems to have a preference for harvested crops. Stores of groundnuts may appear to be mold-free one day, and become infected after a short period of unusual humidity. "In a few instances, bags (of groundnuts) had become accidentally wetted," writes S. S. Bampton, "and it was assumed from previous experience that these would have a high content of toxin." In the field, the yellow or blackened nuts would simply have rotted away. In storage they represented so many milligrams of a carcinogenic toxin which *might* be milled in with healthy nuts, and which *might* be consumed by ducklings, turkeys, pheasants, chickens, hogs, calves, and sheep. And, perhaps, by human beings.

The multiple epidemics of 1960 compelled the governments of many countries to move swiftly and firmly to prevent any further outbreaks. In Britain, as soon as the cause of Turkey "X" disease was known, suppliers of animal feeds adopted a voluntary code of practice which included testing all incoming consignments of groundnuts for toxicity to ducklings, known to be specially sensitive to aflatoxin. In the United States, peanut producers, shellers and processors willingly agreed to a governmental-inspired program designed to keep damaged peanuts "which may contain mold-produced toxin" from being sold as food. The Acting Deputy Administrator of the Agricultural Research Service of the U. S. Department of Agriculture, described some of the Department's activities in an interview held in Washington at the end of 1966:

> Our research program has several aspects. One is to endeavor to develop accurate and reliable methods of detecting the presence of molds, and possibly of toxins, in various agricultural products. Of course, in addition to being accurate and reliable, such methods would need to be as rapid as possible so that they can be used under normal marketing conditions. Another effort is to endeavor to develop methods for removing any toxins that might be present during processing operations, if this is possible.
>
> Yet another area of work that we have under way is trying to determine the conditions under which molds of various

kinds proliferate in agricultural products—the temperatures, the humidities, the moisture contents, the storage conditions, the handling conditions—all the factors that enter into the harvesting and storing and marketing of crops, which might in some way contribute to the development of molds. We have also done surveys to check into the incidence of molds in storage facilities in different locations. Then, we also have under way studies of the effects of toxins on different kinds of animals.

These, essentially, are the research activities the Department has initiated in the past several years in response to this problem. The United States Department of Agriculture has recognized that this research is in the public interest, that it is in the public interest to get the facts and to find out the conditions under which these substances develop and the conditions under which they can be prevented from developing; so that we can continue to insure that the foods marketed in this country are the most wholesome and the safest in the world—we have confidence in this.

Research into the contamination of agricultural products is carried out in twelve laboratories of the Agricultural Research Service at various locations. In addition, the A.R.S. has several contracts for research with other laboratories. "The research, regulatory, service, education, conservation, action, lending, and consumer programs administered by this Department would rank it as possibly the outstanding organization of its kind in the world," the Acting Deputy Administrator said on another occasion; and one cannot help being impressed.

At this interview and at other interviews in Washington, two new aspects of the aflatoxin problem were raised for discussion.

One was that numerous molds besides *Aspergillus flavus* produced toxins capable of causing cancer in animals, if not in man.

The other—obviously, more alarming—was the possibility that our great Midwestern granaries may be contaminated by *Aspergillus flavus* and other toxin-producing molds.

In the penultimate paragraph of their survey for the National Cancer Institute, Dr. Kraybill and Dr. Shimkin have something to say about the first matter:

> Estimates of the number of fungal species in nature may vary from 40,000 to 250,000. While many fungi are presumably not harmful, the striking effect of a toxin produced by one of these, aflatoxin, has stimulated some thoughts on the possible role of other mycotoxins which affect animal and human health through the induction of cancer.

Thus, in the past few years, an almost limitless field of research has opened up: the role of the metabolic by-products of about a quarter of a million different species of little known, almost invisible organisms. Aflatoxin is only the most familiar (but not necessarily the most prevalent or the most virulent) of a totally new spectrum of natural toxins. A report published by the National Cancer Institute in 1966 placed the mycotoxins at the head of a list of research projects:

> Identification of aflatoxin as a cancer-causing agent in trout has emphasized the possible role of natural products in causing cancer in man. In addition to *Aspergillus flavus*, other fungi producing toxins of potential carcinogenic significance include members of the penicillium genus. *Penicillium rubrum* is responsible for acute liver damage in animals, similar to that produced by *A. flavus*. . . . At Temple University, Philadelphia, scientists are studying dermatophytes (fungi which infect the skin) and Alternaria (a genus of fungi producing blight in many fruits, and leaf spots and black mold in many plants) which are widely distributed in nature and known to grow on tobacco. . . . At the City of Hope, Duarte, California, investigators are studying toxins produced by molds added to food by Japanese or other Asian peoples in their homeland or in this country. The Japanese Institute of Fermentation is cooperating with the City of Hope in carrying out important steps in this research.
>
> In many underdeveloped non-industrial societies, natural products such as plants, nuts, and other vegetation, have been shown in certain instances to have carcinogenic constituents. Their role in the causation of cancer is also being investigated.

Some of the issues relating to aflatoxin and food contamination were discussed in a conversation with Dr. Kenneth M. Endicott, Director of the National Cancer Institute at Bethesda, Maryland. Again,[1] the relevant section is given here verbatim:

> ENDICOTT: I think there is a big task ahead for all of us in discovering better ways of storing foodstuffs in humid climates to avoid the growth of molds. It's a fairly obvious, straightforward problem that we ought to be able to solve.
>
> Q: You have a program which is investigating the whole situation?
>
> ENDICOTT: Yes. We are supporting work on a broad front, including studies of the distribution of aflatoxins in Africa, and so on. . . . We have some collaborative programs with the Japanese Institute of Fermentation, studying the production of aflatoxin-like fermentation processes. But as far as I know, we are not collecting milk from lactating mothers in Japan; but we are in Africa. So it's a fairly extensive program.
>
> Q: I was discussing this problem with some scientists, and they came up with the startling suggestion that the Midwestern granaries [of the United States] may be infected with aflatoxin. Do you know anything of that?
>
> ENDICOTT: Well, I would be surprised if they were not. I do know that virtually all our peanut butter, on the market, contains traces of aflatoxin.
>
> Q: Is this being investigated?
>
> ENDICOTT: Oh, yes. But the amounts here are extremely minute and probably constitute no particular hazard. But that there is aflatoxin in American foodstuffs—there is no question about that. It's much worse in tropical climates because the mold grows better there.

The National Cancer Institute has no regulatory powers. That is to say, it cannot ban or seize any material which it considers to be carcinogenic. The U. S. Department of Agriculture is responsible for the inspection (for wholesomeness) of meat and poultry moving in interstate commerce; but the main burden of responsibility for the safety of the nation's food sup-

---

[1] Other points brought up in the course of this conversation appear in Chapter Two.

plies rests with the Food and Drug Administration. In an article entitled "Mycotoxins as a Food Problem" (*Cereal Science Today,* January, 1966), Dr. Daniel Banes, Deputy Director of the Bureau of Scientific Research in the Food and Drug Administration, stated with great clarity and precision how his agency stands on the subject of mycotoxin contamination:

> Many kinds of mycotoxins have long been recognized as baleful substances that must be rigorously excluded from the food supply. Moldy foods have been illegal products in interstate commerce since 1906, when the first Pure Food and Drug Act was passed. Under the present law they are among the articles that are considered adulterated because they "consist in whole or in part of any filthy, putrid, or decomposed substance," or "are otherwise unfit for food." ... Our tissue culture studies indicate that aflatoxin B_1 is a mutagenic agent, and they tend to confirm the view that this is one of the most toxic substances known. ... Because there are as yet no pharmacological data indicating a safe level of aflatoxins in man or in any laboratory test animal (except sheep) and because aflatoxins are carcinogenic, no tolerance can be set for these substances. Any demonstrable concentration of aflatoxins is proof of excessive mold contamination. ... Wherever there is a suspicion that a mycotoxin has contaminated foods, we shall develop biological and chemical tests, as specific as attainable, to determine whether contamination has occurred. If it has, we shall then proceed to remove such adulterated foods from the channels of commerce both by inducing the manufacturers to clear their own houses and by invoking the legal powers granted to us under the FD & C Act.[2] ... The task confronting cereal chemists, both inside and outside of government laboratories, is an awesome one. However, considering the progress we have made in improving food sanitation during the last fifty years, I am confident that we shall succeed in our endeavors.

Some of Dr. Banes' phrases have a Churchillian ring to them: *The task confronting cereal scientists is an awesome one.*

[2] The Pure Food and Drug Act of 1906 was amended in 1912, 1913, and 1919. It was superseded in 1938 by the much stricter Food, Drug, and Cosmetic (FD & C) Act.

What is perfectly clear, though, is that the mycotoxins are becoming more significant in the world's affairs. We have come a long way since May, 1960, when evidence of depravity was noticed in a number of turkey poults.

The possibility that the granaries of the United States might be contaminated by *Aspergillus flavus* arose indirectly from some remarks by Dr. John Higginson, which concluded our talk in the Hotel New Otani in Tokyo. Dr. Higginson had referred to the nitrosamines and then to aflatoxin; and we finally arrived—in Dr. Higginson's words—at the most critical aspect of the whole matter:

> A last point I should mention is that one of the major problems in the world today is undernutrition. It is necessary to feed children in some of the underdeveloped countries with a certain amount of protein supplementation, and it has been suggested that it would be very advisable to choose supplements from various sources. The people responsible for doing this found to their horror that many of these stocks of supplements were contaminated with aflatoxins.
> Now, what do you do? Do you prevent the children from getting their protein supplements, on the theoretical possibility that you might be giving them cancer twenty or thirty years later?
> This is a problem that is right in our lap at the present moment, and we don't have the data to provide the answer.

There was no opportunity on this occasion to go into the question of where and how the contamination of protein supplements might have occurred; the matter was raised during my conversation with Dr. Endicott at the National Cancer Institute:

> Q: I didn't have time, when I was talking to Dr. Higginson, to find out precisely where these contaminated supplements were being stored, or which countries were involved.
> ENDICOTT: Well, I don't know to which he was referring. But the protein supplements tend to be derived from peanuts, from linseed, from cottonseed, from meat scraps, from

fish, and from milk. These are the common sources. The ones that are likely to be contaminated are those in which the basic material is stored in almost field conditions: for example, peanuts in a big pile (on the ground) or cottonseed meal in a big bin. This encourages the growth of molds. . . . Now, my own feeling is that a live child who may subsequently get cancer is infinitely better than a dead one who won't. So I would be all for continuing to provide protein supplements, but I would be careful to screen out those that had heavy contamination.

Dr. Endicott's response to the "startling suggestion" that the great Midwestern granaries of the United States might be infected with aflatoxin was, "Well, I'd be surprised if they weren't." Another scientist at the National Cancer Institute said the same thing, in effect, in a slightly different way: "I have no idea whether they actually are or are not, but on a purely theoretical basis one might reasonably suspect that our granaries are contaminated." A standard reference source, M. Milner and W. F. Geddes, "Storage of Cereal Grains and Their Products" (*Assoc. Cereal Chem.*, St. Paul, Minnesota, 1954) gives *Aspergillus flavus* as a common contaminant of stored cereals.

It is, of course, in the nature of granaries that they attract fungi, as well as insects, rodents and birds; and it is in the nature of fungi, insects, rodents and birds that they seek out stored grain. This is far beyond man's control. But a personal communication from the U. S. Department of Agriculture indicates that in the United States, at least, the authorities are fully aware of the problem and that they are doing whatever they can to overcome it:

When Government-owned grain is placed in commercial storage it is commingled with other stocks. Storage operators rotate their stocks so that there is a progressive "turnover" of the inventory. The operator is obligated, on request, to return to the Government grain of equal quantity and quality to that placed in storage originally. The storage fees paid to the operator force him to operate on a very narrow margin. If he is to realize a small profit, he must be diligent in protecting the

quality of grain the Government stores in his facility. . . .
Through the years, the Department has stored grain in its own facilities located at so-called "bin sites." In operating the bin site program, the Department follows maintenance practices such as those used by prudent warehousemen. The grain is inspected at monthly intervals, and more often if deemed necessary. Most bins are equipped with aeration systems. The grain is turned, screened, or fumigated when necessary as a protection against mold growth and damage.

Surveys, the spokesman for the Department pointed out, have not shown that aflatoxins exist in the grains used for food. In addition, the industries responsible for other products used in protein supplements have been eager to cooperate in reducing the hazard of aflatoxin contamination. The Department's summing-up was, "The public has the maximum assurance of protection and of the maintenance of foods of high quality."

The guardians of the nation's food supplies are clearly on the alert; and this applies to many other countries. In the circumstances, really, that is the best we can expect.

Responsible scientists insist that we do not know if aflatoxin will induce liver cancer, or any other form of cancer, in man. We have evidence that chickens, pigeons, rats, rabbits, cats, pigs, calves, minks, and monkeys, among other animals, are likely to develop hepatomas from a diet of aflatoxin-contaminated food. In the case of man the direct evidence is lacking.

But there does exist a considerable amount of circumstantial evidence which even the most cautious observer is compelled to take into account. Circumstantial evidence lacks the authority of controlled laboratory experiments: it consists of assumptions and speculations. Nevertheless, it is—in this case —remarkably impressive.

Western man is on the whole wary of all species of fungi, with the possible exception of the common mushroom—and he will not even trust these when they are growing in a field; he prefers to buy them in a store. He tends to be revolted by moldy food, and it is not accepted in his culture. He expects his food to be fresh and to be kept in conditions that maintain its freshness. Not for him that Chinese delicacy, the hundred year old egg. Since the passage of the first Pure Food and Drug Act in the United States in 1906 there has been a steady improvement in methods of handling and preserving foodstuffs and, as a result, the American diet is now considered by many experts on nutrition to be one of the best in the world. Taking the nation as a whole, there are only relatively small pockets of poverty where people do not receive enough food.

It is noteworthy, therefore, that in the past quarter of a century cancer of the stomach and cancer of the liver in the United States have decreased by about 50 per cent. Whether this is related in any way to a better diet or to the avoidance of mold-contaminated foodstuffs is unknown. All told, some nine thousand Americans died of liver cancer in 1965, less than the number who died of stomach or duodenal ulcers, and less than 3 per cent of deaths from all forms of cancer.

The story is different elsewhere. The Bantu in Africa, for example, have been studied intensively by a number of researchers (including John Higginson), and we have some disquieting, but still inconclusive, information about their dietary habits and a *possible* correlation to the incidence of cancer. The Bantu are a family of Negroid tribes, with a total population of about fifty million, who occupy most of equatorial and southern Africa. They include the Swahili, Zulu, Kikuyu, Basuto, Matabele and Mashona tribes, but any effective federation is hindered because altogether they speak more than a hundred different dialects and languages.

The Bantu suffer severely from cancer of the liver. Among males, 68 per cent of all cancers are hepatomas, probably the highest incidence of liver cancer in the world. In Denmark, by comparison, only 0.18 per hundred thousand of the male population suffers from cancer of the liver; in America the figure is 1.7 of white Americans; while for the Bantu it is 14. Negroes in the United States, whose forebears may have come from the same territories in Africa, show a ratio of only 3.2 hepatomas per hundred thousand, and even when they have cirrhosis of the liver, hepatomas are far less likely to develop than among the Bantu.

A large part of the Bantu diet, in the villages, in the mining compounds, even in prison, consists of cereal products, and nearly 40 per cent is corn (or maize) which has deliberately been stored in such a way that it becomes moldy, to improve the flavor. The molds usually include *Aspergillus flavus;* and in the prevailing conditions of high humidity and temperature it is more than likely that there is heavy aflatoxin contamination. Cancer of the liver strikes the Bantu early. He contracts it, and dies of it, in his middle thirties.

The disease, and the conditions which may produce the disease, are not confined to Africans who live south of the Congo. Dr. A. Coady, of the Hospital for Tropical Diseases in London, has told of buying a variety of grains in Addis Ababa markets at the end of the rains which proved to be contaminated with *Aspergillus flavus, Penicillium islandicum,* and *Aspergillus ochraceus,* all blacklisted as molds which produce carcinogenic toxins. "Aflatoxin itself was found in a selection bought during the next rainy season—only two of eight samples were free of it, and at least one (sorghum) yielded a quantity which would probably have given a positive duckling assay (a standard test for aflatoxin concentration)." Dr. Coady made the additional point that cirrhosis and hepatoma are as prevalent in North Africa as in other parts of the continent. "The populations of developing countries carry among their many burdens a heavy incidence of liver disease," he concluded: a burden which might be eased by utilizing simple techniques of grain storage.

India, with its fearful twofold problems of overpopulation and famine, faces on an immensely greater scale the same difficulties as the Africans. Peanuts and various grains, principally rice, help to provide the proteins which keep the majority of Indians alive until they reach their early forties. In most villages, about half of the available rice is soaked in lukewarm water for 24 hours or so, a process which makes the rice more appetizing and more nutritious, and also more attractive to molds. The rice is then partially boiled, or steamed, making it still more attractive to molds. The parboiling may be carried out in the home where there are no storage facilities, or in small communal processing plants in the villages, where there may be just the barest storage facilities. The conditions for mold production throughout India—except during periods of drought—are little short of ideal, and one of the results is that widespread aflatoxin contamination has been found there. What also has been found is cirrhosis of the liver among the children. Medically, this provides a grievous but interesting problem. Juvenile cirrhosis is one of the symptoms of kwashiorkor, or protein deficiency. If you give rats a *low* protein diet contaminated with aflatoxin, you will induce cirrhosis, such as these children have. If you give rats a *high* protein diet contaminated with aflatoxin, you will induce cancer of the liver. Thus to increase the daily input of contaminated foodstuffs supplied to these half-starving children might be to doom them to an earlier and more painful death than they can ordinarily expect—a situation described earlier by Dr. John Higginson.

Rice, free of suspicion in the United States because it is dried very quickly and brought down to a moisture level which inhibits molds, is under serious suspicion in Japan and throughout the Orient. Yellowed rice, contaminated by one of the most common of the toxin-producing molds, *Penicillium islandicum*, together with other mold-infected foodstuffs which are considered delicacies, may well be responsible in part or in whole for the extremely high rate of cirrhosis among Japanese adults. The incidence of liver cancer is three times as high as in the United States.

Dr. Kraybill and Dr. Shimkin, near the end of their massive report, refer to a series of experiments which neatly demonstrates some of the pitfalls that lie in wait for scientists studying new aspects of carcinogenesis. In 1935, two Japanese researchers reported that unpolished rice treated with a carcinogenic substance called AAT caused liver cancer in 24 per cent of a number of experimental rats.

American researchers duplicated this experiment, substituting wheat for rice. None of their rats developed liver cancer.

In 1937 the experiment was repeated by another Japanese scientist. Again, he used rice, but treated it with another carcinogen. His rats duly developed liver cancer.

Once more American researchers followed suit, and they again used wheat. Their rats remained healthy.

From these two sets of experiments it was deduced that the relatively high content of B vitamins in the wheat inhibited the development of liver cancer. This finding is often quoted by nutritionists when the relationship of cancer and vitamins is discussed.

But another explanation has now been suggested: that the rice used by the Japanese researchers (like so much of the rice in Japan) may have been contaminated by fungal toxins; and that it was these mycotoxins which induced liver cancer in the rats.

For the people of the Orient, then, our new-found knowledge of the aflatoxins and other substances related to them may be one of the most significant cancer clues that the researchers have yet uncovered. And it arises, simply and directly, from reports by some English farmers that their young turkeys were dying in large numbers of a totally mysterious disease, and the subsequent discovery of carcinogenic toxins whose existence nobody had suspected. In the long run, the catastrophe that led scientists to aflatoxin may be of enormous benefit to mankind.

8

Finale:
The Best of Hopes

FOURTEEN

The Best of Hopes

There is one aspect of the planet Earth—as it might be seen by an astronaut on the moon—in which it appears to be composed almost entirely of water, with slivers of land visible only around its circumference and a few insignificant pinpoints of volcanic rock or coral scattered over its surface. This demi-world of water is the Pacific Ocean, covering 64,000,000 square miles (in fact, about one third of the superficial area of the world); and among the pinpoints are the Hawaiian Islands, not quite midway between North America and Asia. There are eight major islands in the group, of which seven are inhabited; and 114 smaller islands, or islets, of which only a handful are inhabited. In 1778 they were discovered (or, more accurately, re-discovered) by Captain James Cook, who named them the Sandwich Islands; he was killed by natives on a return voyage. The history of Hawaii thereafter was turbulent. In 1959 the Paradise of the Pacific, as it is apt to call itself, held a plebiscite, voted to join forces with the United States, and became the Union's fiftieth State.

The capital of Hawaii is Honolulu, on the south-east coast of the island of Oahu. It is described in travel brochures as famous for its beauty, for its luxury hotels and its excellent housing developments; but these aspects of civilization can be rather depressing. Outside the capital the visitor will find scenes of utterly spectacular beauty; he will be overwhelmed by the marvelous flowers, by the bushes and trees that seem to be growing vigorously as one looks at them, by the volcanic peaks swathed in long sheets of cloud and almost always sporting a rainbow or two. On the north shore of the island, where the waters are dangerous for swimmers, one catches glimpses of the paradise that actually existed here a hundred or even fifty years ago: lovely, deserted, unlittered beaches encircled by dense groves of palm, and wild, incredibly blue seas.

Hawaii has a place in this book because, like India, it serves as a laboratory in which scientists can observe natural forces at work. But the polarities are opposite and quite different. The Indian population is made up of groups of human beings who have remained separate over many centuries. Most of the inhabitants of Hawaii are recent arrivals; intermarriage is common; and the pure blooded Hawaiians, descended from the original Polynesian settlers, now comprises less than 2 per cent of the total population.[1] About one third of the population is Japanese—Tokyo is some four thousand miles west-north-west. About one third of the population is Caucasian—San Francisco is some twenty-four hundred miles east-north-east, Europe is further to the east by six thousand miles. Slightly less than 15 per cent of the population is part Hawaiian, less than 11 per cent is Filipino, 6 per cent is Chinese, less than 1 per cent is Negro, 0.1 per cent is American Indian.

We have, therefore, gathered on these islands in the midst of a stupendous expanse of ocean, a large number of Japanese who have left Japan; we have an equally large number of Caucasians from the United States and Europe; we have large numbers of other ethnic groups. And the cancer epidemiologist, enthralled by this almost perfect set-up, immediately asks, What is the pattern of cancer among these people? Have the Japanese brought the Japanese cancer pattern with them to

[1] Total population of Hawaii in the 1960 Census was 632,772. The estimated total population as of July 1, 1965, was 711,000.

Hawaii? How does the Hawaii Japanese cancer pattern compare with the cancer pattern of the Japanese who have settled in California? Have the Caucasians brought to Hawaii *their* special patterns?

We have only partial answers to some of these questions. Even so, they are of enormous importance and interest.

Kuakini Hospital is not far from the center of Honolulu: ten or fifteen minutes by bus. It is a modest community hospital of 200 beds, maintained principally for Hawaii Japanese. An even more modest hospital existed before Pearl Harbor; but after the war a group of young Nisei physicians decided to improve the facilities; and, among other things, a research institute was set up for the study of disease in the Japanese people of Hawaii. The Director of Laboratories at Kuakini Hospital is Dr. Grant N. Stemmermann, a tall, blond, voluble New Yorker; and on an exceedingly warm and sunny November afternoon he spoke to me for more than three hours about some of the matters he and his colleagues have been investigating.[2]

It is necessary, first, to establish the pattern of the *native* Japanese. On the whole, the people of Japan are very fortunate. Of twenty-four countries around the world, they have the nineteenth lowest cancer death rate for males, the twenty-third lowest for females.[3] Analyzed in more detail, the statistics are very striking. The Japanese have the lowest rate of oral cancer, for both males and females. In lung cancer, the males have the twenty-third lowest rate, females are inexplicably fifteenth. In skin cancer, males are twenty-fourth, females twenty-third. In leukemia, males are twenty-third, females are twenty-fourth. In cancer of the prostate, Japanese males have the lowest rate in the world; in cancer of the breast, Japanese women have the lowest rate in the world. In cancer of the colon and rectum, males and females have the same very low incidence: both are twenty-third.

[2] Dr. Stemmermann was also, at the time I met him, Associate Professor of Pathology, University of Hawaii School of Medicine, Honolulu.
[3] *Cancer Facts and Figures, 1968*, American Cancer Society.

But in cancer of the uterus the incidence is high: Japanese women have the fourth highest rate in the world—a finding that is not altogether unexpected when we recall the curious inverse relationship that seems to exist nearly everywhere between breast cancer and uterine cancer. A similar relationship seems to exist between cancer of the colon and rectum and cancer of the stomach; and it takes effect with great force among the native Japanese. With almost the world's lowest incidence of colon-rectum cancer, they have the highest incidence of stomach cancer for males and the second highest incidence of stomach cancer for females.

At the beginning of our conversation, Dr. Stemmermann made it clear that the Japanese in Hawaii do indeed present a characteristic cancer pattern, different from that of the native Japanese. "There is a tendency for stomach cancer to maintain a rather high level of frequency among the migrant Japanese," Dr. Stemmermann said. "But the frequency is gradually dropping; and Dr. W. Haenszel and others have shown that this drop is greater in the Nisei—that is, the second generation, American-born, American-speaking Japanese—than it is in the first generation Japanese migrant. This suggests to us that the environment is related in some way to gastric cancer.

"At the same time, large intestine cancer (of the colon and rectum), which is quite infrequent in Japan, has become very, very common; it is now found just as frequently in the migrant Japanese as stomach cancer, and this is an indication that something has happened to the migrant Japanese which hasn't happened to the native Japanese.

"What is of great interest is that this increase in large intestine cancer is found almost exclusively in Japanese males, not females; and this is so both in Hawaii Japanese males and California Japanese males.

"There are several possible explanations. One is that the male is exposed to a carcinogen to which the female is not exposed. Another is that both the male and the female are exposed to some carcinogen, but the male is exposed to it for a longer period of time. A third, but less likely possibility, is that the female is more resistant to the carcinogen."

I asked, "Do you have any clues as to its nature?"

"None at the moment," Dr. Stemmermann replied. "We've only just started these particular studies. I think, though, we do have some clues about stomach cancer.

"The first seems to be that this is a tumor with a very long induction period.

"Then, it occurs most frequently in people of the lower economic groups. People who've had a predominantly starch diet. People who live in a society that has a low level of industrialization. It has been shown, for instance, that stomach cancer is inversely proportional to the gross national product:[4] the lower the gross national product, the higher the incidence of stomach cancer; and *vice versa*.

"Now, if one follows the trend of cancer of the stomach in a country like Finland, the rate has gradually decreased over the past sixty years; and with this decrease there has been a corresponding decrease of starch in the diet.

"Presumably, the decrease of starch products in the diet corresponds with an increase in the standard of living; and this would explain the difference between the rates of the tumor in various social or economic groups. Those countries with the highest degree of industrialization have low rates of cancer of the stomach, and in some parts of the United States it has almost disappeared. Japan and Russia still have a high incidence of this malignancy, but we can expect a decrease in the next two or three decades if the patterns of other industrialized nations are followed. At the same time, there are some features of stomach cancer that are difficult to explain and may very well have a genetic basis. For instance, cancer of the stomach in northern Europeans is different in certain ways from the form we see in Japanese; and in all likelihood there is more than one cause of this cancer."

The stomach has been described, in a rather offhand way, as the most dilated part of the digestive tract. It has a deceptively

---

[4] The gross national product is the total market value of a nation's goods and services. It can be used as an index of a nation's overall prosperity—a high gross national product, of course, indicating a high level of material prosperity.

simple, bag-like shape, but like everything else in the human body it is remarkably complex. Structurally, the wall of the stomach consists of four coats. The outer surface is covered by a thin membrane, the serous coat; beneath this is the powerful muscular coat which is constructed of three sets of muscle fibers, longitudinal, circular, oblique. Below this is the submucous coat, connecting the muscular layer to the stomach's innermost coat—the mucous membrane, composed of a variety of different kinds of cells which, in turn, make up a variety of ducts and glands.

What is most astonishing about the stomach is that hour after hour, day after day, year after year, it manages to survive the insults to which it is subjected. In the general scheme of things it is the second sub-station on the digestive route (the first is, of course, the mouth, with its grinding-shredding-rolling apparatus and salivary solvents); and into it pours a torrent of substances of every kind—tannin-laden tea, caffeine-laden coffee, bacteria-laden sausages, raw whisky, and occasionally something quite unexpected like fuel oil.[5] In this respect the stomach, like the mouth, is wide open to the environment. It receives (all too often) a certain amount of air, so that it is not immune even to the atmospheric environment.

Nobody should be surprised, therefore, that environmental factors are believed to play a significant part in the induction of stomach cancer. We cannot point with absolute certainty to any single environmental cause; but we can regard with suspicion, to say the least, a number of factors which *may* play a part in the malignant process.

The first factor, the most obvious factor, is diet. We have already seen that in Japan and in other countries with a high incidence of this disease, the people (and particularly the poor people) rely greatly on such starch foods as rice, or potatoes. Nobody has yet supplied *proof* of a direct relationship between a starch diet and stomach cancer, but it might be added that nobody is *likely* to supply proof. Controlled experiments

[5] In 1959, some ten thousand persons in Meknes, Morocco, were affected with paralysis as a result of poisoning caused by the use of fuel oil which had been marketed as cooking oil.

on human beings to settle the matter are prohibited; they would take, in any case, some thirty or forty years.

An additional factor is a deficiency of fat. The Japanese diet consists of about 10 per cent unsaturated fat, while in the United States the consumption of fat, mostly in saturated form, is more than four times as great. Dr. Ernest L. Wynder has pointed out, also, that cancer of the stomach declined significantly in the United States during a period when there was a reduction in the intake of potatoes accompanied by a rise in consumption of fresh fruits and vegetables.

Another possibility is, in the words of Dr. Stemmermann, "that stomach cancer is caused, not necessarily by something *taken in*, but something that is *not taken:* in other words, that at some period of malnutrition during early life, atrophy (a wasting of tissue or of organs) of the stomach may have occurred, leading to cellular changes which eventually result in the absorption of a carcinogen and the development of a tumor." Pernicious anemia (a condition which, curiously enough, is almost nonexistent among Japanese) appears to be "associated" with stomach cancer; but, here again, we have suspicions, we have evidence, but we have no definite proof.[6]

Gastric ulcers (stomach ulcers) have been implicated as precursors of stomach cancer by some authorities; other authorities have stated that there is no significant relationship between the two conditions. Here we run into what seems to be an international dispute; and Dr. Stemmermann expressed himself with great vigor on the matter. "Many American and European pathologists will say that cancer of the stomach does not occur, to all intents and purposes, in ulcer beds. This is simply not true. I've seen it among Japanese, who have a high

---

[6] Suspicion also extends to various other factors. (1) A condition called achlorhydria, in which there is an absence of hydrochloric acid in the stomach secretions, is often found in patients suffering from stomach cancer, but it is not known whether this plays any part in the induction of the disease or is one of its effects. (2) Both in areas of low or high incidence, cancer of the stomach occurs 20 per cent more frequently in people belonging to blood group A than in people belonging to blood groups O or B. (3) It is uncertain whether gastric polyps may become malignant. (4) Also unexplained is the curious fact that stomach cancer is far more common in human beings than it is in animals.

incidence of gastric ulcer. There haven't been many reports of it in Caucasians, but this may be due to a difference in population, or it may be that it's much more common in Japanese and we have a better opportunity to see it occur. In the Japanese we see ten gastric ulcers to one duodenal ulcer. In the Caucasian it's the other way around, three to one."

I asked, "There's a general belief that the pressures and anxieties of daily life, when they become too great, may lead to a gastric ulcer. In your experience, is this true?"

"That's a hard question," Dr. Stemmermann said. "Everyone has stresses. Everyone has problems. We would have to find out what specific stress causes a specific injury to the stomach, resulting in an ulcer."

"Working too hard? Worrying too much?"

"That's what they say," Dr. Stemmermann said pleasantly. "But I don't know why people get gastric ulcers or duodenal ulcers. Nobody does."

"Could gastric ulcers in the Japanese be related to diet?"

"I wouldn't eliminate diet. But it could be psychological. Let's go back to the question of stress for a moment, and how it might affect a gastric ulcer. We know that the Japanese attitude to stress is different from the attitude of most other people. They are remarkably stoical. A Japanese delivery room is as silent as the tomb. It would be a terrible loss of face for a woman who's bearing a child if she uttered a sound, complaining of pain. The Japanese male bears insults, the worst of insults, in utter silence and with a complete lack of facial expression. Obviously, something must be going on inside; and the unusually high incidence of gastric ulcers in Japan has been attributed to this stoic trait in the Japanese personality." Dr. Stemmermann paused. "Is this true? I don't know."

What happens, then, to the Japanese who leave their native land and settle and raise families in Hawaii—roughly midway between Japan and the United States—is a change in environmental conditions which produces (or, more scientifically, appears to produce) a marked change in the cancer pattern.

Stomach cancer, so typical of Japan, begins to decrease; large intestine cancer, rare in Japan, begins to rise. The migrant Japanese woman may encounter another problem, for when she leaves Japan, where breast cancer is relatively infrequent, she becomes as vulnerable as her American sister.

"Many factors have been put forward to account for the changed incidence of breast cancer in Hawaii Japanese women," Dr. Stemmermann said, "but nothing has been proven. We have only just begun our studies, and I think there are certain aspects we should look into. One is delayed childbearing. Another is a history of infrequent nursing among women who have borne children. Another is a tendency to have few children and to work in jobs outside the home, so that nursing—even if it's started—is ended sooner than it might be. The social pattern of Hawaii Japanese women is that most girls work after marriage; and this is a pattern that results in late childbearing and fewer babies. The new generation of Hawaii Japanese girls do, in fact, have a high rate of gynecological complications that are related to late childbearing; and I suspect that some of the rise in breast cancer is probably related to distortions in reproductive cycles."

On the other hand, the Caucasian going to Japan for a lengthy period of time is not likely to become a victim of stomach cancer, unless he was formerly a native of some country with very similar environmental conditions—where, for example, he suffered from malnutrition throughout his early years because of low living standards, and rice or potatoes were the staple food. The reason, obviously, is that stomach cancer (like most forms of cancer) does not occur suddenly. In adults it is a disease with a very long induction period. Similarly, a Caucasian woman going to live in Japan will not instantaneously achieve the same relative freedom from, say, cancer of the breast, or cancer of the colon and rectum, as the native Japanese woman. The individual's history, heredity, environmental conditions, and perhaps blind chance, all play a part in the induction of malignancies; and nobody can possibly predict the outcome of their interactions.

So the existence of this natural laboratory in Hawaii is of the greatest value, and it is not surprising that the National Cancer Institute is supporting studies there, and also parallel studies in Japan. From the clues picked up in Hawaii and Japan the scientists can add clues picked up in other parts of the world where stomach cancer has been studied intensively: Finland and the Scandinavian countries, the Near East, equatorial and South Africa, Latin America, the United Kingdom. It is now seen that the sum total of this information leads even beyond the eventual control of stomach cancer, vital as this is, and the possibility of larger rewards has been expressed (in very guarded terms) in one of the National Cancer Institute's publications:[7] "Research on identification of the factors involved in the declining incidence of stomach cancer in many countries has implications beyond the narrow confines of this particular body site. Scientists believe that if such factors can be pinpointed, some of the basic questions about malignancy, in general, will also be answered, and will, perhaps, lead to development of preventive measures."

That is, measures *to prevent the occurrence* of cancer of the stomach: not to *control* it after it occurs, not to *cure* it after it occurs, but to prevent it from occurring at all. And, perhaps, in similar ways to prevent the occurrence of other forms of cancer. For the research scientist, as well as for humanity at large, this is the best of hopes.

We cannot really congratulate ourselves on our present situation. It is not satisfactory. We are only just emerging from the Dark Ages of the contest with cancer. Despite our vast resources—all our knowledge, all our superb equipment, all our ingenious drugs, all our skilled and devoted doctors—the disease outwits us too often. Even in the most advanced treatment centers, where every one of the newest technological miracles is available to cure or stem the advance of the disease, our best efforts are too often inadequate. Too many children

[7] *Public Health Service Bulletin*, No. 1237. U. S. Department of Health, Education, and Welfare.

are denied a fair life span, too many adults experience long periods of pain and indignity.

The situation is not altogether black. We have a variety of approaches to the actual physical problem of human cancer, and some of them work well. It is worth looking over them again briefly.

Our first line of attack is surgery (unless the malignancy is leukemia or an allied disease). Particularly if the tumor is *in situ*, but even in later stages, surgery may provide a complete cure. It has saved hundreds of thousands of lives, but in the words of Dr. Sidney Farber, *it takes something away*, it is by its nature mutilatory, and it is the form of treatment human beings fear most.

Our second line of attack is radiotherapy. It cannot be manipulated with the fine precision of the surgeon's scalpel; it can harm healthy tissue; but there are times when surgery is unduly difficult or hazardous, and radiotherapy can save life. Or, where a cancer has spread, it can help to control the malignancy.

Chemotherapy at present will not alone effect a cure, except in two rather rare forms of cancer. Nor will immunotherapy. Their promise lies in the future. Today they serve to extend life, to palliate the disease; they are additional tools for the surgeon or the radiotherapist.

In recent years medical authorities have been instructing the public about the dangers of cancer, and urging regular examinations so that malignant changes might be detected at an early stage and halted before the condition has become too widespread for effective treatment. The "Pap smear" test for uterine cancer is one example of this kind of procedure; another is mammography, a special treatment developed for breast examination by X-ray. Nobody questions the value of early diagnosis, but it is by no means infallible, and one of its most serious limitations is that many forms of cancer are characteristically silent—that is, they are without any apparent symptoms, even at a relatively advanced stage. And only too often the early symptoms are in fact the manifestation of a late stage in a malignant process which has been progressing for twenty, thirty, or forty years from its first beginnings.

Quite clearly, the best hope for the future lies in a planned program that aims at the active prevention of cancer. Every improvement in technology is obviously welcome beyond words; but we have to recognize that surgery, radiotherapy, chemotherapy, immunology, only *treat*, with varying degrees of success, conditions that are a grave peril to the individual. The surgeon or the radiotherapist cannot guarantee that every malignant cell has been removed, that the disease will not return (although increasingly, because of the ever-growing skill of these men, the disease *does not* return). Early detection does no more than provide the individual with a better chance of obtaining treatment before the condition has spread and thus becomes difficult or impossible to treat successfully.

But from what we have learned about the causes of cancer it has now become apparent that if we take the right precautions, *certain forms of cancer need not occur at all;* or their incidence can be greatly reduced. On pages 72 and 109 are listed a few of the agents that have been proven to bear at least some responsibility for inducing malignant changes in human beings. Many of these are chemical substances; some are physical agents such as ionizing radiation from X-rays or nuclear explosions, or the ultraviolet rays of sunlight. Most are termed exogenous—that is, generated or originating outside the body; some, such as hormones, are endogenous, generated within the body. It should be obvious that as far as external agents are concerned they can do us little harm if we avoid exposure to them. This is a strategy we have followed with considerable success in dealing with a number of infectious diseases. If we avoid contact with the tsetse fly in tropical Africa we are unlikely to become infected by the trypanasome that causes sleeping sickness; and this has been accomplished by suppressing the tsetse fly. In the same way, we have drained swamps which were the breeding grounds of malarial mosquitoes, and in many parts of the world we are thus unlikely to become infected by the malaria plasmodium.

Because cancer is not a single disease but a complex of different diseases, we cannot in the near future expect to find ways to prevent the occurrence of all cancer, of cancer in general. The disease occurs in so many forms that we simply cannot expect anybody to discover a wholesale cure for cancer, just as we cannot expect anybody to invent a ball that is suitable for all kinds of ball games, or a musical instrument that can take over any part in a symphony. We have to attack each type of cancer separately: and at present our situation is that in some types we have absolutely no idea how to begin the task of prevention; in some types we have good hopes of, at least, limited success; in some types, if only the human race would listen and behave rationally, we have hopes of enormous success.

We can see how the concept of cancer prevention might be put into practice if we go back to the work of Dr. Stemmermann in Hawaii (and his fellow workers all over the world). One of the peculiarities of cancer of the stomach is that it occurs more frequently among the poor than among those who enjoy better economic condition. This poses problems that are somewhat beyond the scope of cancer prevention: we cannot supply the poor with large sums of money, although in the nature of things the standard of living is rising in many parts of the world. But what seems to be paramount in stomach cancer is not a person's net worth but, to a large extent, his diet in the first twenty or thirty years of his life. A man who has struggled out of the slums of Hong Kong is not immune to stomach cancer because, at the age of fifty, he has a million dollars deposited in Swiss banks. An increase in the consumption of citrus fruits and lettuce; a reduction in starchy foods; prompt attention to pernicious anemia and the correction of achlorhydria—all this would be part of a rational program conducted by the health authorities in any area where the incidence of stomach cancer is unusually high. At the same time a close watch would be kept on all persons suffering from chronic gastric atrophy (or chronic atrophic gastritis), chronic gastric ulcers, gastric polyps or any other benign gastric tumors, and recognition of the slightly greater susceptibility of individuals with group A blood.

Could a program of this kind be instituted in a high risk country like Japan? A few years ago the question would have been laughed out of court as Utopian, impractical, impossible. But Japan has changed very greatly in the past two decades. Television is ubiquitous—an invaluable tool for spreading information. The young people of Tokyo are as lively and uninhibited as young people anywhere else in the world; economic standards have risen sharply; and there is no reason to believe that the cancerophobic Japanese will demand their traditional rice tomorrow and the day after tomorrow if they are convinced of the hazards of a diet that is overloaded with starch. The elderly and the middle-aged would be under no compulsion to take part in any program of prevention: they have already been exposed for lengthy periods of time to the carcinogenic factors involved, and their best hope is a change in their pattern of living that might lessen the likelihood of a proliferating cancer, and constant supervision to detect anything that might be going wrong. A program of cancer prevention in this particular instance would apply principally to the children, the adolescents, the young adults; and it might well become a matter of national determination to take all possible action against an intolerable state of affairs. A high incidence of any form of cancer in any country might very well be considered a national disgrace.[8]

[8] Organized teams of medical workers, mostly volunteers, travel through the Japanese countryside in specially equipped buses, stopping in villages where all the inhabitants are rounded up for intensive questioning, X-ray photographs, internal photographs by means of a gastrocamera and internal examination by means of a gastroscope. In the course of six years (up to August, 1966) 350,000 people had participated in the scheme; some 550 cases of cancer had been found; and of these, two out of three were in an early stage which could be treated successfully by surgery. This program of early detection was started by one man, Toshio Kurokawa, who has described vividly how he began: "I decided to install an X-ray device in a car and go into the mountains. For I painfully realized that if I was merely waiting for visitors, it would be utterly impossible to discover cancer cases in an early stage, which are usually characterized by a lack of symptoms."

Probably the most important statistic to come out of the past half century of cancer research is that 80 per cent, or more, of all cancer is caused by some interaction between the individual and the environment in which he spends his life. *The environment,* as we have already seen, includes the foods he eats, the liquids he drinks, the air and the pollutants he inhales, the peculiar substances he chews; the conditions under which he works and the materials he encounters in the course of his work; what he or she rubs onto his or her skin; the life-giving and death-dealing sun; medications; religious practices, sexual practices, hygienic practices. The list is endless.

Because we can control our environment to some extent, or alter our relationship to it, we can claim that a proportion of all environmental cancers is preventable. Referring specifically to Britain, Dr. Richard Doll writes at the conclusion of his monograph, *The Prevention of Cancer,* "Setting aside the possible benefits of earlier diagnosis, we might now be able to prevent about 40 per cent of the cancer deaths that occur annually in men, and a somewhat smaller proportion—about 10 per cent—in women. In addition, there is good reason to believe that a large proportion of the remaining types is, in principle, preventable, and with continued research we may learn how to prevent them within the next two or three decades." The same possibility holds true for Western Europe generally, and for the United States.

Many of the preventable environmental cancers have been discussed in earlier chapters. It can only be of benefit to draw attention to them again. Cervical cancer—cancer of the cervix of the uterus—seems to be closely related to sexual experience: the age at which sexual intercourse begins, the number of men with whom the woman has had intercourse, sexual hygiene, and so on. The causative agent of cervical cancer may be smegma, a substance produced by glands close to the glans penis in the male. In uncircumcised males the foreskin normally covers these glands, with the result that the smegma may not be cleansed away, and may be deposited in the female's vagina. The epidemiological evidence is strong that a great deal of cervical cancer would never occur if young women were aware of the nature of this hazard and took care to obviate it. Cancer of the penis, which seems to be related to tightness of the foreskin (phimosis) and the retention of smegma, is rare among people who practice circumcision. (Cancer of the penis of horses is seen most often in those animals which have been castrated; and here, too, the evidence strongly suggests that the malignancy is related to the accumulation of smegma.)

Skin cancer provides a good example of what we can hope for when our knowledge and our skills are more advanced. It has, in the United States, the highest incidence of all forms of cancer: 105,000 new cases are reported every year. But it has also by far the highest cure rate—mortality is only about 5,000 every year: that is, of 21 who contract the disease, only one person dies. The reason is, of course, that it occurs on the outer surface of the human body where it is readily seen and readily treated, and also where it can most readily be studied. Cancer of the scrotum in young chimney sweeps was the first occupational skin cancer to be described (by Percival Pott, in 1775). Mule spinner's cancer is another historic skin cancer: the spinning mule, used in twisting and drawing wool or cotton into yarn or thread, was lubricated with shale oil which splashed onto the clothing of operators, penetrated to the skin, and frequently caused cancer of the scrotum or vulva.[9] Coal tar, arsenic compounds, radium and X-rays, are other causes of skin cancer; but virtually all of these hazards, in most countries, are now strictly controlled by legislation.

What is not controlled by legislation is sunlight, and it is now quite clear that excessive exposure to the sun, as in sunbathing, may seriously affect the skin and cause changes

[9] It is strange to learn that a minor epidemic of skin cancer—in particular, cancer of the scrotum—has now become evident among machine workers in the engineering industry who are heavily exposed to mineral oils. In England this epidemic is centered on Birmingham, where there are currently between 10 and 20 new cases of cancer of the scrotum each year.

leading to cancer *many years later*. People with fair skin, and those with the exceedingly delicate light skin that accompanies red hair, are particularly susceptible (it has always been common among fair-skinned farmers and sailors). People with darker skin (such as Negroes and many of the inhabitants of Mediterranean countries) are far less susceptible —the brown color of their skin is due to a pigment, melanin, which serves to filter out the harmful rays of the sun.

Prevention of skin cancer, therefore, is relatively simple. Apart from industrial hazards, one avoids excessive exposure to sunlight, particularly in the middle of a hot summer day and particularly if one's skin is very fair. The physician today is not apt to regard a deep suntan as a sign of bursting health. He is more likely to be suspicious of it as a source of future distress. "Deliberate tanning," the National Cancer Institute reports, "not only increases the chances of skin cancer development but also contributes to the aging appearance of the skin." This additional factor and not the fear of cancer alone, the noted epidemiologist Russell Baker has pointed out in *The New York Times,* may serve to make our age-sensitive society uneasy about the effects of excessive sunlight on the human organism.

More often we find that we have valuable pointers to the cause, or the causes, of a particular malignancy but we are unable to formulate a program of prevention as simple as that for skin cancer because the situation is too complex, and many factors are still not understood or remain unknown. As an example we can take cancer of the esophagus, one of the less common cancers of the digestive system in Western man.

The esophagus is the tube, about nine inches long, leading from the pharynx—at the back of the mouth—to the stomach. To reach the stomach it must pass through an opening in the diaphragm called the esophageal hiatus (or aperture). Occasionally the stomach itself may protrude upward into the opening, a condition called hiatus hernia which often can be corrected by surgery. But if it is left uncorrected, pressure from the hernia may cause a stricture (a narrowing, or constriction) to form in the esophagus and this, as a result of what is believed to be stagnation or retention of various food particles, may lead to malignant changes. Another possible cause—fortunately rare in the United States and Europe, since there is no effective treatment for it—is Chargas' disease, arising from infection by trypanosomes (a protozoan parasite) transmitted by a South American bloodsucking bug, the barbiero. This disease may result in a condition called megaesophagus (*mega* = large) in which the lower part of the esophagus is greatly enlarged, leading (for much the same reason as in hiatus hernia) to the retention of food particles. Alcohol is under suspicion; so are the various chews, such as tobacco, the betel chew in Southeast Asia, and "nass" in the USSR. Corrosive chemicals such as lye, swallowed deliberately or by accident, may cause scars which will become malignant. One investigator (E. E. Hurst, in *Cancer*, No. 17, 1964) has reported that Alaskan women have a high rate of cancer of the esophagus, possibly as a result of chewing sealskin sprinkled with wood ashes, an unusual combination which no doubt has a most delicious taste but, at the same time, is a rather primitive method of manufacturing lye and producing esophageal scars.

Still another cause, suggested by many scientists, may be a condition called sideropenic dysphagia, which means difficulty in swallowing resulting from iron deficiency, one of the major symptoms of a disease called variously Plummer-Vinson's or Paterson-Kelly syndrome. The iron deficiency may occur at puberty, while the malignancy of the esophagus may occur forty or fifty years later. It has been demonstrated that something positive can be done about this, for the syndrome is reported to have been reduced in Swedish women after the Swedish Public Health Service enforced the addition of iron and vitamins to white flour and bread.

Other steps to prevent esophageal cancer are fairly obvious: correction of hiatus hernia and other constrictions or obstructions of the esophagus, the avoidance of scarring, and so on. But much remains to be learned about the disease; and much that we now know is puzzling. Thus, A. G. Oettlé has pointed out that while sideropenia (iron deficiency) is an important factor in European countries, the opposite condition, hemosiderosis (an accumulation of an iron-containing substance in the blood) is frequently seen in Bantu patients with cancer of the esophagus. Similarly, in France there is "good reason" for suspecting alcohol as a factor, yet in one district in China with an unusually high incidence of the disease there is practically no consumption at all of alcohol and, in fact, no alcohol had been drunk by any of 276 patients suffering from this cancer.

The situation is to some extent similar in bladder cancer. Historically, the bladder has almost the same appeal for the cancerologist as the scrotum. In 1895 Louis Rehn, a German surgeon, described cancer of the bladder among men who worked in the aniline dye industry—then fairly new but highly successful and prosperous. At first it was suspected that aniline itself, "the starting point for all the brilliant dyes that play so large a part in our modern life," as Charles Oberling described it, was responsible for causing the tumors; subsequent research showed that the danger arose from a group of chemical compounds known as aromatic amines,[10] and that these compounds could be found not only in the aniline dye industry but throughout a wide range of industries—the chemical industry in general, the rubber industry, the cablemaking industry, and even some sections of the textile and printing industries. Some of the compounds were freely used in hospitals for certain blood tests, and—almost at the other end of the spectrum—by ratcatchers as an ingredient in rat poison.

Prevention, in this case, was effected by legislation, so that to a large extent the industrial danger has been controlled. But this may not be the end of the story. "To assess the pro-

[10] The most potent of the carcinogens responsible for bladder cancer is beta-naphthylamine; others are benzidine, and possibly orthotolidine. They only affect the bladder and urinary tract, it is thought, because they are converted into carcinogens as they pass through the body, and then become concentrated in the urine. Stasis—that is, stagnation, a stoppage of the flow of urine carrying carcinogenic materials—may also contribute to the induction of malignancies.

portion of all bladder cancer which is due to environmental conditions is difficult," says Professor E. Boyland,[11] "but the known facts indicate that it must be substantial. Cancer of the bladder is caused in man by chemical substances which are not confined to the factories where they are made." In other words, some of these substances may be in circulation in forms that are available to the public (for example, in cosmetics, in foodstuffs, in various manufactured goods), and it is of great importance that public health officials stay alert to this hazard.

Recently there has been an increase in this type of cancer, for which no precise cause has been found. Although the association has not been proven, strong evidence exists to link the increase with cigarette smoking. One scientist has suggested, most ingeniously, that since the disease is occurring more frequently in younger *city* men, the carcinogen might be found in the hair creams so greatly favored by the sophisticated young male, once referred to by the late President John F. Kennedy as "that greasy kid stuff." In fact, some of these hair creams have, in the past, contained a well-known carcinogen, butter yellow, a yellow azo dye derived from aniline.

Many other forms of cancer are so little understood that there is virtually no positive action we can take to prevent them from occurring at present, and we must therefore place our hopes in early detection. It will be enough to mention only a few, to illustrate the point.

Liver cancer has often been associated with cirrhosis[12]

---

[11] *The Biochemistry of Bladder Cancer*, Thomas, Springfield, Ill., 1963.

[12] Cirrhosis (from the Greek, meaning tawny or orange-colored) of the liver has a great many symptoms, such as inflammation, atrophy, fatty infiltration, hardening, degeneration, all of which disturb liver functions and interfere with the circulation of blood and bile. There are numerous kinds, arising from alcoholism, prolonged congestive heart failure, and nutritional deficiencies such as kwashiorkor. Other organs—the gall bladder, stomach, kidney, lungs—can develop cirrhotic conditions of their own.

which—in Western man—results with great frequency from overindulgence in alcohol. It is also associated with certain food toxins—aflatoxins, other mycotoxins, and cycasin; but not enough is known for any rational program of prevention. Another hazard is malignant changes arising from infestation by liver flukes;[13] and in the Far East, particularly China, this is a serious health problem. One theory is that, as in many forms of cancer, the process occurs in two stages: liver *damage*, due to alcoholism, malnutrition, infection, or poisoning, which is followed by the intervention (perhaps many years later) of a secondary agent, setting off the actual malignancy. Prevention of stage one is a very, very remote possibility— who is going to keep the martini drinker from his third martini, the *sake* drinker from his third cup of *sake*? Prevention of stage two is still more remote for we have no idea of its nature—we do not really know, indeed, if there *is* a stage two.

Cancer of the pancreas is also associated with alcohol,[14] with inflammation of the pancreas (pancreatitis), with gall stones, and with the presence of pancreatic tissue (known as ectopic pancreas) outside the pancreas itself—a malignancy may arise in the ectopic pancreas. The physician will regard any pancreatic disturbance with suspicion; but ectopic pancreas is only likely to be discovered in the course of surgery.

Cancer of the rectum is known to be related to a hereditary condition called familial polyposis; but there is no strong evidence that it is related to the use of purgatives (notably medicinal paraffin, or mineral oil, which has frequently been

---

[13] *Fluke* is the common name for certain flatworms (trematodes) which are parasites in man and animals. They may live in various parts of the blood stream, in the intestines, in the lungs and elsewhere. Some have chosen to reside in the liver.

[14] To put this subject to rest, the consumption of alcohol is known to have damaging effects on the cell, in particular on the mitochondria which are the source of cellular energy; alcohol also affects the cell membrane, possibly enabling carcinogens to enter more easily. Alcohol itself is not believed to be a carcinogen, but it is "associated" with liver cancer, cancer of the pancreas, oral cancer, cancer of the larynx, cancer of the esophagus, rectal cancer, and—in brief—with cancer of *any part* of the gastrointestinal tract (which is some thirty-two feet in length) and the associated organs of the digestive system.

implicated in the past); and there is no strong evidence that it is related to hemorrhoids. At the same time, there is some reason to suspect certain salves and suppositories used by persons suffering from hemorrhoids; and scientists have strongly recommended that special studies should be made of these products.

A large number of cancers have so far remained completely obscure; their origin is totally unknown; and so we cannot propose any means for preventing them. The most prominent of these is leukemia in its various forms: ionizing radiation can only be responsible for a relatively small proportion of cases. The lymphomas are unexplained, but for at least one form, Hodgkin's disease, effective treatment and a very significant extension of life is now possible. Cancer of the brain and central nervous system is unexplained; but the work of Professor Druckrey and other scientists is beginning to throw light on it, and we may find in the near future that the nitrosamines or some similar substances are implicated. The causes of bone tumors are unknown.[15] We have no satisfactory explanation for cancer of the prostate, of the testes, of the ovaries, of the breast: hormones are almost certainly involved, but we have not learned the mechanism of the malignant change. For these cancers, our best hope at the present time is early detection and prompt treatment.

So we come to the cancer we understand best, the cancer that kills more human beings in Western Europe and the United States than any other; the cancer we can most easily prevent, the cancer we seem impotent to prevent; the cancer we can rarely cure: lung cancer.

Everything that needs to be said about it has been said over and over again, with magnificent persistence and pa-

[15] An exception, of course, is the bone cancer developed by radium dial painters and others who have been exposed to radium or radioactive products.

tience, by the American Cancer Society and the Canadian Cancer Society and the British Empire Cancer Fund and the French National League Against Cancer and the Japan Cancer Society and all the other organizations around the world that are concerned about malignant disease. There are many causes of lung cancer: asbestos dust is known to be implicated, war gases are implicated, and so are oil mists used on certain machine tools. Workers in the chromate industry are more susceptible than the general population; and uranium miners, exposed to radioactive ores, respond predictably with a high rate of lung tumors. But the principal cause of lung cancer is the smoking of cigarettes; and although other factors may be involved—as in the theory that cigarette smoke merely acts as a co-carcinogen in conjunction with some other agent (perhaps a virus) to initiate a tumor—*the principal cause of lung cancer still remains the smoking of cigarettes.* In the United States, sixty thousand people now die *in a year* as a result of lung cancer, and of these fifty-four thousand will be cigarette smokers. In Great Britain, 40 per cent of all cases of cancer are lung cancer; and this, the highest rate in the world, is probably due to additional encouragement given to the induction of the disease by widespread bronchial ailments. One of the senior administrators of an American cancer hospital told me recently, "Half of all our beds are now occupied by lung cancer cases," and it was quite clear that he really did not know what to do about the situation. Only 5 per cent of lung cancer patients survive for five years after surgery—the most radical surgery; the great majority of patients die within a year after surgery; and apart from the steady increase of the disease in men, every hospital administrator must be aware that women are now—after some twenty-five years of intensive smoking since World War II—appearing with greater and greater frequency in the gruesome statistics.

A safer cigarette? Milder tobacco? More effective filters?

The answer is, a safe cigarette is no more possible than safe cyanide. Every time a more effective filter has been devised it has been necessary to strengthen the flavor of the tobacco in some manner, by using coarser cuts or different blends, so that the fastidious smoker can *taste* the carcinogens he is taking into his respiratory system. Otherwise—cigarette manufacturers have learned from long and costly experience—the fastidious smoker feels he is being robbed of something infinitely precious and he will immediately switch to another brand. A safer cigarette today would probably arouse such widespread consumer resistance that it would almost certainly be followed by a far more dangerous cigarette tomorrow; and the truth of this statement is shown by the constant increase in the *length* of cigarettes, from the so-called normal or regular size (which were carcinogenic enough) to king-sized (which are ten or fifteen per cent more carcinogenic) to still longer kinds (which are proportionately more carcinogenic than their predecessors).

There is little hope that anything can be done about this particular insanity. It may be, indeed, part of some intricate evolutionary process, whereby at a time when populations are increasing rather too rapidly for comfort, Nature supplies the means—an insatiable craving for a destructive toxin—to check the rate of increase. Lung cancer, and cancer of the bladder, and emphysema, and heart disease, and circulatory diseases such as Buerger's disease: all arise from tobacco tars and nicotine, all serve to reduce the population. Even in Japan and India, where lung cancer was unknown until recently, it is now known only too well; and today there are no unshaded areas left on the lung cancer map of the world.

It is preventable. It need not happen. And that, perhaps, is where one should leave it. Or one can repeat it, just for the ears of young people, *It really is preventable.* One wishes the same could be said here and now about every other kind of malignancy.

The cancer men and women still have a lot to do. They are very special human beings, and the observer is likely to find them strangely innocent. They have fifty years of work ahead of them or (as Sir Ernest Kennaway predicted) two hundred and fifty—nobody can tell for certain. But they are totally engrossed in what they are doing: in their enzymes, or their nucleic acids, or their cell membranes, or in the statistics of liver cancer among the Bantu, or the effects of sealskin chewing among Alaskan women. They seem to think of nothing else. They are completely committed. When I saw Dr. Eva Klein in her laboratory in the Karolinska Institutet in Stockholm one Saturday afternoon (she had driven in specially to see me and to talk to me for more than three hours about the mysteries of immunology, leaving her children in the country with Dr. and Mrs. Stjernswärd) I tried to explain to her what was in my mind about all these people I had met in so many laboratories, in so many countries; people who had impressed me so deeply and whom I had come to respect so much. I said, "I think the real purpose of the book I am writing is to say the human race is not so bad, after all. It can produce cancer researchers. I have tremendous admiration for them; I think they are doing absolutely marvelous work; and I am very proud to be a member of the same race."

She seemed a little surprised by this outburst. I daresay I was a little surprised myself. She did not reply for a moment. Then she smiled, and said, "I'll remember that the next time I feel blue."

Index

AAT (carcinogenic substance), 321
Abbottempo (London), 6 n., 14 n., 22 n.
Abercrombie, Prof. Michael, 84
Aboul-Nasr, Dr. Ahmed Lofty, 179
Accidents, as a cause of death, 28
Accra, 14
Achlorhydria, 331 n., 337
Acid-mucopolysaccharide, 267
Acrocentrics, 79–80
ACS, *see* American Cancer Society
Actinomycin D, 231–35, 237–38
Acute Leukemia Task Force (National Cancer Institute), 54
Addis Ababa, 320
Addison's disease, 4
Adenoids, 249 n.
Adrenals, 6
Advances in Cancer Research, 305
Afghanistan, 152, 153
  cholera in, 92
Aflatoxins, 275–82, 292–322, 345
  food contamination by, 314–16, 318
  discovery of, 167
  response to in animals, 308
Aflatoxin B_1, 315
Africa, 3, 4, 5, 6, 8, 10, 13, 14, 16, 19, 40, 168
  choriocarcinoma in, 258
  incidence of cancer in, 103
  lung cancer in, 93–94
  see also East Africa, South Africa

Africans, 113
Agra University, 152, 153
Agricola, 96 n.
Agriculture Research Service, 311–12
Alcohol, 342, 345
Alcoholism, 345
Alexander, Peter, 23, 59, 97, 198 n., 210, 249–50 n., 255–56
Alternaria, 313
Altona, 93 n.
Amazon River, 176
Ambrose, Prof. E. J., 84, 149–50, 267
America, *see* United States
American Association for Cancer Research, 1966 Meeting, 180
American Cancer Society, 41–50, 230, 237, 327 n., 347
  estimate of incidence of leukemia, 181
  report of special committee on Society's performance and policies, 47–48
  statistics of cancer incidence and mortality, 106–7
American Society for the Control of Cancer, 41
Amethopterin, 198, 231
Amiel, J. L., 212 n.
Amines, aromatic, 343
Aminopterin, 231
Anabolism, definition of, 82 n.

Anaphase, 68
Anaplasia, 75 n.
Anatomical pathology, 71 n.
Andhra Pradesh, India, 137, 140
Anemia, pernicious, 331
Anesthetics, 91
Angina pectoris, 112
Animals, cancer in, 117–20
Animal Health Society, London, 294
Anopheles mosquito, 117 n., 173–74, 194
Anthracene, 95 n., 110
Antibiotics, 28
Antibodygen, 251
Anti-carcinogens, 95 n., 110
Antigens, 251, 253–55, 270
Antimitotic drugs, 213
Antimony, 295
Areca catechu, 137
A.R.S., *see* Agricultural Research Service
Arsenic, 110, 295
  compounds, 340
  poisoning, 168
Arthropod, 17
Arua, Uganda, 12
Asia, Southeast, 92, 153, 176
Asian 'flu, 28
Aspergillus, varieties of, 308–11
  A. carneus, 309
  A. flavus, 301–3, 305, 320
  A. fumigatus, 309
  A. glaucus, 309
  A. niger, 308
  A. ochraceus, 320
  A. ruber, 309
  A. versicolor, 309
Asthma, 112
Ataxia, locomotor, 196
Atomic Radiation and Life (Alexander), 97 n.
Atrophy, gastric, 337
Audubon's warbler, 4
Australia, incidence of cancer in, 104
Austria, incidence of cancer in, 103

Bacillus Calmette-Guérin, *see* BCG
Bacteria, 65, 247
Bacteriophages, 190 n.

Bagshawe, Dr. K. D., 161, 165–66, 219, 258, 259–65, 266
Baker, Russell, 341
Bampton, S. S., 311
Banes, Dr. Daniel, 315
Bang, Dr. Olaf, 188
Bantus, 112, 319–20, 343, 349
Barbiero, 342
Barium, 295
Barr, Dr. Evelyn, 172
Barry, Martin, 71 n.
Basuto tribe, 319
Bateson, William, 68
Bauer, George, *see* Agricola
BCG, 197 n., 197–98, 200, 208–10
Bedford, England, 301
Belfast, Ireland, 275
Belgium, 179
  incidence of cancer in, 103
Bell, T. M., 169
Bell's palsy, 4
Benjamin, W. A., 56 n.
Bennet, John Hughes, 182 n.
Benzidine, 343 n.
Berenblum, Dr. Isaac, 179
Bergel, Franz, 238
Bergkrankheit, *see* Mountain disease
Beta-naphthylamine, 343 n.
Betel chew, 137–38, 155, 342
Betel palm, 137
Beveridge, Dr. William I. J., 55–56, 118
Biafra, 299 n.
Bidis, 136–37, 143
Bihar, State of, 130
Biology, 82
  cellular, 70
  molecular, 207
Biology of Cancer, The, 220, 220 n., 223 n., 255 n.
Biochemistry, 206
Biochemistry of Bladder Cancer, The (Thomas), 344 n.
Birds, 30
Biris, *see* Bidis
Birmingham, England, 228
Bland Sutton Institute, London, 172
Blastocyst, 261 n.
Blokhin, Dr. Nikolai, 179

INDEX

Blood, group A, 338
Blood-brain barrier, definition of, 185, 185 n.
Blount, W. F., 293–303, 310
Bluecomb, 296
Bombay, 129
 University of, 131, 142
Bone marrow, transplants of, in leukemia, 216–17
Bonn, University of, 117–18, 284 n.
Borneo, incidence of cancer in, 94
Boston, 230–40
Boveri, Theodor, 79
Bowen's disease, 110
Bowles, Chester, 156
Boyd, Dr. T. R., 97–100
Boyland, Prof. E., 344 n.
Boyse, Dr. Edward A., 255
Bracken, 110
Braganca, Dr. Beatriz M., 144–45, 156
Brahmans, 142
Brain, 87
Brazil, 195, 297–99
Breast malignancies, 78
Bright's disease, 4
Brill, 97 n.
British Army, 8, 21
British Commonwealth, 112
British Empire Cancer Fund, 347
British Journal of Cancer, 116
British Journal of Pathology and Bacteriology, 286 n.
British Medical Journal, The, 143 n., 144, 175
British Medical Research Council, London, 12, 97
British Turkey Federation, 293
Brodey, R. S., 119 n.
Bronchitis, 131
Bubonic plague, 27, 154, 246
Bucalossi, Dr. Pietro, 179
Buerger's disease, 348
Bunsen burner, 4
Burchenal, Dr. Joseph Holland, 3, 4, 18, 180–201, 213
Bureau of Scientific Research (FDA), 315
Burkitt, Dr. Denis P., 5, 6–23, 46, 195, 257, 275

Burkitt's lymphoma, 4, 17, 20, 160, 176, 177, 186 n., 231, 257
 see also Burkitt's tumor
Burkitt's Lymphoma: A Study in Medical Detection, 22 n.
Burkitt's tumor, 3–23, 167–70, 175, 194–96, 199
 see also Burkitt's lymphoma
Burkitt's Tumor as a Stalking Horse for Leukemia (Burchenal), 194, 197
Burma, 152
Butler, Samuel, 69
Butter yellow, 344

Caceres, Dr. Eduardo, 179
Caecum, 249 n.
Cairo, 114
California, University of, 45, 119 n.
Cambridge University, 118
Canada, 103, 144
Canadian Cancer Society, 347
Cancer, 61–84
 anaplastic, 75
 in animals, 117–20, 283–90
 of the bladder, 103, 343–44, 348
 of the blood, 288
 of the brain and central nervous system, 78, 105, 239, 283, 285, 346
 of the breast, 104, 105, 126, 234, 327
 as a cause of death, 312
 causes of, 114
 cell division in, 80
 circumcision as a factor in, 123
 of the cervix, 104, 120 n., 123, 339
 and chromosomal changes, 79
 of the colon and rectum, 103–4, 327–28, 345–46, 345 n.
 detection of, 335
 dietary factors in, 230
 in domestic pets, 118
 environment as a factor in, 95–96, 339–46
 environmental biology of, 281
 epidemiology of, 94–108
 of the epipharynx, 112
 of the esophagus, 103, 112, 143,

Cancer (cont'd)
  281, 283, 285, 288, 341, 342, 345 n.
  female, 104, 105–6
  gastric, 115
  of the gastrointestinal tract, 234
  genetic factors in, 106
  hereditary causes of, 72, 95
  incidence of, 96, 103–8, 347–48
  infective agents of, 170
  of the kidney, 61, 78, 106
  of the larynx, 345 n.
  of the liver, 78, 103, 106, 112, 239, 281, 288, 319, 320–22, 344–45, 345 n., 349
  of the lung, 77, 96, 103, 104, 106, 110, 135, 239, 285, 288, 327, 346–49
  male, 103–4, 105
  mortality from, 103, 106–7, 348
  of the mouth, 103, 142, 143, 155, 345 n.
  natural remedies for, 227
  of the nasopharynx, 112–13
  of the neck, 30
  occupational, 96
  of the oropharynx, 143
  of the ovaries, 81, 346
  of the pancreas, 345, 345 n.
  pathology of, 167
  of the penis, 104, 124, 340
  of the pharynx, 143
  prevention of, 334, 336–38
  of the prostate, 103, 104, 288, 327
  in rabbits, 31
  due to radiation, 96
  in rainbow trout, 306–7
  of the rectum, 345–46, 345 n.
  relation of to geographical conditions, 17
  remissions in, 231
  research, modern era in, 31–57
  of the retina, 78
  of the scrotum, 30, 340
  of the skin, 59, 76, 77, 103, 104, 106, 139, 168, 227, 327, 340–41
  of the stomach, 103–4, 107, 127, 140, 234, 309, 328–32
  superstitions about, 114–17
  of the testes, 346
  of the throat, 133
  of the thyroid, 106
  of the tongue, 143
  of the tonsils, 143
  treatment of, 159–77, 243, 334–36
  of the uterus, 103, 104, 120, 126, 133, 328
  see also Leukemia, Lymphomas, Pap smear test, Mammography, Tumors
Cancer (R. J. C. Harris), 277 n.
Cancer (E. E. Hurst), 342
Cancer, Chromosome Theory of (Boveri), 79
cancer à deux, 117, 120–26
Cancer Chemotherapy National Service Center (U. S. Public Health Center), 220
Cancer Facts and Figures, 1968 (American Cancer Society), 327 n.
Cancer houses, 114–15
cancer, la guérison de, 60
Cancer Programs of the U. S. Public Health Service, 192
Cancer Research Institute, Paris, 138
Cancerology, 120, 179
Cancerophobia, 104
Canine Neoplasia: A Prototype for Human Cancer Study (Prier and Brodey), 119 n.
Capsicum annum (Guinea pepper), 140
Capsicum frutescens (Chile), 140
Carcinogenesis, 171, 207, 281, 288–91
Carcinogens, 77, 94, 109–11, 137–38, 287, 343 n., 344, 345 n.
  chemical, 79, 95 n.
Carcinogenic material, 72, 113
Carcinogenic metals, 110
Carcinoma:
  Lucké, 171
  of the penis, 125
  in situ, 83
  squamous cell, 168
  of the tongue, 77
  see also Cancer, of the skin

INDEX

Carter, 286 n.
Carver, George Washington, 299
Cassava, 112
Castiglioni, Arturo, 124 n., 246 n.
Castor oil, 112
Catabolism, definition of, 82 n.
Cattan, A., 212 n.
Cattle, 30
Cauterization, 30
Cell differentiation, 69
Cells:
  blood, 81, 98, 183–85
  bone marrow, 76, 81
  cancerous, 70, 81, 83–84
  connective tissue, 69
  contact inhibition of movement of, 84
  division of, 68
  germ, 68, 69
  of the intestines, 68, 76
  kidney, 83
  leukemic, 72
  of the liver, 66, 83
  male reproductive, 68
  malignant, 61, 70–87
  muscle, 69
  nerve, 69
  normal, 61–70, 76, 81
  skin, 66, 68, 69
  totipotent, 69–70
  tumor, 78
Centre National de la Recherche Scientifique, 206
Centriole, 65
Cereal Science Today, 315
Cerebral hemorrhage, 29 n.
Cervical cancer, *see* Cancer, of the cervix
Cervix, 120 n.
Ceylon, 8, 142, 152, 153
Chargas' disease, 342
Charcot's joints, 4
Chaucer's Doctor of Physic, 30
Chemical Defence Experimental Station, Wiltshire, 295
Chemotherapy, 18–20, 40, 51–52, 54, 151, 163–66, 180, 220–1, 222–29, 230–31, 243, 288, 335
  of the central nervous system, 212 n.

geographic, 180–81
  in leukemia, 181, 213–14
Chemotherapy of Cancer, The (Stock), 220, 227
Chemotherapy of Cancer: First Report of an Expert Committee, 180
Chester Beatty Research Institute, England, 4, 111, 138, 149, 160, 198 n., 219, 223, 238, 253 n., 255, 267
Chesterman, Dr. F. C., 188
Chicago, 79 n.
Chickenpox, 117 n.
Children, malignancies of, 77
Children's Hospital, Boston, 230
Chile, 104, 126
Chili pepper, 140
China, 112, 252, 343, 345
  incidence of cancer in, 103–4
Chinar, 139, 139 n.
Chinese in Singapore, 112
Chloroform, 91
Chloroquinine, 196
Cholera, 27, 91–95, 100, 246, 283
  epidemic of 1854, 91
  in India, 131, 133, 153
Cholera Inquiry Committee, England, 92
Choriocarcinoma, 40, 160–61, 162, 166 n., 219, 257–61, 270
Chromosomal abnormalities, 80–81
Chromosomes, 61, 67, 69, 78–81, 87
  Ph^1, *see* Philadelphia chromosome
Cigarettes, *see* Smoking
Circumcision, 123–26
Cirrhosis, 320–21, 344–45, 344 n.
City of Hope, California, 313
Clifford, Dr. Peter, 112, 198
Clinical pathology, 71 n.
Coady, Dr. A., 320
Coal tar, 31, 110, 340
Cobra venom, 145–51
Co-carcinogens, 77, 77 n., 109
Colchamine, 227
Colchicine, 227
Cold Spring Harbor Laboratory of Quantitative Biology, Long Island, N.Y., 56

Collagen, 140, 140 n.
Colombia, 195
Colon, malignancies of, 78
Colonial Office, British, 9, 10
Colonial Service, British, 8
Columbia University, 142
Committee on Tumor Nomenclature, 4
Comparative pathology, 71
Congo, 12
Conjunctivitis, 111
Connors, T. A., 220
Consumption, 245
    see also Tuberculosis
Contagion, definition of, 117 n.
Cook, Sir Albert, 11 n.
Cook, Captain James, 325
Coombe, Reginald G., 38
Copts, 124
Cornea of the eye, 83
Corti, organs of, 4
Cortisone, 209
Cowpox, 245
Cramer, W., 105
Crick, Francis, 56 n.
    see also Watson-Crick
cri du chat syndrome, 80
Croton oil, 112, 295
Curie, Madame, 96
Currie, Dr. G. A., 258, 266, 271
Curtis, Brian, 306
Curtis, Helena, 189
Cyanides, 295
Cycad palm, 109
Cycasin, 109, 345
Cyclophosphamide, 19, 212
Cytoplasm, 61, 65, 66, 82, 94
Cytoplasmic fluid, 65
Cytosan, 19
Cytotoxic drugs, 19
Czechoslovakia, 96

Davies, Dr. J. N. P., 16
Davies, R. I., 116
Datura stramonium, 295
DDT, 295
de Gaulle, Charles, 277
Death, causes of, 28 n., 29 n.
Deccani Hindus, 143
De Re Metallica (Agricola), 96 n.
Denmark, 126 n., 140, 142, 319
    incidence of cancer in, 104
Demecolcine, 227
Denoix, Dr. Pierre, 179
Denver, 180
Deoxyribonucleic acid, see DNA
Department of Scientific and Industrial Research, London, 295
Dermatitis, 96
Dermatophytes, 313
Deucalion, 4
Diamond, L. K., 230 n.
Diet, 330, 337
Digitalis, 228, 295
Digitalis purpurea, 228
Diospyros melanoxylon, 136
Diphtheria, 210, 246
Diseases:
    Addison's, 4
    Bright's, 4
    Buerger's, 348
    degenerative, 28, 56
    epidemic, 28, 94-95
    heart, 28, 29 n., 131, 228, 237, 348
    Hodgkin's, 4, 5, 30, 346
    infectious, 28, 56, 131, 153, 163-64, 283
    Newcastle, 296
    parasitic, 118
    prevention of, 284
    respiratory, 118
    Turkey "X," 293-303, 308, 311
Dimethylnitrosamine (DMNA), 286 n.
DNA (deoxyribonucleic acid), 67, 82, 237-38, 237 n.
Doll, Dr. Richard, 71, 97, 115, 115 n., 339
Double Helix, The (Watson), 16
Down's syndrome, 81
Dropsy, 228
Druckrey, Dr. H., 281, 282-91, 346
Drugs, anti-cancer, 164
Duarte, California, 313
Dublin, Ireland, 7, 275
Dublin University, 7
Dyes, 110
Dysentery, 131
Dwarfism, see Turner's syndrome

INDEX

East Africa, 11 n., 15, 17, 18, 114, 194, 302, 305, 334
East African Research Institute, Entebbe, 176
Ebers Papyrus, Thebes, 30
Ebony tree, 136
EB virus, 177
ECHO viruses, see Reoviruses
Edinburgh, 7
Egypt, incidence of cancer in, 103
Egyptians, 124
Ehrlich, Paul, 244, 267
Ehrlich ascites tumor, 267
El Tor cholera, 92
Elbe River, 93 n.
Electron Microscopy of Cancer Cells (de Harven), 171 n.
Ellermann, Dr. Wilhelm, 188
Elution, 110
Embryomas, 78
Emphysema, 348
Endicott, Dr. Kenneth M., 52-55, 314, 316-17
Ender, Prof., 286
Endocrinology, 206
Endoplasmic reticulum, 65
Endoxan, 19
England, 7, 55, 60, 77, 106, 110, 112, 167-68, 179, 195, 258, 261, 277, 278, 302, 305, 334, 347
 incidence of cancer in, 93, 104
Enniskillen, Ireland, 7, 21
Entebbe, Africa, 14, 169, 176
Enzymes, 82, 87, 248
Epidemics, 92, 94
Epidemiology, 4, 94-108, 192
Epipharynx, 112
Epstein, Dr. M. A., 6, 15, 172
Erythema *ab igne* (or *caloricum*), 139 n.
Erythrocytes, 183-84
Erythroleukemia, 184
Erz Gebirge mines, 96
Esophageal cancer, see Cancer, of the esophagus
Esophagus, description of, 341-42
Ethiopians, 124
E39, 213
Etiology, definition of, 168 n.
Eucalyptus oil, 110

Eunuchoidism, 80
Euphorbia:
 E. ingens, 111, 112
 E. pilulifera, 112
 E. resinifera, 112
 E. tirucalli, 111, 112
Euphorbiaceae, 112
Europe, 6, 55, 105, 132, 144, 196
Eustachian tubes, 249 n.
Evening Standard, The (London), 159
Ewing, Dr. James R., 37, 132
Ewing's sarcoma, 4

Fallopian tubes, 4, 120
Fallopius, 4
Far East, 345
Farber, Dr. Sidney, 230-40, 282, 288, 335
Fat, deficiency of in diet, 331
Fawcett, Dr. J. S., 112
FD & C Act, see Food, Drug, and Cosmetic Act
Fibrosis, submucous, 140
Figaro, Le, 60
Fiji Islands, incidence of cancer in, 105
Finland, 116, 179, 329, 334
Fluke, 345, 345 n.
5-fluorouracil, 234
Folic acid, 230
Food and Drug Administration, 314-15
Food, Drug, and Cosmetic Act, 315 n.
Forschergruppe Praeventivmedizin am Max Planck Institut für Immunbiologie, 282
Forster, E. M., 129
Fowl pest, see Newcastle disease
Foxglove, 228
France, 60, 100, 103, 128, 179, 198, 276, 277
Freiburg im Breisgau, 282, 288 n.
French National League Against Cancer, 347
French Revolution, 130
Fruit fly, 30
Fulham Hospital, London, 259
Fundus, 120
Furth, Dr. Jacob, 72

Gall stones, 345
Ganges river delta, cholera in, 92
Garrison, Fielding H., 244, 246 n.
Gastrocamera, 338 n.
Gastrointestinal disorders, 131
Gastroscope, 338 n.
Geddes, W. F., 317
General Motors Corporation, 32, 35, 37
Genetics, 207
Geneva, 5 n., 55, 180
Geographic Chemotherapy—Burkitt's Tumor as a Stalking Horse for Leukemia (Burchenal), 180
German measles, 190 n.
Germany, 100, 179, 277, 282
  incidence of cancer in, 103
Ghana, 14
Gilmour, Dr. Mavis, 104–5
Glandula preputialis, see Tyson's glands
Glands, salivary, 6
Glasgow, 275
Golgi bodies, 65
Granulocytes, 183, 249
Great Britain, see England
Great Ormond Street Hospital, London, 168, 170
Groundnuts, 298–303
Groundnut meal, 297
Groupe européen de Chimiothérapie anticancereuse, 212 n.
Guinea pepper, 140
Gujaratis, 133, 143
Guy's Hospital, London, 30
Gyanylhydrazone, 213

Haddow, Prof. Sir Alexander, 14, 16, 95, 160–62, 165, 176, 179
Haenszel, Dr. W., 328
Haffkine Institute, 145
Hamburg, 93 n., 96
Hamperl, Dr. Hedwig, 117, 179, 284 n.
Hansemann, D., 79
Harijans, 142
Harris, Dr. R. J. C., 22, 190, 277 n.
Harvard Medical School, 230
Harven, Dr. Etienne de, 171
Hawaii, University of, 327 n.

Hawaiian Islands, 325–34
Heart disease, 28, 29 n., 131, 228, 237, 348
Hedgerow, 111
Heidelberg, 112
Hellebore, 295
Hellen, 4
Hematopoeisis, 165
Hemorrhoids, 346
Hemosiderosis, 343
Henle, Drs. W. and G., 177
Hepatitis, in animals, 296
Hepatoblastoma, 78
Hernia:
  as a cause of death, 28
  hiatus, 342
  strangulated, 10
Herpes, 169
Hertz, Dr. Roy, 161, 259
Hess, W., 96
Heterochimeras, 216
Heyssel, 97 n.
Higginson, Dr. John, 275–82, 216, 319, 321
Hindus, 132–33
Hippocrates, 30, 114
Hiroshima, 32, 97
Histamines, 248, 250
History of Medicine, A (Castiglioni), 124 n., 246 n.
History of Medicine (Garrison), 246 n.
Hodgkin, Thomas, 30
Hodgkin's disease, 4, 5, 30, 228, 240, 346
  see also Lymphogranuloma
Hohenheim, Philippus A. T. B. P. von, 96
Hong Kong, 8, 113, 337
Honolulu, 325
Hookworm, 10
Hôpital Broussais, 206
Hôpital Paul Brousse, 205, 212 n.
Hormones, 66, 346
Hormone therapy, 47
Hospital for Tropical Diseases, London, 320
Howard, Frank, 33, 40
Huggins, Dr. Charles B., 46, 230
Hurst, E. E., 342
Hürting, F. H., 96

INDEX 359

Hydrazines, 287
Hydrocele, 10
Hyperplastic masses, 75, 75 n.
Hypothesis (Currie, Lond, and Bagshawe), 258

Iceland, 103
Ichikawa, Prof. K., 31
Immunity, definition of, 243
Immunogenetics, 206
Immunology, 82, 207, 243–72, 268–71, 336
Immunotherapy, 210, 214–17, 243, 255–56
Imperial Cancer Research Fund, Entebbe, 22, 169
India, 127–56, 179, 320, 348
  cholera in, 91–92, 131, 133, 153
  choriocarcinoma in, 257
  life in, 128–31
Indian Cancer Research Center, 131, 135, 137–41
Indian Cancer Society, 128
Indians, South America, 174
Indonesia, 152, 258
Infection, 345
  definition of, 117 n.
Influenza, 28, 108, 117 n., 131, 187, 246, 247
Inoculation, 246 n.
Insects, 65
INSERM, 206
Institute of Cancer Research, 223
Institut de Cancérologie et d'Immunogénétique, 205, 212 n.
Institut Gustav Roussy, Villejuif, 206, 212 n.
Institut National de la Santé et de la Recherche Médicale, 206
Interferon, 248
International Agency for Research on Cancer, France, 276–78
International Journal of Cancer, The, 277
International Union Against Cancer, 4, 4 n., 125, 131, 160
  Mexico Symposium (1964), 125
Iran, cholera in, 92
Ireland, 7, 102, 104, 296
Iron, deficiency of in diet, 343
Irradiation, 76, 114, 235

  see also Radiation therapy, Radiotherapy
Isaacs, Alick, 248
Island of Dr. Moreau, The (Wells), 217
Isonicotinic acid hydrazide, 109
Israel, 103, 123, 126, 179
Istituto Regina Elena, Rome, 55
Italy, 60, 100, 103, 179, 277

Jamaica, Chinese population in, 105
James Ewing Hospital, 138
Japan, 55, 97, 100, 106, 116, 126, 127, 179, 258, 275, 327–29, 338, 348
  incidence of cancer in, 104
Japan Cancer Society, 347
Japanese in Hawaii, 327–34
Japanese Institute of Fermentation, 314
Jatropha curcus, 295
Jaws, 6
Jenner, Edward, 244–46
Jimson weed, 295
Jinja, Uganda, 10
Joachimsthal, 96
Johannesburg, hospitals in, 114
John of Arderne, 30
Journal of Tropical Medicine, 11 n.

Kampala, 3–4, 10, 14, 15, 23, 170, 180
Kangri, 139
Kansas, University of, 276
Kano, Nigeria, 14, 15
Karolinska Institutet, Stockholm, 3, 112, 349
Karyotype, 79
Kashmir, 139
Kennaway, Sir Ernest, 31, 348
Kennedy, John F., 344
Kenya, 8, 13, 113, 114, 287, 301
Kenya, Mount, 112
Kenyatta National Hospital, Nairobi, 114
Kettering, Dr. Charles F., 33–36
Khanolkar, Dr. Vasant Ramji, 131–38, 143 n., 156, 179
Kidneys, 6, 61, 75, 78, 252
Kikuyu, 113, 286

Kingston Public Hospital, Jamaica, 105
Kirby, Dr. D. R. S., 265–66
Klebs, Edwin, 79, 79 n.
Klein, Dr. Eva, 3, 112, 180, 349
Klein, Dr. George, 112, 179, 180
Klinefelter's syndrome, 80
Koch, Robert, 91, 93 n., 215–16
Kraybill, Dr. H. F., 305–13, 321
Kshatriyas, 142
Kuakini Hospital, Hawaii, 327
Kununka, Dr. B., 9
Kurokawa, Toshio, 338 n.
kwashiorkor, 299, 299 n., 321

Lack, David, 7
Lambaréné, 11 n.
Lancet, The (Great Britain), 258, 271
Landsteiner, Dr. Karl, 188
Langerhans, islets of, 4
Lasker, Mary (Mrs. Albert D.), 43
L-asparaginase, 219, 239
Latin America, 128, 334
Lead, 295
Lederle Laboratories, 18
Leprosy, 41, 133, 150
Leprosy Institute, India, 134
Leucocytes, 183, 249–52
Leukemia, 18, 21, 40, 72–73, 78, 81, 97, 103, 177, 180–94, 208–9, 253, 256, 327, 335, 346
  acute, 181
  in animals, 187–88
  bone marrow in transplants, 214–16
  chemotherapy in, 212–14
  chronic, 81, 240
  definition of, 182
  in domestic animals, 118
  epidemiology of, 192
  granulocytic, 81 n.
  immunotherapy in, 214–17
  incidence of, 103
  lymphatic, 230
  lymphoblastic, 212 n.
  lymphocytic, 184–85
  methods of classification of, 182–83
  mortality rate of, 103–4
  myelocytic, 81 n., 184

myelogenous, 81 n.
  periwinkle cure for, 227–29
  treatment of, 180, 217–29
  viruses, 215–17
  see also Erythroleukemia
Leurocristine, 227
Life Story of the Fish, The (Curtis), 306
Liver, 6, 78, 87, 103
Liverpool, 168
Lira, Uganda, 9–10
Lond, M. B., 258
London, 4, 6 n., 30, 31, 59, 77, 97, 111, 138, 159, 160, 167–68, 172, 217–29, 259, 278 n., 294, 297, 300, 320
  University of, 223 n.
London Hospital, 112
Lourenço Marques, 13
Loustalot, Dr. Prosper, 179
Lucké, Dr. Balduin, 171
Lucké carcinoma, 171
Lucké virus, 171
Lumiére, A., 115
Luminizers, 98–100
L'Union Internationale Contre Le Cancer, see International Union Against Cancer
Lungs, 77, 87
  malignancies, 78
Lwoff, André, 66
Lye, 342
Lymph:
  glands, 87
  nodes, 5, 183
Lymphocytes, 183, 249, 253, 269
Lymphomas, 4, 6, 78, 167, 177
  see also Burkitt's lymphoma, Burkitt's tumor
Lymphogranulomas, 5
Lymphosarcoma, 195, 240
Lyons, France, 276

Macromolecules, 66
Magee, P. N., 284 n.
Maisin, Prof. J. R., 179
Makarere University, 166
Malaria, 10, 27, 117 n., 153, 173–75, 176, 196, 196–97
  as an agent, 170

INDEX 361

Malarial plasmodium, 117 n., 172 n., 173–75, 336
Malariotherapy, 196
Malaya, 111, 258
Malays in Singapore, 112
Maldive Islands, 152
Malignancies, 107
Malpighian bodies, 4
Malnutrition, 10, 331, 345
Mammography, definition of, 335
Manchester Children's Tumor Registry, England, 168, 170
Manchuria, 8
Manhattan Project, 55
Manioc, see Cassava
Mansonia mosquito, 194
Margerison, Dr., 302
Mashowa tribe, 319
Masking of Antigens on Trophoblast and Cancer Cells, 258
Matabele tribe, 319
Mathé, George, 198, 206–17, 218, 255
Matthias, Dr. J. Q., 77
Meadow saffron, 227
Measles, 28, 117 n., 187, 246
Medical Clinics of North America, The, 157 n., 255 n.
Medicine, preventive, 284
Megaesophagus, 342
Meiosis, 68
Meknes, Morocco, 330 n.
Melanin, 341
Melanoma, definition of, 119 n.
Memorial Hospital for Cancer and Allied Diseases, New York, 18, 32, 37, 39, 180, 194
Mercer, Dr. R. D., 82, 230 n.
Mercury, 295
Mesothelioma, 110
Mesothorium, 98
Metabolism, definition of, 82, 82 n.
Metaphase, 68
Metastases, 71
  pulmonary, 232
Metchnikoff, Elie, 250
Methotrexate, 18, 19, 161, 212, 231
Methyl-glyoxal-bis, 213
Methyl-nitroso-urea, 289, 290
Mexico, 141
Milner, M., 317

Min Chiu Lin, Dr., 161, 259
Mitochondria, 65, 82
Mitomycin C, 236
Mitotic apparatus, 68
MLD (Minimum Lethal Dose), 146
Modest, Dr. E. J., 238
Molecular Biology of the Gene (Benjamin), 56 n.
Molybdenum, deficiency of in soil, 286
Mongolia, 152
Mongolism, see Down's syndrome
Monocytes, 183
Morocco, 330 n.
Moselle valley, 110
Mountain disease (*Bergkrankheit*), 96, 96 n.
Mouse, laboratory, 76
Mozambique, 13
Mucopolysaccharide, 267, 269–70
Mühlbock, Dr. Otto, 179
Mulago Hospital, Kampala, 10
Mumps, 117 n., 246
Murphy, J. B., 209
Mycotoxins, 314–16, 322, 345
"Mycotoxins as a Food Problem" (Banes), 315

Nairobi, 3, 18, 112, 114, 198
Nasopharyngeal cancer, see Cancer, of the nasopharynx
Nasopharynx, 112, 249 n.
"nass" (USSR), 342
National Advisory Cancer Council, 42, 51 n.
  annual report (1966), 186
National Cancer Institute, Bethesda, 38, 45, 50–55, 60, 110, 138, 161, 163, 190 n., 218 n., 221, 221 n., 288, 305, 313–14, 316, 317
  Acute Leukemia Task Force, 193
  chemotherapy development program, 288
  report on tanning, 341
  support of studies in Hawaii, 333–34
  and virus-leukemia research, 186
National Cancer Day (England, 1967), 160

National Institutes of Health, 43, 51, 259
Nature, 300, 302
Necrosis, 236 n.
Nelson, Dr. Clifton, 12
Neoplasms, 75
Nepal, 152
  cholera in, 92
Nephroblastomas, 78
Nephroma, embryonic, 5
Nervi, Dr. Carlo, 55
Netherlands, 179
Neuraminidase, 270
Neuritis, peripheral, 240
Neuroblastomas, 78
Neurotoxins, 145–46
New Delhi, 130, 151
"New Directions in Cancer Research" (American Cancer Society), 50
New England Journal of Medicine, 230 n.
New Guinea, 6, 176, 194–95
New Jersey, 98
New York, 72, 207
New York Times, The, 56, 159, 341
New Zealand, 193
Newcastle disease, 296
Newton, 56
Newton's rings, 4
Ngu, Dr. Victor, 179
Nigeria, 14, 179, 198
Ninth International Cancer Congress, 180, 279
Nisei, *see* Japanese
Nitabuch, Dr. Raissa, 265
Nitabuch, layer of, 265–66, 267, 269
Nitrogen mustard, 239
Nitrosamines, 275–91, 316, 346
Nobel prize, 56, 82
Norway, incidence of cancer in, 103
Nuclear membrane, 65
Nucleic acids, 56, 67
Nucleus of a cell, 65, 67
Nuffield Provincial Hospital Trust, The, 115 n.
Nyasaland, 13, 14

Oahu, 325
Oberling, Charles, 115, 244, 343
Oettgen, Dr. Herbert F., 18
Oettlé, A. G., 11, 342
Ohio State Penitentiary, 257
Old, Dr. Lloyd J., 197, 255
Oleander, 295
Oncology, definition of, 207, 207 n.
O'nyong-nyong fever, 16–17
Oral cancer, *see* Cancer, of the mouth
Orange oil, 110
Organelles, 66, 82, 87
Orthotolidine, 343 n.
Osler, Sir William, 96
Osteomyelitis, 98
Osteosarcoma, 119
Ova, origin of, 68, 79
Ovaries, 6, 120
Oxford University, 265

Pacific Ocean, 325
Palsy, 240
  Bell's, 4
pan, chewing of in India, 141
Pancreas, 345
Pancreatitis, 345
Pandemic, 28
Pap smear technique, 120, 335
Papilla, definition of, 120 n.
Papillomas, definition of, 120 n.
Papuans (New Guinea), 174–75
Paralytic ileus, 240
Paratyphoid, 246
Paris, 5, 138
Parkinson's syndrome, 4
Parsis, 132
Paterson-Kelly syndrome, 342
Pathology, 4, 71, 71 n.
  definition of, 166 n.
Pathologisches Institut, Bonn, 117
Peanut meal, *see* Groundnut meal
Peanuts, *see* Groundnuts
Pearl Harbor, 327
Penang, 8
Penicillin, 279
Penicillium islandicum, 320, 321
Penicillium rubrum, 313
Penis, 124
Pennsylvania, University of, 119 n., 171

INDEX

Percival, 286 n.
Periwinkle, 227–29, 240
Pernicious anemia, 337
Persia, 132
Perth, Australia, 169
Peru, 179
Pesticides, 110
Ph¹ chromosome, 81
Phagocytes, 183, 250
Pharmacology, 228
  definition of, 282
Pharyngeal tonsil, 249 n.
Phenanthrene, 95 n.
Philadelphia, 166, 177
Philadelphia chromosome, 81, 185
Philippines, choriocarcinoma in, 258
Phimosis, 124, 340
Phipps, James, 245–46
Phosphorus, 295
Physical injuries as a cause of cancer, 77
Pike, M. C., 17 n.
Pituitary gland, 39
Plant pathology, 71
Plants, 30, 65
Plasma membrane, 65, 66
Plasmodium, types of, 173
Plasmodium falciparum, 176
Plummer-Vinson's syndrome, 342
Pneumonia, 131
  bacterial, 28
Podophyllotoxin, 228
Poliomyelitis, 172, 181, 186, 246
Polyposis coli, familial, 72, 345
Polyps, gastric, 337–38
Portugal, incidence of cancer in, 103
Pott, Percival, 30, 31, 95, 340
Pratique Cancérologique, 207
Prednisone, 198, 209, 210, 212
President's Commission on Heart Disease, Cancer, and Stroke, 237
Prevention of Cancer, The (Raven and Roe), 166 n., 189 n., 223 n.
Prevention of Cancer: Pointers from Epidemiology (Doll), 115 n., 339
Prier, J. E., 119, 119 n.

Printer's ink, 110
Progress Against Cancer (National Advisory Cancer Council, 1966), 52 n., 61 n., 186 n.
Prophase, 68
Proteins, 67
Protoplasm, definition of, 82 n.
Protozoa, 30 n.
Public Health Service, 50, 75 n.
Public Health Service Bulletin, 334 n.
Pulmotor, invention of, 91
Pure Food and Drug Act (1906), 315 n., 319
Purgatives, 345
Purkinje cells, 4
Pyrene, 95 n.
Pyretotherapy, 196
Pyrrolizidine alkaloids, 109

Rabbits, 31
Rabies, 246
Radiation, 18, 139 n., 181, 192, 346
  atomic, 96, 97 n.
  of the central nervous system, 212 n.
  effects on the human organism, 97–100
  and the incidence of leukemia and cancer, 97
Radiation therapy, 40, 41, 54, 162–63
Radiobiology, 97, 206
Radiotherapy, 18, 113–14, 162, 234, 239, 243, 335
  see also Radiation
Radium, 96, 97–100, 340
"Radium water," 98
Ramachandran, T. R., 136–37
Rao, K. C. M., 143 n.
Rats, 109
Rauwolfia, 228
Raven, Ronald W., 70, 110, 113, 189 n., 223 n.
Rectal cancer, *see* Cancer, of the colon and rectum
Red blood cells, *see* Erythrocytes
Rehn, Louis, 343
Remission, definition of, 208 n.
Reoviruses, 169, 172–73

Reticuloendothelial system, 250
Retina of the eye, 78
Retinoblastoma, 72, 78
Rheumatic fever, 28
Rhoads, Dr. Cornelius Packard, 32, 34–40, 55, 230
Rhodesia, 13, 114, 194
Ribosomes, 65
Riddle of Cancer, The (Oberling), 115
RNA (ribonucleic acid), 237 n.
Roe, Dr. Francis J. C., 61, 110, 111–12, 189 n., 220, 223–27, 228–29, 286 n.
Rockefeller family, 37
Rockefeller University, 48
Rolando and Sylvius, fissures of, 4
Role of Tumor-Specific Antigens in the Genesis, Development and Control of Malignant Disease, 255 n.
Röntgen, 96
Roswell Park Memorial Institute, 46
Rous, Peyton, 230
Royal Botanic Gardens, Kew, 295
Royal Cancer Hospital, London, 31
Royal Dental College, Denmark, 140
Royal Marsden Hospital, London, 223 n.
Rubella virus, 190 n.–191 n.
Rush Medical College, Chicago, 79 n.
Russell's viper, 145
Russia, *see* USSR

Sahara Desert, 15
St. Bartholomew's Hospital, London, 30
St. Mary's Hospital, London, 259
Salisbury, Rhodesia, 114
Salk and Sabin vaccines, 186
San Francisco, 326
Sanghvi, Dr. L. D., 142–44, 156
Santonin, 295
Sarcoma, 11 n.
  Ewing's, 4
  Yoshida, 149–51
Sartre, Jean-Paul, 277
Saxen, Dr. Erkki, 179
Scandinavia, 123, 128, 334

Schlemm, canal of, 4
Schlumberger, J. R., 212 n.
Schneeberg, Germany, 96
Schneider, M., 212 n.
Schwarzenberg, L., 212 n.
Schweitzer, Dr. Albert, 11 n.
Science and Cancer (Shimkin), 75
Scotland, 103, 296
Scots, 110
Scrotum, 30, 95
Sealskin chewing, 349
Seckel pear, 4
Selenium, 295
Senecio plants, 109
Shabad, Dr. L. M., 179
Shanghai, 8
Sheep-dip, 110
Sheffield, England, 168
Shimkin, Prof. Michael B., 75, 166, 226, 305–13, 321
Shope, Dr. Richard E., 48–50, 230
Sialic acid, 267
Sideropenia, 343
Sideropenic dysphagia, 342
Singapore, 8, 112
Singer, Charles, 31
Sirsat, Dr. (Mrs.) Satyavati M., 125, 156
6-mercaptopurine, 198, 212
Skin, 72
Sleeping sickness, 16, 27, 336
Sloan, Jr., Alfred P., 33, 35
Sloan-Kettering Institute for Cancer Research, 18, 32–40, 42, 45, 138, 180, 257
Smallpox, 27, 153, 245, 247
Smegma, 124–25, 339
Smoking, cigarette, 77, 94, 114, 344, 347–48
Smoking and Chewing of Tobacco in Relation to Cancer and the Upper Respiratory Tract (Sanghvi, Rao, Khanolkar), 143 n.
Snow, John, 91, 95, 100, 125, 244
Soil, character of, 115–16
Somaliland, 8
South Africa, 11, 13, 142, 275, 286, 334
  incidence of cancer in, 104, 111

South African Institute for Medical Research, 11
South America, 38, 176
Southam, Dr. Chester M., 256
Soviet Union, *see* USSR
Special Report: Cancer Chemotherapy Program (Public Health Center), 221 n.
Specific Antigens of Tumors and Leukemias of Experimental Animals, 255 n.
Spermatozoa, 68
  origin of, 79
Spleen, 183
Squill, 295
Standard Oil of New Jersey, 33
Stanley, Prof. N. F., 169
Stasis, 343 n.
Stedman's Medical Dictionary, 94, 236 n.
Steinbeck, John, 35
Stemmermann, Dr., 327-34, 337-38
Stjernswärd, Dr. Jan, 112-13, 349
Stock, Dr. J. A., 219, 240
Stockholm, 3, 180
Stocks, Dr. P., 116
Stomach, 329-30
Storage of Cereal Grains and Their Products (Milner and Geddes), 317
Stroke, 237
Strontium 90, 295
Suicide, 28
Sundarbans, cholera in, 92
Sunlight, exposure to, 340-41
Surgeon General of the U.S., 43
Surgery, 40, 54, 162, 181, 233, 243, 335
Swahili tribe, 319
Swaziland, 13, 14
Sweden, 112, 179
  incidence of cancer in, 103
Swedish Public Health Service, 342
Switzerland, 179
Swinepox, 245
Sylvester, Jr., R. F., 230 n.
Sylvius, *see* Rolando and Sylvius
Symbionts, 82
Symptom, definition of, 285 n.
Syndrome:

cri du chat, 80
  definition of, 80 n.
Down's, 80-81
Klinefelter's, 80
Parkinson's, 4
Paterson-Kelly, 342
Plummer-Vinson's, 342
Turner's, 80, 81
Syphilis, 196, 279

T.A.B. vaccine, 196
Taiwan, 112, 258
Tanganyika, 13, 16
Tata Memorial Hospitals, India, 135, 138, 141-42, 152
Telophase, 68
Temburni leaf, 136
Temple University, 166, 313
Temporary Remissions in Acute Leukemia in Children Produced by Folic Acid Antagonist, 4-aminopterolyglutamic acid (Aminopterin), 230
Testing of Carcinogens in Relation to Cancer Etiology, 138-39
Tetanus, 246
Texas, University of, 46
Thailand, 152
Thallium, 295
Thebes, 30
3,4-benzpyrene, 31, 113
Thymus, 183
Times, The (London), 160
Timmis, Dr. Guy, 7
Tobacco, 137, 342
  smoke, 31, 96
  see also Smoking
Tokyo, 127, 180, 275, 279, 316, 326, 338
  University of, 31
Tomonaga, 97 n.
Tongue, carcinoma of, 77
Tonsilla intestinalis, 249 n.
Tonsils, 183, 249 n.
Toxicology, definition of, 282
Transkei, Africa, 286
Trisomy, 80
Tropical Products Institute, London, 295, 300, 301, 309
Trophoblast, 261-65, 270, 271
Trophoblastic necrosis, 165

Trout, rainbow, 306–22
Trowell, Dr. Hugh, 10, 21
Trypanosome, 16
Tsetse fly, 16, 336
Tuberculosis, 27, 107, 117, 153, 246, 247, 288
Tumors, 5, 76, 77, 113
  abdominal, 21
  benign, 75
  bone, 98, 100, 346
  cancerous, 30
  of the jaw, 167
  of the kidney, 5
  malignant, 70–71, 77
  and oils, 112
  of the retina, 72
  see also Burkitt's tumor, Ehrlich's ascites tumor, Wilms' tumor
Tungsten, 295
Turkeys (British Turkey Federation), 293
Turkey "X" disease, 293–303, 307, 311
"Turkey 'X' Disease" (Blount), 293
Turner's syndrome, 80, 81
Turpentine oil, 110
Typhoid, 131, 246, 247, 288
Typhus, 117 n.
  epidemic, 246
Tyson's glands, 124

Uganda, 9, 10, 12–13, 16, 18, 167, 176, 198
UICC, see International Union Against Cancer
Ulcers:
  as a cause of death, 28
  gastric, 331–32, 337
Unilever Research Laboratory, England, 301
United Arab Republic, 179
United Kingdom, see England
United Nations, 278
United States of America, 28 n.–29 n., 55, 60, 93, 97, 105, 127, 128, 144, 179, 195, 196, 219, 276, 277, 278, 278 n., 296, 305, 317, 319, 321, 329, 331, 339, 342, 347
  Department of Agriculture, 317
  Department of Defense, 42
  Department of Health, Education, and Welfare, 43, 50, 75 n., 192, 221 n., 334 n.
  Public Health Center, 220
USSR, 55, 92, 100, 116, 128, 142, 143, 154, 179, 277, 278, 278 n., 342
  incidence of cancer in, 103
Uterine cancer, see Cancer, of the uterus
Uterus, description of, 120

Vaccination, 246, 247–49
Vaccine, 28
Vaccinia, 246
Vaisyas, 142
VAMP, 198
Van der Waals' forces of interaction, 268
Vector, definition of, 172 n.
Vesalius, 4
Vespucci, Amerigo, 4
Veterans Administration, 43
Vibrio cholerae, 91
Vibrio comma, 91, 93, 93 n.
Victoria, Lake, 16
Victoria, Queen, 91
Vigne, P., 115
Villejuif, France, 201, 205–17
Vinblastine, 213, 227
Vincaleukoblastine, 227
Vincristine, 19, 198, 212, 240
Vinleurosine, 212
Virchow, Rudolph, 30, 71, 71 n., 182
Virology, 206
Viruses, 65, 72, 79, 114, 169
  as a cause of leukemia, 186, 189–92, 215–17, 247, 252
Viruses, The (Curtis), 189
Virus Hunters (Williams), 244
Virus Research Institute, Entebbe, 14, 16
Vitamin B_2 complex, 230

Wales, England, 296
Warburg, Otto, 81
Washington, D.C., 50, 278 n.
Water supply, character of, 115–16

Waterhouse, Benjamin, 246 n.
Watson, Dr. James D., 16, 56, 56 n.
Watson-Crick model of DNA, 238
Weiss, L., 268
Weisses Blut, 182
Wells, H. G., 217
Welsh, 110
West Country, England, 296
West Germany, 60
    see also Germany
Whales, 30
White blood cells, *see* Leucocytes
Whooping cough, 246
Williams, E. H., 17 n.
Williams, Greer, 244
Williams, Ted, 12
Wilms, Dr. Max, 5
Wilms' tumor, 4, 5, 78, 231, 233–35, 238–39
    see also Embryomas, Neuroblastomas
Wilkins, Maurice, 56 n.
Wirth, 77
Wisconsin, University of, 46
Withering, Dr. William, 228
Woglom, Dr. William H., 115 n.
Wolff, J. A., 230 n.
World Health House, 152
World Health Organization, Geneva, 55, 92, 118, 140, 151, 153–55, 180, 227, 278, 290
Regional Office for Southeast Asia (New Delhi), 142, 151, 152
report on chemotherapy in cancer (1962), 164–65
World War I, 98
World War II, 8, 31, 38 n., 97, 99, 111, 128, 163, 197, 276, 347
Wright, B., 17 n.
Wright, Dr. Dennis, 5, 11 n., 166, 175–77, 195
Wynder, Dr. Ernest L., 331

Xenopus, 171
X-rays, 18, 340
    exposure to, 96
    see also Irradiation, Radiation, Radiation therapy, Radiotherapy

Yamagiwa, Prof. K., 31
Yellow fever, 27, 246
Yoshida, Dr. Tomizo, 149–50, 179, 279

Zinc, 295
Zubrod, Dr. C. Gordon, 218 n.
Zulu tribe, 319
Zymosan, 210